Complementary Therapies for Health Care Providers

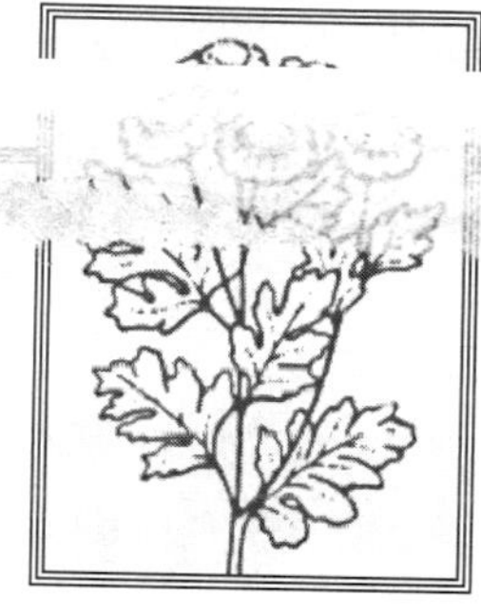

Complementary Therapies for Health Care Providers

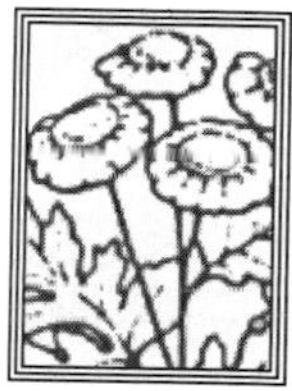

Merrily A. Kuhn, RN, PhD
ND PhD Student

Lippincott Williams & Wilkins
A **Wolters Kluwer** Company
Philadelphia • Baltimore • New York • London
Buenos Aires • Hong Kong • Sydney • Tokyo

Editor: Lisa Stead
Editorial Assistant: Claudia Vaughn
Marketing Manager: Jean Rodenberger
Production Editor: June Choe

351 West Camden Street
Baltimore, MD 21201-2436, USA

530 Walnut Street
Philadelphia, PA 19106, USA

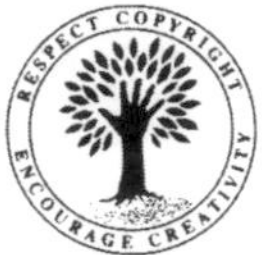

Printed in the United States of America.

Library of Congress Cataloging-in-Publication Data

Kuhn, Merrily A., 1945-
Complementary therapies for health care providers / Merrily A. Kuhn.
p. cm.
Includes bibliographical references and index.
ISBN 0-7817-1919-4
1. Alternative medicine. I. Title.
[DNLM: 1. Alternative Medicine. WB 890 K955c 1999]
R733.K83 1999
615.5—dc21
DNLM/DLC
for Library of Congress 99-10977
CIP

To purchase additional copies of this book, call our customer service department at **(800) 638-3030** or fax orders to **(301) 824-7390**. International customers should call **(301) 714-2324.**

00 01 02
2 3 4 5 6 7 8

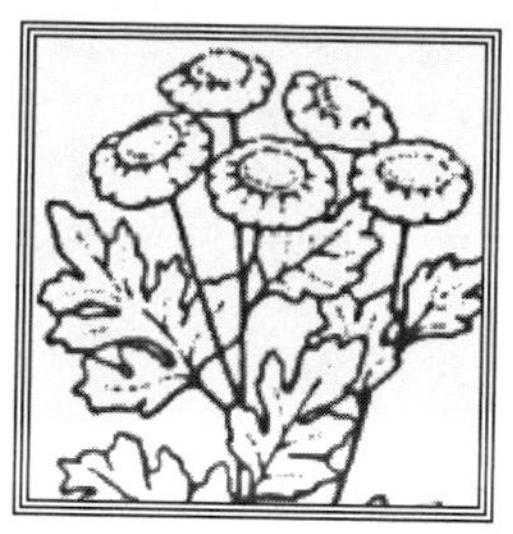

DEDICATION

To my parents, Audrey and Norbert Kuhn,
who taught me perseverance;

To my husband, James, the love of my life,
for his devotion, care, and daily concern;

To Susan Doherty, my administrative assistant,
for her organization and typing of this manuscript; and

To all readers who are willing to take a step beyond
their comfort zone into complementary medicine!

Merrily A. Kuhn
RN, PhD
ND PhD Student

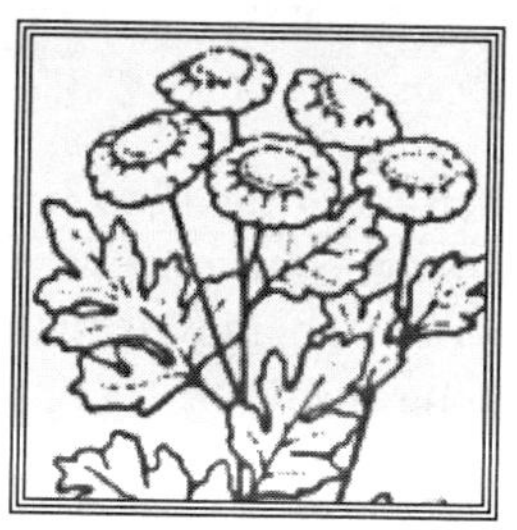

PREFACE

Socrates once said, "There is only one good: knowledge; and one evil: ignorance." Certainly this statement should guide us as health professionals to learn as much as we can about the complementary therapies that our patients are flocking to!

Complementary therapies have come of age. According to recent research, people are making more visits to complementary therapy providers than to traditional health care practitioners. Health care practitioners must understand these therapies and be able to counsel their patients about the advantages and disadvantages, or pros and cons, of complementary therapies.

This text presents information on more than 100 complementary therapies, provides detailed monographs regarding 33 of the most commonly used herbs, details holistic nutrition (including 20 different diets claimed to treat cancer or other medical conditions), and provides detailed monographs regarding 31 phytochemicals. The text is research-based and attempts to separate media hype from research-based truths.

A similar format is used to describe each complementary therapy. For each therapy, I provide a description, history, what the therapy can treat or improve, what happens during a visit, the risks involved with the therapy, and the training that is required of the practitioner. There is always a section on the existing research about the therapy. Information was obtained through a Medline search from research performed during the last 10 years. Whenever possible, placebo-controlled trials were evaluated; however, these studies were often lacking or poorly performed.

There is a great need for more scientific and medical research on the effectiveness of complementary therapies. Research is ongoing, so it is important for practitioners to continually consult scientific journals. Science will continue to increase our understanding of how these therapies work. Each complementary therapy section concludes with a bibliography and a further reading list.

This book is NOT designed as a "how-to" text. Additional education and training are necessary for someone interested in learning how to administer complementary therapies. Resources for further information and Web sites are included for each complementary therapy.

Let us all enhance our own healing and health, and share our knowledge with our patients. The ultimate goal of this book is to place health and healing within the grasp of all people!

Enjoy maximal health and longevity!

Merrily A. Kuhn

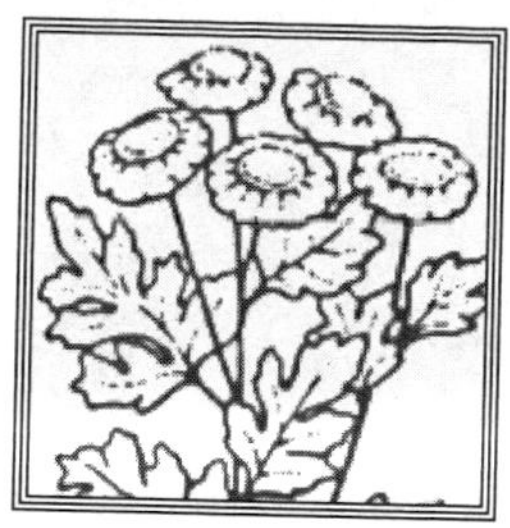

ACKNOWLEDGMENTS

This book would never have come to be without the foresight of Lisa Stead, Editor, at Lippincott Williams & Wilkins. My thanks to Claudia Vaughn, Editorial Assistant, for organizing this text and readying it for production. Also, my thanks to all the production staff at Lippincott Williams & Wilkins, particularly June Choe, Production Editor.

My thanks also go out to the reviewers of this book for their knowledge and encouraging comments. All of the Complementary Therapy Providers that I worked with were willing to share their knowledge and expertise with me and the medical community.

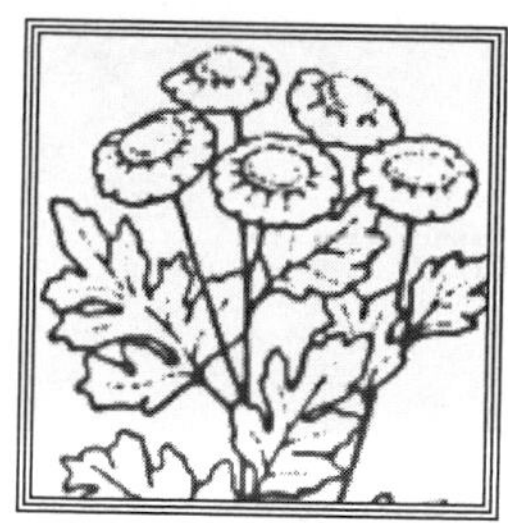

List of Reviewers

Laurie Azzarella, LMT, CRR
IIR Certified Registered Reflexologist and Authorized Instructor
Nationally Certified Massage Therapist
Board of Directors of RAA
Daphne, Alabama

Amanda McQuade Crawford
MNIMH, Diploma of Phytotherapy
The National College of Phytotherapy
Ojai, California

Paula J. Defendorf-Tenz, MSED, LMT
Dynamic Touch Massage Therapy
Hamburg, New York

Carol Lou Eisenhardt, RNC, BSN
Therapeutic Touch Practitioner and Lecturer
Acute Geriatric Unit at Buffalo General Hospital
and Buffalo Hospice, Inc.
Buffalo, New York

Pamela A. Gay, NC
Private Practice
Buffalo, New York

Nancy T. Holbrook
Hypnotician
Westfield, New York

Nancy Leone
Certified Advanced Rolfer
Orchard Park, New York

Michael Scholes
President, The Michael Scholes School of Aromatic Studies
Los Angeles, California

Norman E. Smith
Registered Acupuncturist, Diploma in Acupuncture, N.C.C.A.O.M.
The Acupuncture and Therapy Center
Colorado Springs, Colorado

Ray Watson, BA, ACH, CI
Certified Instructor and Executive Director, T'ai Chi Chih
Hypnosis Training and Wellness Center
Batavia, New York

Sally A. Williams, RSHom
Healing Arts Association of Western New York
Buffalo, New York

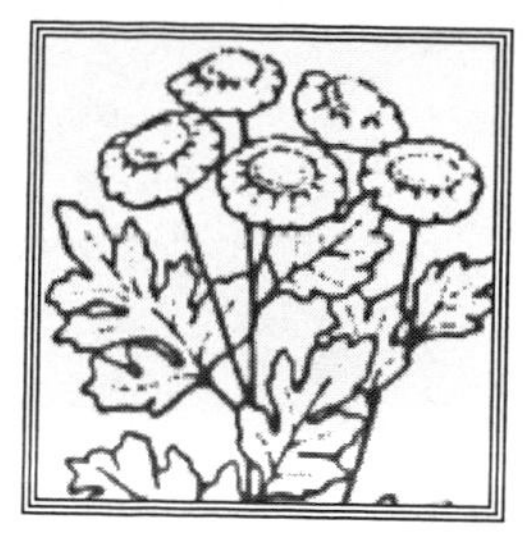

Contents

CHAPTER 1

The Role of Complementary Therapies

YESTERDAY AND TODAY

It is no secret that the U.S. medical system is in a state of disarray. Although conventional medicine excels in the management of medical emergencies, certain bacterial infections, and trauma care with many—often heroically complex—surgical techniques, it seems to have failed in the areas of disease prevention and the management of the myriad new and chronic illnesses afflicting the patients who are filling our hospitals and physicians' offices. In addition, as a nation, we pay more for our medical care, but accomplish less than most other nations of comparable living standards. Our health care costs continue to spiral out of control. Treatment of chronic disease accounts for 85% of the national health care bill. This state of affairs has resulted because we spend almost nothing to treat the causes of chronic disease before major illness develops.

Former Surgeon General, C. Everett Koop, in his 1988 Report on Nutrition and Health, points out that "dietary imbalances" are the leading preventable contributors to premature death in the United States and recommends the expansion of nutrition and lifestyle-modification education for all health care professionals. This is borne out by the Centers for Disease Control and Prevention, which state that 54% of heart disease, 37% of cancer, 50% of cerebrovascular disease, and 49% of atherosclerosis is preventable through lifestyle modification.

Greater recognition and acceptance of "alternative" methods was demonstrated by the National Institute of Health with the creation of its Office of Alternative Medicine (OAM). Established in 1991 and funded

TABLE 1-1 ALTERNATIVE MEDICINE UPDATE

Center	Location	Specialty
Bastry University	Seattle, WA	HIV/AIDS
Beth Israel Hospital/Harvard Medical School	Boston, MA	General medicine
Columbia University of Physicians and Surgeons	New York, NY	Women's health
Kessler Institute/University of Medicine and Dentistry	W. Orange, NJ	Stroke, neurologic conditions
Hennepin County Hospital Minnesota Medical School	Minneapolis, MN	Addictions
Stanford University	Palo Alto, CA	Aging
University of California at Davis	Davis, CA	Asthma, allergy, immunology
University of Maryland School of Medicine	Baltimore, MD	Pain
University of Texas Health Science Center	Houston, TX	Cancer
University of Virginia School of Nursing	Charlottesville, VA	Pain

with $2 million in 1992, this office received 452 grant applications and funded 30. In 1995, this budget was increased to $5 million. The purpose of the OAM research is to allow validated therapies to be further integrated into conventional medical practice. There are now 13 OAM-funded centers to evaluate various holistic therapies (Table 1-1) and there are 50 different research projects being conducted. The centers and the trials together will provide new opportunities for training researchers in complementary medicine studies.

The annual OAM budget was increased to $20 million in 1998. Small grants, awarded to universities, clinics, and practitioners, cover a variety of treatments. For example, antioxidant vitamins are being studied to see if they enhance the ability of anticancer drugs to eradicate cancer cells. Guided imagery, also known as visualization, is being tested for its ability to boost the immune system and help the body resist or fight disease. Acupuncture is being tested with women as a treatment for depression, and the dietary supplement glucosamone is being studied for the treatment of arthritis. While not comprehensive, these studies represent the start of "official" acceptance of what is already a reality. Some 60% of the inquiries the OAM receives deal with cancer. The National Cancer Institute has joined the OAM to help determine the best methods of research. Ongoing research includes work with shark cartilage and a complex nutritional program.

Congress has approximated $50 million for 1999 to establish the National Center for Complementary and Alternative Medicine, an outgrowth of the OAM. This center will be able to fund research grants and other projects directly.

The underlying concepts of alternative medicine are not new. They represent a return to the principles that have been a part of human understanding of health and disease for thousands of years. Over the centuries, medical wisdom evolved within a framework that linked health to a state of harmony or balance, and disease to a state of disharmony or imbalance, and took into account the factors that contributed to both.

In addition, Hippocrates recognized that life forces that pervade all of nature have multiple expressions. He taught that health depended on living in harmony with these forces. Recognition of these life forces is also vital to Traditional Chinese Medicine and Ayurvedic Medicine from India.

> *I would rather know what sort of person has a disease than what sort of disease a person has.*
>
> —HIPPOCRATES, 500 B.C.

SEVEN FIELDS OF PRACTICE

NIH has categorized alternative modalities and therapies into seven specific fields of practice:

Herbal medicine encompasses herbal approaches for pharmacologic use. It is derived from practices in European, Asian, and Native American traditions.

Diet, nutrition, and lifestyle changes promote study of the effects of various food groups, vitamins, and minerals on acute and chronic disease. There is also a focus on health maintenance and disease prevention.

Mind/body or behavioral interventions includes such therapies as biofeedback, relaxation, imagery, meditation, hypnosis, psychotherapy, prayer, mental healing art, dance, music therapy, and yoga.

Alternative systems of medical practice includes traditional Oriental medicine, Ayurveda (a system of healing from India relying on diet, exercise, and meditation), homeopathy, naturopathic medicine, environmental medicine, and community-based heath care practices (such as those practiced in shamanic or Native American cultures).

Manual healing methods use techniques such as osteopathy, massage therapy, chiropractic, physical therapy, and therapeutic touch as diagnostic and therapeutic tools.

Bioelectromagnetics explore how living organisms interact with electromagnetic fields for a variety of applications, including bone repair, wound healing, and immune system stimulation.

Pharmacologic and biologic treatments include drugs and vaccines not yet accepted by mainstream medicine.

This handbook uses the NIH categories to present information.

ALLOPATHIC VERSUS TRADITIONAL MEDICINE

Western medicine practices "allopathic medicine." Allopathy has two definitions in the dictionary: Derived from Greek roots, the term means "other than disease"; derived from German roots, it means "all therapies." Therefore, allopathy is a system of medicine that embraces all methods of proven value in the treatment of disease. In our society, until recently, allopathy was the only form of medicine taken seriously. Backed by vast sums of money and the intellectual prestige of great universities and supported by impressive records of clinical success, allopathic medicine is dominant.

Traditional medicine (complementary or alternative medicine) is the primary health care of the world, used by 65% to 85% of the world's population. The OAM has recently been designed as a collaborating center in traditional medicine by the World Health Organization (WHO). This alliance is a major undertaking to bring more information about traditional healing systems to this country, where they can be researched for the purpose of benefitting the American public.

WHO is interested in the safety and efficacy of indigenous and traditional practices because of the extent that they are practiced around the world. WHO's mission is "the attainment by all peoples of the highest possible level of health."

COMPLEMENTARY VERSUS ALTERNATIVE THERAPY

The definition of complementary and alternative medicine has been debated in recent years. In 1995, the OAM proposed a definition.

Alternative Medicine: Modalities used instead of conventional medicine. This type of health care is neither widely taught in U.S. medical schools, nor generally available in U.S. hospitals.

Complementary Medicine: The use of modalities together to complement offerings of conventional medicine (Panel Definition and Description, 1997).

Integrative Medicine: A term suggested by Dr. Andrew Weil at the University of Arizona Health Science Center. Used to define a hybrid of complementary and conventional medical treatments: a synergistic combination of therapies that incorporates acupuncture, herbal medicine, manipulation, and Ayurvedic and conventional measures such as antibiotics and surgery.

Doctors in the University of Arizona's medical program are taught to identify the acute medical conditions that require immediate conventional care. They then study 12 areas of complementary care, including mind/body medicine and the study of medicinal plants and energy medicine, exploring each treatment's strengths and weaknesses. All students on the Arizona program complete intensive study in guided imagery, acupuncture, basic homeopathy, and osteopathic manipulative therapy. They may choose further education in these areas or study other healing approaches approved by the program directors.

The doctors in this program staff an outpatient Integrative Medical Clinic, where the doctors learn practical treatment techniques from complementary practitioners in a clinical setting. As part of their hands-on, holistic education, they experience how a person's emotional, psychological, and spiritual makeup affects illness and treatment. Clinical research at these centers will eventually push integrative medicine into the national spotlight.

Fontanarosa and Lundberg (1998), in an editorial in *The Journal of the American Medical Association*, suggest there is no alternative medicine. There is only scientifically proven, evidence-based medicine supported by solid data, or unproven medicine for which scientific evidence is lacking. Fonterosa and Lundburg further suggest that whether a therapeutic practice is "Eastern" or "Western," unconventional or mainstream, involves mind-body techniques or molecular genetics, is largely irrelevant, except for historical purposes and cultural interest. Fonterosa and Lundburg suggest that it is important to evaluate all therapies using explicit, focused research methods (controls, effective blinding procedures, state-of-the-art-techniques for systemic reviews), incorporating measurable, objectively assessed end points, and reporting meaningful patient outcomes. If complementary therapies demonstrate efficacy and safety, they should be used; if they demonstrate no benefit, they should be abandoned.

For the purpose of this handbook, the term "complementary therapies" is preferred. Many of the therapies discussed within this handbook, however, can stand alone as treatment modalities. Thus, to improve diagnosis, treatment, cure, and prevention, take the best from each therapy and use them in combination to promote health.

PUBLICLY FUNDED INTEGRATED MEDICAL CENTER

While several medical centers around the country combine allopathic and complementary medicine, only one facility, the King County Natural Medicine Clinic, just outside Seattle, WA is publicly funded. The idea for this clinic originated with Seattle residents Merilee Manthey and Joe Pizzorno, ND, President of the Bastry University, a naturopathic medical school. Together they went before the King County Council to propose an Integrative Medical clinic for low-income and uninsured residents of the Seattle area. That every member of the council had personally consulted complementary practitioners smoothed the way for approval of the plan. Consequently, three institutions—Bastyr University, the Kent Community Health Center, and the Statistical and Epidemiological Research Corporation—collaborated in securing a $750,000 grant provided by the state of Washington.

In October 1996, the King County Natural Medicine Clinic opened with a staff of doctors, a physician assistant, and a nurse practitioner together with naturopaths and naturopathic residents, an acupuncturist, a nutritionist, a mental health counselor, off-site chiropractors, and massage therapists. To make the collaboration complete, the clinic is codirected by medical doctor Mary Ross and naturopathic physician Jane Guiltinan.

The local population's familiarity with "natural" medicine has aided the clinic's success. Plus, the region's immigrant communities of Southeast Asians, Hispanics, Russians, and Ukrainians are comfortable being advised to take herbs such as ginkgo biloba, burdock root, or celery seed. However, those uncomfortable with natural medicine can choose to learn more about complementary therapies, or consult with a "standard" practitioner.

CULTURAL DIVERSITY, FOLK MEDICINE, AND COMPLEMENTARY THERAPIES

Complementary medicine, a relatively new term, has important connections with folk medicine (e.g., herbs). The ethnic and cultural diversity of the U.S. population has grown constantly throughout history. The linguistic, religious, and cultural patterns of American society are more varied than ever before. And, it makes sense that medical needs must also become more diverse. Immigrants bring with them a variety of treatments: acupuncture from China, yoga from Indians, and some herbal therapies from Native American culture. Folk medicine is the future of complementary medicine.

EFFECTIVENESS OF COMPLEMENTARY THERAPIES

Do complementary therapies work because we think they will? Is it possible that it is just a placebo effect and we feel better because we want to? The psychiatrist authors of "The Powerful Placebo" (Shapiro & Shapiro, 1998) require viewing a placebo as more than a sugar pill that we've come to associate with the term placebo. We need to consider placebo as "any treatment or component thereof, which is knowingly used for its non-specific physiological or psychophysiological therapeutic effect, but without specific activity."

There are four significant concerns to be considered with placebo-controlled trials of the complementary systems. First, usually persons seeking an alternative to the standard orthodox medical care expect a positive result from their treatment and therefore experience an intense placebo effect. Second, persons often overreport their signs and symptoms when first going for treatment, thereby ensuring they will receive the treatment they desire. They also underreport the negative signs and symptoms after receiving treatment as a way of justifying receiving treatment in the first place. Third, a significant aspect of complementary therapies is that each therapy is tailor-made for each patient, thereby undermining the control situation used with any standardization of treatment. Fourth, measuring the subjective response is just that: subjective, and can be easily biased by the person providing the information. These four concerns stress the need for double-blind and controlled studies with consideration of no treatment as part of the study.

Complementary therapies are designed to be used alone or in addition to traditional medical care. Consider treating a sinus infection that includes lots of mucus: it can be treated with over-the-counter decongestants to treat the stuffy nose, but that is only temporary relief. A conventional physician may provide an antibiotic to cure the infection, but it will not prevent further infections. A naturopathic physician will ask, "Why the infection?" The naturopath identifies that there is excessive mucus. Increased mucus provides a nutrient base for bacteria, but why is there mucus? An allergy will provide increased mucus, so if you avoid the allergen, you avoid the mucus; thereby avoiding future sinus infections.

WHO IS USING COMPLEMENTARY THERAPIES?

The first qualitative study was published in the *New England Journal of Medicine* by Eisenberg in 1993. The large national survey found 36% of those surveyed used alternative medicine, but only 3% used only alternative medicine. Persons with more education and higher incomes were likely to use alternatives. In a study published by Austin in the *Journal of the American Medical Association* in 1998, the author found that 30% to 34% of those surveyed used alterative therapies, and that 4% used alternative therapies only. Austin found the following variables were significant predictors of alternative medicine use:

- Distrust of conventional physicians and hospitals
- Desire for control over health matters
- Dissatisfaction with conventional practitioners
- Belief in the importance and value of one's inner life and experiences

Austin also identified that persons chose alternative therapies because of their perceived benefits: "I feel better," "I get relief from my symptoms," or "The treatment works better for my health problem." In addition, most people stated, "The treatment promotes health rather than just focusing on illness." Austin also found users tended to be better educated and have higher incomes. In addition, users tended to have a more "holistic" approach to health care and to be more likely to report a poor health status to their traditional provider. Thus, alternative medicine is a choice for persons with more chronic health problems, for whom conventional medicine does not offer much in the way of a cure or symptom relief.

Eisenberg and collaborators (1998) conducted a telephone survey of 2,055 U.S. adults in 1997 about their health practices. The first study was conducted in 1991, and published in 1993. In 1997, 46% of those surveyed said they had visited a complementary practitioner, compared to 36% in 1991; 42% used at least one alternative therapy in the previous year compared to 34% in 1990. Extrapolating their results to the entire U.S. adult population, the Harvard researchers estimated that Americans made 629 million visits to complementary medicine practitioners in 1997, compared to 386 million visits to primary care doctors. A conservative estimate of out-of-pocket expenditures for complementary medicine in 1997 is $27 billion, compared with $29 billion out-of-pocket for all U.S. physician services. People from 30 to 50 years of age are most likely to seek complementary therapy. This generation is used to having choices and questioning authority. Eisenberg, et al. found that persons who saw their medical doctor for a chronic condition were also more likely to seek out at least one complementary therapy provider. Eisenberg, et al. also found a 380% increase in the use of herbal remedies, and a 130% increase in high-dosage vitamins. Herbal sales are increasing at a rate of 25%/year. (Cirigliano & Sun, 1998).

Another study by Furnham, et al. (1995) suggests that persons visiting complementary practitioner were not a homogenous group. They consult different practitioners based on a combination of their level of skepticism about medicine, their life style, and other health benefits.

Vincent (1996) found in his survey that most people choose alternative therapy because they believe that alternative medicine will "enable me to take a more active part in maintaining my health," and that conventional medicine was not able to treat or control symptoms of their current condition.

Furham and Kirkcaldy (1996) found that most people in their surveys chose alternative medicine from a belief that it was more effective than conventional medicine.

HEALTH INSURANCE COVERAGE

Complementary therapies are now being reimbursed by some insurance companies that are slowly beginning to recognize that there are lowered health care costs from the benefits of these therapies and improved physician-supervised preventive care. The insurance companies vary widely in terms of modalities covered. At least 40 states mandate that health plans provide at least some coverage for chiropractic; 6 mandate some coverage for acupuncture, and 3 for naturopathy. The chance of reimbursement is increased if conventional and alternative providers are under one corporate umbrella. Several insurance reimbursement policies are discussed.

Washington State

The state of Washington is one of the most friendly environments for complementary medicine. In 1995, a law mandated health insurance plans in the state to provide access to every category of health care provider to treat conditions that are covered under the state's basic health care plan. Regency Blue Shield of Washington offers members the option of choosing a naturopath as their primary care physician, and 1% of the eligible 358,000 members have done that.

Blue Cross

Starting in 1994, Blue Cross of Washington and Alaska covers complementary therapies at 50% of the cost, up to $500/year.

Mutual of Omaha

Since 1993, Mutual of Omaha has covered Dr. Dean Ornish's program for reversing heart disease in any of the facilities around the country that offer the program. (See Nutrition chapter for more information on the Ornish program.) Ideally, Mutual of Omaha would like to see a patient who needs heart surgery to get involved with the program and avoid surgery; and that has been the case in approximately 50% of the patients who participate in the Ornish program.

Wellness Health Plans

In 1993, Wellness Health Plan established a plan (available in 13 states) that encouraged consumers to manage their own preventative care. Subscribers are required to visit an M.D. yearly, but can then use complementary therapies of their choice. The Wellness Health Plan (American Western Life) was purchased in 1996 by Prime Care Health Network, Inc. Prime Care plans to extend this plan to other states.

Kaiser Foundation

Kaiser Foundation of California offers acupuncture, relaxation training, and acupressure for patients with chronic pain. In addition, nutrition counseling is available.

Oxford Health Plans

Oxford Health Plan offers a complementary medicine program to members in Connecticut, New York, and New Jersey. Oxford developed its network of accredited providers by establishing three advisory boards to develop the quality standards. The criteria for admission include:

- A license in the state
- Graduation from a fully accredited college
- Demonstration of 2 years of continuous clinical experience
- Pursuit of continuing education credits
- Proper malpractice insurance

Members also have access to special rates on vitamins and herbs through a natural products mail-order plan.

Health Partners

Health Partners is a new managed care company in Arizona that covers acupuncture, Trager therapy, and guided imagery. Herbs are reimbursed as part of the initial health assessment, but not as an alternative to prescription drugs. Patients may avail themselves of services at the Arizona Center for Health and Medicine, which offers acupuncture, homeopathy, therapeutic message, therapeutic touch, osteopathic manipulation, cranial sacral manipulation, guided imagery, herbal therapy, yoga, and Tai chi classes.

MEDICAL EDUCATION

Medical schools are beginning to recognize the need to teach doctors about complementary therapies. In 1996, 60 medical schools included the subject in existing, required courses, while another 56 offered it as an elective, according to the Association of American Medical Colleges. Only 37 offered no instruction in complementary medicine. Few nursing schools include any content on complementary medicine, and fewer still teach herbal therapies.

MELDING PRACTICE

It is necessary to discuss the use of complementary therapies and herbs with one's health care provider. Keeping mum can cause real risks. It is best to discuss the idea of complementary therapy with your provider before therapy is started, and to keep the provider updated with progress. If your primary care provider seems open, ask if he or she would be willing to speak to your complementary provider. Complementary practitioners are usually willing to share information and progress about their patients and to work with the primary care provider to develop a combined plan of care. This technique may safe-guard your health and perhaps bring the two worlds of medicine a little closer together.

In a conventional medical practice, the use of holistic modalities does not fit, so such practices are viewed as contrary to accepted medical practice. Possibly, medicine could concentrate on its traditional strong points and allow useful treatments to be used where appropriate. Practitioners of complementary therapies are often willing to work with medical supervision.

SUMMARY

Insurance companies are increasingly willing to examine ways to reduce health care costs. Complementary therapies may be one such option. The process of including complementary practitioners in health care has created a new industry: credentialing practitioners. Credentialing needs to be examined carefully. Standardization, fairness, and management of the process are serious issues that have yet to be universally addressed. Regulation should serve the needs of the patients; not the needs of regulators or insurance companies.

BIBLIOGRAPHY

Astin, J. (1998). Alternative medicine. Journal of the American Medical Association. 279, 1549–1554.

Astin, J. (1998). Why patients use alternative medicine. Journal of the American Medical Association. 279, 1555–1561.

Bower, H. (1998). Double standards exist in judging traditional and alternative medicine. British Medical Journal. 316, 11694.

Bratman, S. (1997). Alternative medicine: how well does it live up to its own ideals? Alternative therapies. 3, 127–128.

CAM Research Methodology Conference. (1997). Defining and describing complementary and alternative medicine. Alternative Therapies. 3, 49–57.

Cirgliano, M. & Sun, A. (1998). Advising patients about complementary therapies. Journal of the American Medical Associaton. Nov. 11;279:1565–1566.

Davis, P. A., Gold, E. B., Hackman, R. M., Stern, J. S., & Gershwin, M. E. (1998). The use of complementary/ alternative medicine for the treatment of asthma in the United States. Journal of Investigative Allergology and Clinical Immunology. 8, 73–77.

Dossey, B. (1998). Holistic modalities and healing moments. American Journal of Nursing. 98, 44–47.

Eisenberg, D. (1993). Unconventional medicine in the United States. New England Journal of Medicine. 328, 246.

Eisenberg, D., Davis, R., Ettner, S., et al. (1998). Trends in alternative medicine use in the United States, 1990–1997. Journal of the American Medical Association. Nov. 11; 279:1569–1575.

Fahey, C. (1998). Medical decisions. Energy Times. March, 49–53.

Furnham, A., Vincent, C., & Wood, R. (1995). The health beliefs and behaviors of three groups of complementary medicine and a general practice group of patients. Journal of Alternative and Complementary Medicine. 1, 347–359.

Furnham, A. & Kirkcaldy, B. (1996). The health beliefs and behaviors of orthodox and complementary medicine clients. British Journal of Clinical Psychology. 35, 49–61.

Green, J. (1996). Integrating conventional medicine and alternative therapies. Alternative Therapies. 2, 77–81.

Hufford, D. (1997). Integrating complementary and alternative medicine into conventional medical practice. Alternative Therapies. 3, 81–83.

Kelner, M. & Wellman, B. (1997). Who seeks alternative health care? A profile of the users of five modes of treatment. Journal of Alternative and Complementary Medicine. 3, 127–140.

Moore, B. (1997). A review of reimbursement policies for alternative and complementary therapies. Alternative Therapies. 3, 26–92.

Rossman, M. (1997). Managed care and alternative medicine: who will manage what and how? Alternative Therapies. 3, 63–66.

Seligson, S. (1998). Main Line medicines. Health. May/June, 64–70.
Shapiro, A. & Shapiro E. (1998). The powerful placebo: from ancient priest to modern physician. British Medical Journal. 316, 1396.
Vincent, C. & Furnham, A. (1996). Why do patients turn to complementary medicine? An emprical study. British Journal of Clinical Psychology. 35, 37–48.
Vincent, C., Furnham, A. (1998). Complementary medicine: a research perspective. British Medical Journal. 316, 1396.

INTERNET

University of Pittsburgh Alternative Medicine homepage
www.pitt.edu/~cbw/internet.html
Provides links to many other alternative medicine resources.

Quackwatch
www.quackwatch.com
Homepage with National Council Against Health Fraud.

Alternative Medicine Connection
arxc.com/hotlinks.html
Links to numerous medical libraries and research center's pages.

Health World Online
www.health.net/library/journals/index.html
Consumer and professional information. Full journal articles available.

Alternative Care
www.sky.net/~ngt/welcome.html

Natural Medicine and Alternative Therapy
www/amrta.org/~amrta

Oregon Health Sciences, University of Holistic and Alternative Medicine
www.ohsu.edu/ohmig.cam.html

Infoseek-Alternative Medicine
infoseek.com/health/alternative_medicine

CHAPTER 2

Responsibilities of Health Care Providers Whose Patients Are Participating in Complementary Therapies

As health professionals, there are several responsibilities that we must be alert to when a patient whom we are caring for, or consulting with, decides to participate in complementary therapies. As health care providers, we must:

- Understand the purpose of the complementary therapy
- Understand what the complementary therapy is capable of treating
- Identify the symptoms or disease of the patient
- Attempt to ascertain if the complementary therapy will treat or cure the patient's symptoms or disease
- Identify the contraindications and adverse effects of the complementary therapy and discuss these with the patient
- Determine why the patient is seeking complementary therapy (Have traditional therapies failed?)
- Identify allergies of the patient and determine if there are any problems with the therapy. (This is particularly important for aromatherapy and herbal therapy.)

- Help the patient prepare a list of current drugs and encourage the patient to share them with the complementary therapy provider
- Encourage the patient to tell the health care provider about this choice of complementary therapy
- Encourage the patient to have the complementary therapy provider talk to and discuss treatment with the traditional practitioner
- Help the patient determine if the complementary practitioner is qualified (education, certification, license)
- Help the patient determine if there is insurance reimbursement for the complementary therapy and how to obtain such
- Assess for the patient the research that supports or does not support the complementary therapy. (Most complementary therapists are doing or beginning to do evidence-based, controlled, placebo trials to determine the effectiveness of the therapy.)
- Monitor the progress of the patient, determining if symptoms or disease is improving. If not, encourage the patient to seek other treatments.
- Share with the patient and family any personal interest that you may have with the complementary therapy
- Periodically consult with the patient. (This may be weekly, monthly, or every several months, depending on the patient's condition.) Review current therapies and determine if there are any interactions between their traditional therapy and current therapy such as diet, herbs, and so on
- Identify if the patient is an alcoholic or a recovering alcoholic, addicted to any prescription drug or recreational chemical, or taking drugs that may interact with alcohol (e.g., antibiotics, Antabuse). Teach the patient to be aware of tinctures made of alcohol that may further complicate his or her condition. Teach that there are tinctures made with glycerin, which may be more appropriate.
- Help the patient make dietary and lifestyle changes that may be necessary when using some complementary therapies such as Ayurvedic or Oriental medicines.
- Teach the patient that complementary therapy herbs or remedies should not be shared with others. (Most complementary therapists believe in individuality of the human body. Even though two persons may have the same symptoms, because of their individuality, they are treated differently.)
- Teach the patient as much as possible about his or her illness and the need to avoid, if any, causative foods or lifestyles with traditional and complementary therapies
- Discuss with the patient that trial and error testing is often necessary with complementary therapy to develop and correct treatment protocols

- Suggest the keeping of a daily log or journal of treatments and symptom relief or progression
- Understand the contraindications to the complementary therapies (see individual sections under risks) and review with patient
- Encourage the patient to progress slowly with lifestyle changes such as a new exercise and diet program
- Explain to the patients that if they have any chronic lung disease, they may have difficulties with breath control for yoga, meditation, imagery, Tai Chi, and so on
- Advise patients with a history of schizophrenia, attention deficit disorder, and psychosis that they should be cautious when participating in mind-body therapies
- Advise the patient that if unpleasant sensations, thoughts, or physical signs occur during the complementary therapy to discuss these with the practitioner
- Encourage the patient not to substitute complementary therapy for traditional therapy
- Provide resources to the patient—books, Internet addresses, support groups—about the complementary therapy
- Always maintain patient confidentiality
- Recommend appropriate clothing for yoga, Tai Chi, Qigong dance therapy—loose shirt and pants and sneaker-type footwear to prevent slipping
- Recommend caution with various complementary therapies for pregnant women and children younger than 6 years
- Remind patients with pacemakers and implantable defibrillators to tell their complementary therapist
- Advise your patient to seek instruction from a qualified teacher when learning activities such as meditation, Tai Chi, and Qigong.

CHAPTER 3

HERBOLOGY

Herbs have always been integral to the practice of medicine. Approximately 25% of all prescription drugs are still derived from trees, shrubs, or herbs. Some are made from plant extracts; others are synthesized to mimic a natural plant compound. There are an estimated 250,000 to 500,000 plants on the earth today (the number varies depending on whether subspecies are included). Only approximately 5,000 of these have been extensively studied for their medicinal applications. This illustrates the need for modern medicine and science to turn its attention to the plant world once again to find new medicine that may cure cancer, AIDS, diabetes, and many other diseases and conditions. The World Health Organization notes that of 119 plant-derived pharmaceutical medicines, approximately 74% are used in modern medicine in ways that correlated directly with their traditional uses as plant medicines by native cultures. Eighty percent of the world's population still use herbal therapy as their primary treatment.

Because of the dissatisfaction with traditional medicine, more people are turning to complementary therapy, particularly herbs. It is estimated that half of all Americans use herbs, and the growth of the herb industry in the past few years is phenomenal! (See Table 3-1.) A study published in HerbalGram in Spring 1998, looked at the characteristics of an herb user (Table 3-2). Most people do not or will not tell their physician that they are taking herbs. There are herb/drug, herb/herb, and herb/vitamin interactions (see Table 3-3 for a selected list of possible interactions). So it is important to stress to people that they need to tell their physician about herb use.

Yet, for the most part, modern medicine has veered from the use of pure herbs in its treatment of disease and other health disorders. One of the reasons for this is economic. Herbs, by their very nature, cannot be patented. Since herbs cannot be patented and drug companies cannot hold the exclusive right to sell a particular herb, they are not motivated to invest any money in that herb's testing or promotion, although this is changing. The collection and preparation of herbal medicine cannot be as easily controlled as the manufacture of synthetic drugs, making its profits less dependable. In addition, many of these medicinal plants grow only in the Amazonian rain forest or other politically and economically unstable places, which also affects the supply of the herb.

As interest in herbs is increasing, research in the United States is being funded. National Institutes of Health (NIH) began funding research on St. John's wort in Spring 1998. There was a research study published in the Journal of the American Medical Association on Ginkgo and Alzheimer's in Fall 1997. Today, the general public probably knows more about herbs than the medical profession does!

TABLE 3-1 TOP SELLING HERBALS—MASS MARKET (FDM)[a] 52 WEEKS—JULY 12, 1998

	In U.S. Dollars (millions)	% of Growth
Ginkgo	$128	140+
St. John's wort	$121	2801++
Ginseng	$ 98	26+
Garlic	$ 84	27+
Echinacea	$ 33	151+
Saw palmetto	$ 27	138+
Grapeseed	$ 11	38+
Kava	$ 8	473++
Evening primrose	$ 8	104+
Echinacea/Goldenseal	$ 8	80+
Cranberry	$ 8	75+
Valerian	$ 8	35+
All others	$ 31	
Total:	**$663.4 million**	

[a]*Food, Drug, and Mass Merchandise.*
Source: IRI Scanner Data, *FDM (Food, Drug, Mass Market combined), Total US, 52 weeks and 12 weeks, 7, 12, 98.*

TABLE 3-2 CHARACTERISTICS OF HERB USERS

Education	Average of 1 year of college
Health insurance	95% have insurance
Used for	84% used for disease prevention and wellness 15% used for treatment of disease
Prescription drug use	50% taking prescription drugs concurrently
Mostly self-taught about herbs	
Tell MD about herb intake	98% did not tell MD

TABLE 3-3 SELECTED DRUG, HERB, AND VITAMIN INTERACTIONS

Herbal Products	Drug/Vitamin/ Mineral Product	Results In
Ginseng	Vitamin C	Decreases ginseng absorption,
Bromelain, Cayenne pepper, Cinchona bark, Dong quai, Green tea, Ginseng, Garlic, Ginger, Gingko, Willow bark, Vitamin E (above 1200 IU), Feverfew, Chamomile (English), Sweet clover, Horse chestnut	Coumadin	Increases bleeding tendency, INR may elevate
Ginseng	Coffee, tea, cola	Increases stimulation with caffeine
Ginseng	Phenelzine sulfate	Increases likelihood of headache, tremulousness, and manic episodes
Ginseng	Steroids and birth control pills	Increases side effects of steroids; decreases effectiveness of birth control pills
Gingko	ASA and vitamin E (greater than 1200 IU/day)	Decreases platelet stickiness; may increase bleeding
Flaxseed	Niacin	Increases flushing
Iron	Pancreatic enzymes and vitamin E	Decreases absorption of iron
Zinc	Selenium, vitamin C	Decreases zinc absorption
Vitamin C	Tricyclic antidepressants	Decreases effectiveness of tricyclics
Vitamin C	Coumadin	Reduces anticoagulant effect
Zinc	Tetracyclines	Interferes with tetracycline absorption
Kava kava	Alcohol, barbiturates, benzodiazepines	Increases sedative effect, may result in coma
Echinacea for longer than 8 weeks	Anabolic steroids, amiodarone, methotrexate ketoconazole	Increases liklihood of liver toxicity
Feverfew	NSAID, ASA, Tylenol	Negates the usefulness of drugs
Licorice, plaintain, hawthorn, ginseng, buckhorn (bark/berry)	Digoxin	Interferes with or intensifies effect of digoxin
Echinacea, zinc, vitamin E, astragalus	Corticosteroids and cyclosporine	Decreases the effectiveness of drugs
St. John's wort, saw palmetto	Iron	Inhibits iron absorption (separate by at least 2 hours)
Kelp	Thyroid products	Alters effectiveness of thyroid drugs
Karela, ginseng	Antidiabetes drugs	May affect blood glucose levels
Senna pod	Antiarrhythmics, cardiac glycosides, thiazide diuretics, corticosteroids	Increases K^+ loss, thus potentiating listed drugs
Brewer's yeast, Scotch broom	MAO inhibitors	Causes high blood pressure
Sulfonylureas, insulin, metformin	With chromium	Increases hypoglycemia (decreases drug dose)

Continued

TABLE 3-3 SELECTED DRUG, HERB, AND VITAMIN INTERACTIONS—CONTINUED

Herbal Products	Drug/Vitamin/ Mineral Product	Results In
Marshmellow, aloe vera, flaxseed (mucilage), psyllium seed, fenugreek, locust bean gum, oat seed, citrus peels, slippery elm bark	All drugs	Decreases the absorption of the drug (separate by 2 hours) due to shortened transient time; also, insulin-dependent diabetics may need to lower insulin dose due to slower absorption of carbohydrates
Alfalfa, St. John's wort, motherwort, parsley, celery	Chlorpromazine, tetracycline	Increases photosensitivity
Diuretic herbs—dandelion (often found in products to treat PMS and diet products)	Lithium	May potentiate lithium toxicity due to sodium depletion
Evening primrose oil/borage (both sources of GLA)	All anticonvulsants, also with anabolic steroids, phenothiazines, ketoconazole	Increases liklihood of liver toxicity
Hawthorn	Digitalis products	Increases likelihood of digitalis toxicity
St. John's wort, saw palmetto	Iron	Inhibits the absorption of iron
Dong quai	Calcium channel blockers	Synergistic with Ca^{++} channel blockers
Ma huang (*Ephedra*)	Cardiac glycocides, anesthetics	Increases liklihood of dysrhythmias
	Quanethidine	Enhances sympathetic activity
	MAOI	Possible hypertensive crisis
	Beta blockers	Elevates blood pressure
	Theophylline	Can elevate blood pressure, tachycardia, anxiety
Meadowsweat, poplar, willow	Probenecid	Inhibits urosuric activity of probenecid
Black cohosh, cola, St. John's wort	Beta-blocking drugs	Increases risk of hypertension
Bayberry, blue cohosh	Nitrates and Ca^{++} channel blockers	Antagonizes the hypertensive effect
Black cohosh, licorice	Oral contraceptives	Reduces effectiveness of oral contraceptives
Black cohosh, goldenseal, hawthorn	Anesthetics	Causes possible hypotensive effect
Broom, cornsilk	Muscle relaxants	Causes possible potentiation of muscle relaxant if hypokalemia occurs
Hawthorn, fig wort, cola	Depolarizing muscle relaxants	Increases risk of arrhythmia
Ginseng	Antipsychotics	Increases insomnia, headache, tremulousness
Goldenseal	Berberine	Interferes with the colon's manufacture of B vitamins
		Decreases their absorption
		Can antagonize heparin

TABLE 3-3 SELECTED DRUG, HERB, AND VITAMIN INTERACTIONS—CONTINUED

Herbal Products	Drug/Vitamin/ Mineral Product	Results In
Saw palmetto	Hormone therapy Oral contraceptives	Has been demonstrated to have anti-androgen and anti-estrogen activity
Aloe, buckthorn, cascara sagrada, castor bean, horsetail, licorice, rhubarb, senna	Cardiac glycosides, antiarrhythmics, diuretics, or laxatives	Increases K^+ loss and all listed drugs may have increased toxicity and lead to confusion, weakness, and arrhythmia
Lemon balm (*Melissa*) calendula, California poppy, hops, passion flower, valerian, black cohosh, German chamomile, kava kava, lavender leaves/flowers, motherwort, Siberian ginseng, skullcap, St. John's wort	Barbiturates and other sedatives	Increases hypnotic effects
Licorice	Corticosteroids	Interferes with steroid elimination thus increasing side effects and toxic effects
St. John's wort	Cough and cold products containing dextromethorphan	Increases likelihood of serotonin syndrome
Saw palmetto	Estrogen (HRT & BCP)	Causes an additive estrogen effect increasing side/toxic effects
Valerian	Barbiturates	Causes excessive sedation
Licorice, plaintain, uzara root, hawthorn, ginseng	Digoxin	Interferes with both monitoring and its pharmacodynamic activity
Hops, kava kava, passion flower, valerian, scopolia	Hismanal, Atarax, Viseral, Claritin	Causes sedative action and exacerbates drowsiness and fatigue side effects
Guggul as guggulipid	Beta blockers, Ca^{++} channel blockers	Diminishes the effectiveness of drugs
Ginseng	Ca^{++} channel blockers	Increases side effects of swollen and tender breasts
Licorice, yohimbe, Asian ginseng	Antihypertensives	Interferes with blood pressure control

Brinker, F. Herb and Drug Contraindication and Interaction. Eclectric Institute, Inc. *Oregon, 1997.*

Brooks, S. (ed.). Botanical toxicology. Protocol J. Bot. Med. *1:147–148, 1995.*

DeSmet PAGM et al (eds.). Adverse Effects of Herbal Drugs 2, Berlin: Springer-Verlag.

Facts & Comparison. Review of Natural Products—Potential and Specific Herb-Drug Interactions. Dec. 1998.

Herb Interactions you should know. Environmental Nutrition. *22(1):1, 6, 1999.*

Miller, LG: Herbal medicinals: selected clinical considerations focusing on known or potential drug-herb interactions. Arch Intern Med *Nov 9;158(20):2200-11, 1998.*

Wichtl, M. (ed.) Herbal Drugs and Phytopharmaceuticals, *CRC Press, Boca Raton, 1994.*

WHAT IS AN HERB?

The word herb as used in herbal medicine (also known as botanical medicine or, in Europe, as phytotherapy or phytomedicine) means a plant or plant part that is used to make medicine, food flavors (spices), or aromatic oils for soaps and fragrances. An herb can be a leaf, a flower, a stem, a seed, a root, a fruit, bark, or any other plant part used for its medicinal, food flavoring, or fragrant property.

Do these natural remedies really work? There's every reason to think they may. For one thing, plants already give us approximately a quarter of all drugs. Analgesics such as morphine or codeine, for example, are derived from the opium poppy. Atropine, a muscle relaxant, comes from belladonna; and the cancer drugs vincristine and vinblastine from periwinkle and taxol from the pacific yew. Even aspirin is derived from the salicin in spirea or willow bark. What's more, at least 16 herbs have been judged by the U.S. Food and Drug Administration (FDA) to be safe and effective, allowing these herbs to carry health claims and be sold as over-the-counter drugs. Among them are slippery elm bark (sold as Throat Coat Tea) and laxatives, such as senna (Senokot) and psyllium seeds (Metamucil).

Drugs have undergone extensive testing. Herbal remedies often rely on testimonials and tradition. For most herbs, scientific proof is difficult to come by. Of the approximately 600 botanicals sold in the United States, fewer than a dozen have been tested in costly, controlled clinical trials, which determine whether an herb is safe and works better than a placebo. Researchers say there is sketchy clinical trial evidence regarding another 50 or so botanicals.

Are There Different Herbal Systems?

There is diversity and richness in the various herbal traditions of the world, most of which still thrive today. Native American cultures contain a cornucopia of healing wisdom as do European traditions, from the Welsh to the Sicilian. There are many highly developed medical systems around the world that use medicinal plants in their healing work. These include ancient systems such as Ayurveda from India and Traditional Chinese Medicine. The essential differences between these various systems of medicine are their cultural contexts rather than their goals or effects. (See individual sections for more information regarding the philosophy of treatments.)

Traditional herbalists use combinations of herbs to subdue or enhance specific effects. However, much of today's western herbalism is based on the use of a single herb that provides a standardized dose of the constituent thought to be responsible for a plant's benefits. Traditional herbalists argue that standardization changes the very essence of a whole plant, making it more like a pharmaceutical. In the quest for the "active" constituent, researches may overlook lesser ingredients that still may enhance potency of a plant or modify its toxicity.

How Does Herbal Medicine Work?

In general, herbal medicines work in much the same way as do conventional pharmaceutical drugs, i.e., through their chemical makeup. Herbs contain many naturally occurring chemicals that have biologic activity. In the past 150 years, chemists and pharmacists have been isolating and purifying the "active" compounds from plants in an attempt to produce reliable pharmaceutical drugs.

Herbs and plants use an indirect route to the bloodstream and target organs. Their effects are usually slower in onset and less dramatic than those of purified drugs. Herbalists use herbs effectively (in the proper dose and frequency) to treat acute and chronic conditions. Herbal medicine also has much to offer when used to facilitate healing in chronic ongoing problems. By skillful selection of herbs for the patient, a profound transformation in health can be effected with less danger of the side effects inherent in drug-based medicine. However, the common assumption that herbs act slowly and mildly is not necessarily true. Adverse effects can occur if an inadequate dose, a low quality herb, or the incorrect herb is taken.

In addition to possessing understood pharmacologic activity, many herbs possess pharmacologic actions that are inconsistent with modern pharmacologic understanding. For example, many herbs appear to impact homeostatic control mechanisms to aid normalization of many of the body's processes: when there is a hyperstate, the herb exerts a lowering effect and when there is a hypostate the same herb has a heightening effect. This action is baffling to orthodox pharmacologists but not to experienced herbalists, who have used terms such as *alterative*, *amphoteric*, *adaptogenic*, or *tonic* to describe this effect. The whole plant contains hundreds of compounds. The lesser constituents may also be active. Until we have more definitive research, it is difficult to say whether we should be taking herbs that have been standardized for specific active ingredients or the whole herb.

What advantages do herbal medicines possess over synthetic drugs? As a rule, herbal preparations are less toxic than their synthetic counterparts and offer less risk of side effects (obviously, there are exceptions to this rule). In addition, the mechanism of action of an herb is often to correct the underlying cause of ill health. In contrast, a synthetic drug is often designed to alleviate the symptom or effect without addressing the underlying cause. It has also been demonstrated with many plants that the whole plant or crude extract is more effective than isolated constituents.

To date, as mentioned previously, there have been few clinical trials in the United States to examine efficacy of herbs and fewer yet to study pharmacokinetics. Because herbs have a complex mixture of active ingredients, the study of pharmacokinetics in herbs should be termed "ethnopharmacokinetics."

When one active ingredient is studied, the pharmacokinetic data may be different than when the whole plant is studied. In addition, the quality of the herb may also affect the results. Because herbs process pharmacokinetic activities, it is important to conduct more research to determine the herb's pharmacokinetics, but also how herbs and drugs can affect each other.

IS THERE QUALITY CONTROL OVER HERBS?

Quality control refers to processes involved in maintaining the quality or validity of a product. Regardless of the form of herbal preparation, some degree of quality control should exist. Currently, no organization or government body certifies the labeling of herbal preparations.

The U.S. Pharmopia (USP), a private nonprofit organization, sets legal recognized standards for medications—purity, quality, and strength. The USP has 18 such standards for vitamins and minerals and is working on standards for 30 herbs. The label of the vitamin/mineral or herb will then carry the USP stamp of approval.

The motto for herb buying seems to be "Buyer beware!" Quality varies between products and between companies. The American Herbal Products Association and The American Botanical Council work with the FDA and within its membership to assist with issues of quality control. There is no guarantee that what is on the label is in the bottle. Within the last few years, bottles of St. John's wort and Ginseng were found to contain no St. John's wort or Ginseng, and some mixtures were found contaminated with digitalis. To be safe, herbs should be purchased from companies with well-developed quality control standards.

The solution to the quality control problem that exists in the United States is for manufacturers and suppliers of herbal products to adhere to quality control standards and good manufacturing practices. With improvements in the identification of plants by laboratory analysis, consumers should at least be guaranteed that the correct plant is being used. Consumers, health food stores, pharmacists, and physicians who use or sell herbal products should ask for information from the suppliers of herbal products on their quality control process. What do they do to guarantee the validity of their product? As more consumers, retailers, and professionals begin asking for quality control from the suppliers, it is possible that more quality control processes will be used by manufacturers.

Only a few manufacturers adhere to complete quality control and good manufacturing procedures, including microscopic, physical, chemical, and biologic analyses. Companies supplying standardized extracts offer the greatest degree of quality control; thus, these products typically offer the highest quality.

TABLE 3-4 FDA EXAMPLES OF ACCEPTABLE AND UNACCEPTABLE CLAIMS FOR DIETARY SUPPLEMENTS

Acceptable Structure/Function Claims	
Helps maintain a healthy cholesterol level for men older than 50 years old	Reduces stress and frustration
Helps maintain regularity to meet nutritional needs during pregnancy	Inhibits platelet aggregation
Supports the immune system	Improves absentmindedness
Promotes relaxation	Use as part of your weight loss plan
Helps promote urinary tract health	Cardiohealth
Helps maintain cardiovascular function and a healthy circulatory system	Heart tabs
Helps maintain intestinal flora	Energizer
Helps maintain healthy intestinal tract	Rejuvenate
	Revitalizer
	Adaptogen
Disease Claims/Unacceptable for Dietary Supplements	
Lowers cholesterol	Alzheimer's disease
Improves urine flow in men older than 50 years of age	Decreased sexual function
Alleviates constipation	Hot flashes
Toxemia of pregnancy	Herbal Prozac
Supports body's ability to resist infection	Carpaltum
Supports the body's antiviral capabilities	Raynaudin
Protective against the development of cancer	Heptacure
Reduces the pain and stiffness associated with arthritis	Use as part of your diet when taking insulin to maintain a healthy blood sugar level
Reduces joint pain	Reduces nausea associated with chemotherapy
Relieves headache	Helps avoid diarrhea associated with antibiotic use
Decreases the effects of alcohol intoxication	To aid patients with reduced or compromised immune function, such as patients undergoing chemotherapy
Premenstrual syndrome	
Presbyopia	

Derived from Notice of Proposed Rulemaking, Federal Register, *April 29, 1998; FDA 1998a; Anon, 1998.*

What Is on the Labeling of an Herb?

The FDA regulations that assure safety and effectiveness of prescriptions and over-the-counter drugs do not apply to botanicals, which were deemed dietary supplements by Congress in 1994. The Dietary Supplement Act of 1994 stated that the herb could not make any specific medical claims on the label, but only state structure and function in the body, so feverfew, helpful for migraine headache prevention can only print "maintains a sense of well being"; echinacea, helpful for colds and flu, can only print "helps to maintain a healthy microbial balance in your body"; and saw palmetto, helpful for prostatic hypertrophy, can only print "maintains a healthy urinary system." Be wary of marketing brochures or labels that promise a cure for anything, such as weight loss. Claims that look too good to be true, probably are.

Some in the herb industry are calling for separate regulations for herbal remedies to improve the quality control and monitoring. In early 1998, new FDA guidelines were recommended and became effective March 1999, which include new labeling directions:

1998 FDA New Label Proposal

Types of claims not allowed under FDA's proposed new rules:

1. Statements about the formulation of the product, including a claim that the product contained an ingredient that has been regulated by FDA as a drug and is well-known to consumers for its use in preventing or treating a disease (e.g., aspirin, digoxin, or laetrile).
2. Citation of a title of a publication or other reference if the title refers to a disease use.
3. Use of the terms "disease" or "diseased."
4. Use of pictures, vignettes, symbols, etc. (e.g., Rx) that suggest an effect on a disease. Whole human body is OK.
5. Product class names strongly associated with diagnosis, cure, mitigation, treatment, or prevention of a disease or diseases, e.g., "antibiotic," "laxative," "analgesic," "antiviral," "diuretic," "antimicrobial," "antiseptic," "antidepressant," or "vaccine."
6. Statement implying that a dietary supplement (DS) has an effect on a disease by claiming that effect of the DS is the same as that of a recognized drug or disease therapy ("Herbal Prozac" or "use as part of your diet when taking insulin to help maintain a healthy blood sugar level").
7. A statement that may contain an expressed or implied disease claim if it suggests that the product cures, mitigates, treats, or prevents a disease or diseases by augmenting the body's own disease-fighting capabilities: "supports the body's antiviral capabilities," "supports the body's ability to resist infection."

8. Claims that the DS is intended to counter adverse events resulting from medical intervention are considered claims that the product is intended as part of the treatment program and, as such, are claims that the DS is intended to mitigate, treat, or cure the disease:
   "reduces nausea associated with chemotherapy"
   "helps avoid diarrhea associated with antibiotic use"
   "to aid patients with reduced or compromised immune function, e.g., patients undergoing chemotherapy"

(Source: derived from Notice of Proposed Rulemaking, *Federal Register,* April 29, 1998; FDA, 1998a; Anon, 1998.)

WHAT HERBAL PRODUCTS ARE AVAILABLE?

Many forms of herbs are available. Herbalists still prefer the whole herb, but most herb manufacturers are using only one or two parts of the plant that are thought to be the most active. The types of herb products that are available include: the whole herb, teas, capsules and tablets, extracts, tinctures, essential oils (discussed in aromatherapy) and salves, balms, and ointments.

Whole Herbs

Whole herbs are plants or plant parts that are dried and then cut or left whole (cinnamon, bay leaf, slippery elm). Bulk herbs lose their potency quickly. When buying whole herbs, insure their freshness—herbs should have good color and strong aroma. They should be in their whole form—flowers, leaves, roots, and so on. Herbs should be protected from light because light decreases potency. Herbs should be stored in opaque containers and protected from heat, air, and insects. Whole herbs are usually made into a tea, but remember that some of the active ingredients may not be water soluble. Those considered most active in water are milk thistle and echinacea.

Teas

Teas come in either loose or tea bag form. Because of the obvious convenience, most Americans prefer to purchase their herbal teas in tea bags, which include one or a variety of finely cut herbs. When steeped in boiled water for a few minutes, the fragrant, aromatic flavor and the herbs' medicinal properties are released. Teas are as medicinal as any other preparation if properly prepared. However, many herbs have undesirable flavor profiles (valerian root smells and tastes like old sweaty socks), from intensely bitter (not all bitter herbs contain alkaloids) as a result of the presence of certain compounds such as alkaloids, to highly astringent as a result of the presence of tannins (oak bark). Tannins in tea are medicinally desirable and common in varying amounts in many teas, including common tea. As a general rule, most teas are consumed for three reasons:

1. As alternatives to caffeinated tea or coffee (although some herbal teas contain caffeine)
2. As a component to a meal for the flavor or for their digestive properties (peppermint, spearmint, rosehips, lemon grass, anise)
3. For their medicinal effects (peppermint and chamomile for upset stomach or to improve digestion, chamomile or hops as a nighttime sleep aid or insomnia remedy, cinnamon tea as a home remedy for diarrhea).

Capsules and Tablets

One of the fastest growing markets in herbal medicine in the past 15 to 20 years has been capsules and tablets. These offer consumers convenience and, in some cases, the bonus of not having to taste the herbs. To create a capsule or tablet, the herb is powdered, exposed to heat and oxygen, or freeze dried or heated and has binders and fillers added. Is the herb still active? More research needs to be done to determine potency.

Extracts and Tinctures

These offer the advantage of high concentration in low weight and space. They are also quickly assimilated compared to tablets, which take more time to disintegrate and ingest. Extracts and tinctures almost always contain alcohol. The alcohol is used for two reasons: as a solvent to extract the various non–water-soluble compounds from an herb, and as a preservative to maintain shelf life. Properly made extracts and tinctures have virtually an indefinite shelf life. Tinctures usually contain more alcohol than extracts (sometimes up to 70–80% alcohol, depending on the particular herb and manufacturer). It is important for persons to understand that because extracts and tinctures contain alcohol, there may be drug interactions that can provoke an antabuse reaction. Glycerine-based tinctures are available for those who want to avoid alcohol.

Salves, Balms, and Ointments

For thousands of years, humans have used plants to treat skin irritations, wounds, and insect and snake bites. In prehistoric times, herbs were cooked in a vat of goose or bear fat, lard, or some vegetable oils and then cooled to make salves, balms, and ointments. Today, many such products, made with vegetable oil or petroleum jelly, are sold in the United States and Europe to treat a variety of conditions. These products often contain the following herbs: aloe, marigold, chamomile, St. John's wort, comfrey, and gotu kola.

WHAT CONDITIONS ARE BENEFITTED BY HERBAL MEDICINE?

Herbal medicine, used by an educated herbalist or naturopath, can be used to treat all conditions, both acute and chronic. Herbal medicine may be more effective than traditional medicine in treating chronic conditions. Herbal remedies can be used for a wide range of ailments that include stomach upset, the common cold, flu, minor aches and pains, constipation and diarrhea, coughs, headaches, menstrual cramps, digestive disturbances, sore muscles, skin rashes, sunburn, dandruff, and insomnia. Other conditions that respond well to herbal medicine include: digestive disorders such as peptic ulcers, colitis, and irritable bowel syndrome; rheumatic and arthritic conditions; chronic skin problems such as eczema and psoriasis; problems of the menstrual cycle and especially premenstrual syndrome and menopausal concerns; anxiety and tension-related stress; bronchitis and other respiratory conditions; hypertension; and allergies. An increasing number of American health consumers use herbal remedies for these conditions, which have been traditionally the domain of the nonprescription or over-the-counter drugs.

Herbal medicines can also be used for several conditions normally treated by prescription only, for example, milk thistle seed extract for use in cirrhosis and hepatitis; hawthorn as a heart tonic; St. John's wort for minor depression; and ginkgo biloba to improve memory. Hawthorn is highly recommended for cardiac patients by physicians in Germany.

When treating chronic illness with herbal medicine, it is important to treat the entire body because the illness may be simultaneously affecting many systems of the body at various levels. The course of the treatment must include nutritional, tonic, and restorative plants in conjunction with herbs that support the body's elimination functions. Alterative and adaptogenic plants can be effective. Digestive function is also an important consideration in most chronic diseases. The duration of treatment with herbs is often longer than it is with drugs, with a changing dose of the herb or herb combinations being administered over a longer period of time.

The uniqueness of each individual is important in evaluating any holistic therapy, whether it be homeopathic, herbal, or nutritional. For the therapy to be effective, the provider must be knowledgeable and adaptable to each patient's situation.

ARE HERBS SAFE?

Generally speaking, herbs are safer than drugs—most of which have potentially serious side effects. Illnesses associated with herbal use are relatively uncommon, and deaths are rare. Still, even the safest herbs carry risks. Herbal medicine is like any other medicine. It should be used with discretion.

Products also can contain harmful or undesirable substances, whether added by mistake or design. Ayurvedic herbs, imported from India, are boiled down in clay or metal pots, often leaving residues of lead, mercury, arsenic, gold, or cadmium. Chinese herbal remedies (typically blends of many different herbs brewed into teas) are sometimes laced with prescription drugs. Misidentified plants can also be a problem. From 1991 to 1993, 48 Belgian women suffered severe kidney damage after taking a Chinese herbal preparation for weight loss that mistakenly contained a toxic plant instead of the herb Stephania.

Toxicities that build up over months or years are another worry, although more difficult to predict. Centuries of use can rule out herbs that are acute poisons, but they cannot always identify those that cause cancer or other chronic illnesses. Only in the last 30 years, for instance, have researchers learned that comfrey, coltsfoot, germander, and borage—herbs used for hundreds of years for a variety of illnesses—contain toxins called pyrrolizidine alkaloids that, over time, damage the liver as an idiosyncratic reaction (usually in persons with a history of liver disease). Similarly, six cases of liver failure reported in the past few years have been linked to the long-term use of chaparral, an herb used for everything from arthritis to cancer. Additional unsafe herbs include: comfrey, coltsfoot, basil, borage (carcinogenic), and yohimbe (causes hypertension and tachycardia).

How Are Herbs Used Safely?

Most experts say it is best to take herbal remedies on your own only for minor, short-term discomforts such as colds. For everything else, see an herbalist, naturopathic doctor (ND) or a doctor educated in the use of herbs—if only to make sure you are not simply alleviating the symptoms of a potentially serious illness. All trained herbal providers refer a patient to a traditional provider for conditions outside their scope of practice. The following are some basic guidelines:

DO NOT TAKE HERBS CASUALLY

Medicinal herbs should only be taken when needed. There are other herbs that are best used on a regular basis for health maintenance and disease prevention (garlic, peppermint, turmeric).

TABLE 3-5 CONTRAINDICATIONS OF SELECTED HERBS

Contra-indicated in All Persons	Contra-indicated in Pregnancy	Contraindicated in Selected Persons	
		Herb	When
Comfrey: carcinogenic	Pennyroyal	Lemon balm	hypothyroid is enhanced
Coltsfoot: carcinogenic	Feverfew	Black cohosh	estrogen + tumors
	Vitex	Dong quai	estrogen + tumors
Germander: liver toxicity	Ginseng	Ginseng	estrogen + tumors
Chaparral: liver toxicity	Dong quai	Ginseng	Acute illness, liver asthma
Skull cap: liver toxicity	Black cohosh root	Echinacea	Autoimmune disorders
Yohimbe: lupus-like symptoms	Aloe latex		
Ephedra (Ma Huang): hypertension		Belladonna/aloe	Glaucoma, any abdominal pain or discomfort of unknown origin
	Echinacea (Augustifolia/Pallida)		
	Basil oil		
	California poppy		
	Comfrey		
	Buckthorn (bark and berry)		
	Kava kava		
	Rhubarb		

[a]*Sometimes herbs are contraindicated in pregnancy because experimental information is unavailable and because of the known activity of the herb. Some contraindications are made as a measure of caution, without direct evidence of risk.*

DO NOT TAKE HERBS IF YOU ARE PREGNANT, TRYING TO BECOME PREGNANT, OR NURSING

Do not give herbs to your baby. Fetuses and babies lack some of the liver enzymes needed to detoxify harmful chemicals in herbs. (See Table 3-5 for a selected list of herbs contraindicated during pregnancy.)

DO NOT OVERDO IT

Start with less than the recommended dose and monitor progress, particularly if you are young, older than 60, or below average weight. Damage to the liver, kidneys, and other organs occurs more often when botanicals are consumed in large amounts or over a long period of time. Generally, early symptoms of liver damage resemble the standard flu or cold symptoms; jaundice may show up a little later (see Table 3-6).

DO NOT REGULARLY USE A LARGE VARIETY OF HERBS

Start with single herbs rather than combinations. Multiherb formulas ("kitchen sink" combinations are readily available from herbal companies) increase the risk of reactions and may contain ingredients with dubious benefits. As yet, few botanicals have been checked by drug standards for safety when combined with other herbs or drugs (they have been combined for centuries in well-developed traditions), whether

TABLE 3-6 ADVERSE REACTIONS WITH SELECTED HERBS

Allergic Reaction Often Occurs	With	Specific Adverse Effect
Anise seed	Ma Huang (ephedra)	Hypertension/cardiac arrhythmia
Bromelain	Licorice root	Water retention in specific people
Cinnamon bark	Willow bark	Salicylism (when other ASA products are also taken)
Dandelion	St. John's wort	Photosensitivity
Echinacea Purpurea	Eucalyptus leaf, oil	Diarrhea
Garlic	Ginkgo biloba	Headache
Kava kava	Sweet clover	Headache
Mistletoe herb	Chaste tree fruit	Hives
Parsley herb and root	Paprika	Hives
Psyllium seed/husks	Aloe, Cascara Sagrada	K^+ deficiency
Tansy	Senna leaf, pod	K^+ deficiency
Yarrow	Kava kava	Yellow skin

prescription or over-the-counter. Get advice from knowledgeable people. Good sources include educated herbalogists, physicians or pharmacists who have taken courses on herbal remedies, and licensed naturopaths, who take extensive course work in botanical medicine. (For referral, call the American Association of Naturopathic Physicians, 206-323-7610.) If you're looking for Chinese herbs, get them prescribed by a licensed acupuncturist trained in Chinese medicine. (For more information, call the National Commission for the Certification of Acupuncturists, 202-232-1404.)

DO NOT SELF-DIAGNOSE

Self-treatment with herbs is appropriate only for minor, self-limiting conditions. Proper medical care is critical to good health. If symptoms are suggestive of an illness, consult a physician, preferably a naturopath, holistic MD or DO, chiropractor, or other natural health care specialist.

WORK WITH YOUR DOCTOR

If taking a prescription medication, the patient must work with the doctor before discontinuing any drug.

BE PATIENT

Many herbs take longer than traditional drugs to have an effect. Other herbs, such as peppermint and kava kava, work more quickly.

USE A GOOD SOURCE BOOK

Many good source books are available. Before trying an herb, discuss it with your physician. Because your physician is most likely unaware of the herb you want to use, you may need to educate him or her. Remember, although many herbs are effective on their own, they work better if they are part of a comprehensive natural treatment plan focusing on diet and lifestyle factors.

LEARN AS MUCH AS YOU CAN ABOUT THE HERBS YOU'RE TAKING

The more you know, the better you can judge quality, effectiveness, and side effects. Buy herbs from companies with good quality control. Learn about potential interactions between other herbs, drugs, and foods. Stop taking an herb immediately if you experience an unpleasant or unusual reaction. If you have an adverse reaction, such as fever, nausea, or headache, report it (see Table 2-5). Call the FDA at 800-332-1088 and the American Herbal Products Association at 512-469-6355.

HERB SOURCES OF VITAMINS, MINERALS, AND TRACE MINERALS

Many botanical plants contain vitamins, minerals, and trace minerals. The body can usually digest vitamins and minerals much easier through plant origin than those of fish or animal origin. Therefore, herbs are excellent to impart the vitamins and minerals needed by the body. Following is a list of some of the best herb sources of vitamins and minerals. Remember, these herbs are not meant to be a substitute for whole foods, and if vitamin and mineral supplementation is required, seek help from an educated provider.

Vitamins

Vitamin C: bee pollen, chickweed, echinacea, garlic, juniper berries, peppermint, rose hips

Vitamin F: red raspberry, Slippery Elm

Minerals

Calcium: chamomile, fennel, marshmallow, sage, white oak bark

Cobalt: dandelion, horsetail, juniper berries, lobelia, parsley, red clover, white oak bark

Iodine: kelp

Iron: Burdock, chickweed, ginseng, hops, mullein, nettles, parsley, peppermint, rosemary, sarsaparilla, yellow dock

Magnesium: alfalfa, catnip, ginger, gota kola, red clover, rosemary, valerian, wood betony

Potassium: aloe, blue cohosh, cascara sagrada, dandelion leaf, fennel, parsley, rose hips, slippery elm, valerian, yarrow

Zinc: burdock, chamomile, dandelion, eyebright, hawthorne, licorice, marshmallow, sarsaparilla

Trace Minerals

Alfalfa, black cohosh, burdock, cascara sagrada, chaparral, dandelion, hawthorne, horsetail, kelp, lobelia, parsley, red clover, rose hips, sage, sarsaparilla, valerian, yellow dock

HOW ARE HERBS TAKEN?

In general, the dosage listed on the bottle has been developed for a 150 lb person. For children 6 to 12 years, use half the suggested dose; for children 1 to 5 years, a third of the suggested dose, and do not administer to children younger than 1 year of age.

In addition, herbs and drugs and vitamins and minerals can react with each other. Table 2-5 has a selected list of possible combinations. There are probably many more undetermined interactions.

BIBLIOGRAPHY

American Botanical Council, Austin, TX. 512-331-8868. www.herbalgram.org. Accessed August 10, 1998.

Astin, J. (1998). Alternative medicine. Journal of the American Medical Association. 279(19):1549–1554.

DeSmet, P. A. G. M. (1997). Adverse effects of herbal drugs. Vol. 3. Berlin: Springer-Verlag.

DeSmet P. A. G. M., et al. (1997). Pharmacokinetic evaluation of herbal remedies. Basic introduction, applicability, current status and regulatory needs. Clinical Pharmacokinetics. 32, 427–436.

Duke, J. A. (1997). The green pharmacy. NY: Pharmaceutical Products Press.

Ernst, E. (1998). Harmless herbs? A review of the recent literature. The American Journal of Medicine. 104, 170–178.

Fugh-Berman, A. (1997). Clinical trials of herbs. Primary Care. 24, (4), 889.

German Commission E Monographs. *Fall 1998. (Considered by professionals outside of the United States to be flawed, and should be used only for historic interest.)*

Herbal Gram. American Botanical Council. Austin, TX. All issues.

Herb Research Foundation. Boulder, CO. 303 449 2265.

Mills, S. The Essential Book of Herbal Medicine. MA. London: FNJMN.

Newall, C., Anderson, L., & Phillips, J. (1996). Herbal medicine: a guide for health care professionals. Rocklin, CA: Prima Health.

The American Herb Association Newsletter. Rescue, CA.

The Lawrence Review of Natural Products. Facts and Comparisons. St. Louis, MO. 1990–present.

Weiss, R. Herbal medicine, ESCOP monographs. (European Scientific Cooperative on Phytotherapy—contact info in U.K. 011 44 1392 264498: Centre for Complementary Health Studies, University of Exeter.)

Young, T. & McCaleb, R. (1998). American Herbal Products Association seeks modification of herbal extract provisions. Herbal Gram. No. 42, 23.

SELECTED HERBS

The following is a selection of the most commonly used herbs in the United States. Every effort has been made to obtain as much scientific information available about each herb. A bibliography follows each herb.

Aloe *(Aloe vera)*

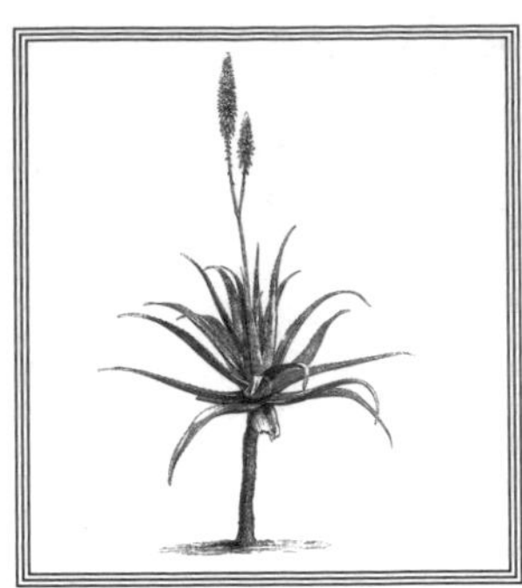

DESCRIPTION

- More than 500 species exist
- Name means "bitter and shiny substance"
- Perennial succulants grow throughout the world except in rain forest and arid desserts
- Short plant has 15 to 30 tapering leaves approximately 20 inches long and 5 inches wide
- Leaf has three layers: outer–tough, middle–corrugate lining, and inner layer–a colorless mucilaginous pulp–the aloe gel
- Mature plant is 1.5 to 4 feet high and 3 feet or more in diameter at the base

TERMINOLOGY

- Aloe vera gel. Naturally occurring, undiluted gel obtained by stripping away the outer layer of the aloe vera leaf
- Aloe vera concentrate. Aloe vera gel from which the water has been removed
- Aloe vera juice. An ingestible product containing a minimum of 50% aloe vera gel
- Aloe vera latex. The bitter yellow liquid derived from the pericyclic tubules of the rind of Aloe vera, the primary constituent of which is aloin.

PART OF PLANT USED FOR MEDICINAL PURPOSES

- Aloe gel: inside each leaf
- Aloe: solid residue obtained by evaporating the latex beneath the skin

FOLK USE

- Ancient Egypt (1500 BC) and Middle East, to heal the skin
- In United States, since 1820, as a laxative

ACTIVE INGREDIENTS

- Aloe latex—anthraquinone barbaloin (local irritant)
  o-glycosides of barbaloin
  resin (63%)
  aloin

- Aloe gel (obtained by crushing the mucilaginous cells found in the inner leaf)
  - polysaccharides glucomannan (contributes to the emollient effect)
- Aloe vera extract—(pulverized whole leaves of the plant)
  - All contain tannins, organic acids, enzymes, vitamins, steroids, bradykininase (protease inhibitor, which decreases pain and swelling), magnesium lactate (antipruritic), prostaglandins.

ACTION

Gel
- Emollient
- Antiprostaglandin activity, therefore topically relieves pain, decreases swelling and redness
- Blocks histamines
- Antibacterial, antifungal activity (conflicting research exists regarding effectiveness)
- Inhibits bradykinins and thromboxane

Latex: irritates gastrointestinal (GI) mucosa

USES*

- Enhances immune function
- Enhances healing of burns
- Decreases psoriasis
- Enhances wound healing (one study suggested it slowed healing)
- Reduce symptoms of fibromyalgia and chronic fatigue syndrome

Latex:
- For constipation
- Healing bowel in inflammatory bowel diseases

DOSAGE

- Gel: apply topically
- Processed aloe vera may not be as active in its antibacterial/ antifungal activity
- Juice: up to maximum of 1 quart/day
- Latex: no more than 1 to 2 tbsp/day

TOXICITY

- Topical: skin rashes

---

*FDA panel recently found aloe not useful for anything.

CONTRAINDICATIONS

Topical
- In deep, vertical wounds
- Hypersensitivity

Internally
- Bowel obstruction
- Inflammatory bowel disease

SIDE EFFECTS

Topically
- Contact dermatitis
- May delay wound healing

Internally
- May cause fluid and electrolyte imbalances
- Cramp-like GI symptoms

LONG-TERM SAFETY

- Gel: safe
- Latex: unsafe for daily long-term dosing of more than 1 to 2 weeks because it may cause intestinal sluggishness

PREGNANT/LACTATION/CHILDREN

- Latex: contraindicated in pregnant or lactating women and in children
- Topical use: safe

DRUG INTERACTIONS

- Aloe latex: binds all drugs. Separate by at least 2 hours from all drugs.
- With chronic use causes loss of K^+ and may increase effectiveness of cardiac glycosides and antiarrhythmics.

Bibliography

Dykman, K. D., Tone, C., Ford, C., & Dykman, R. A. (1998). The effects of nutritional supplements on the symptoms of fibromyalgia and chronic fatigue syndrome. Integrative Physiological and Behavioral Science. 33, (1), 61–71.

Klein, A. D. & Penneys, N. S. (1998). Aloe vera. Journal of the American Academy of Dermatology. 18, (4 Pt 1), 714–720.

Lawrence Review. The Review of Natural Products. Facts and Comparisons. St. Louis, MO. 1997–1998.

Odes, H. S. & Madar, Z. (1991). A double-blind trial of a celandin, aloe vera and psylium laxative preparation in adult patients with constipation. Digestion. 49, (2), 65–71.

Phillips, T., et al. (1995). A randomized study of an aloe vera derivative gel dressing versus conventional treatment after shave biopsy excision. Wounds—A Compendium of Clinical Research & Practice. 7, (5), 200–202.

Sato, Y., et al. (1990). Studies on chemical protectors against radiation. XXXI Protection Effects of Aloe Arborescens on Skin Injury Induced by X-irradiation. Yakugaku Zasshi. 110, (11), 876–884.

Schmidt, J. M. & Greenspoon, J. S. (1991). Aloe vera dermal wound gel is associated with a delay in wound healing. Obstetrics and Gynecology. 78, (1), 115.

Syed, T. A., et al. (1996). Management of psoriasis with aloe vera extract in a hydrophilic cream: a placebo-controlled, double-blind study. Tropical Medicine and International Health. 1, (4), 505–509.

Visuthiokosol, V., et al. (1995). Effect of aloe vera gel to healing of burn wound a clinical and histologic study. Journal of the Medical Association of Thailand. 78, (8), 403–409.

Bilberry *(Myrtillus fructus)*

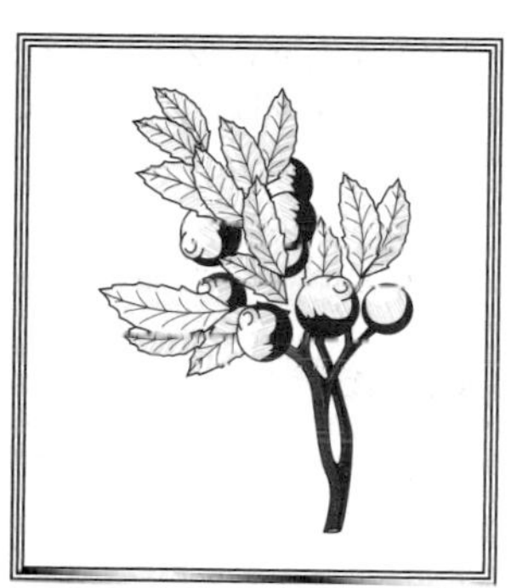

DESCRIPTION

- Originates in northern and central Europe
- Shrubby perennial: grows in meadows and woods
- Produces black, coarsely wrinkled berries containing many small, shiny, brownish-red seeds
- Berries have a caustic and sweet taste
- Vaccinium species contains nearly 200 species of berries including cranberry and American blueberry.

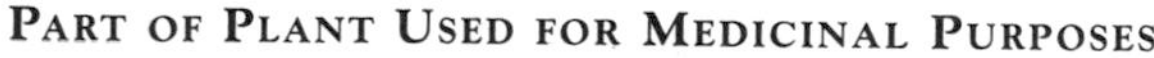

PART OF PLANT USED FOR MEDICINAL PURPOSES

- Fruit

FOLK USE

- Used as food for its nutritive value
- Used to treat scurvy, urinary infections, and stones
- Used to treat diarrhea and dysentery
- British World War II pilots were said to have improved night vision
- Used to treat diabetes

ACTIVE INGREDIENTS

- Anthocyanins
- Tannins
- Flavonoid glycosides

ACTION

- Stabilizes collagen in connective tissue, ligaments, cartilage
- Acts as free radical scavengers
- Stimulates regrowth and reproduction of collagen
- Stabilizes capillary membrane
- Decreases platelet aggregation
- Improves the delivery of oxygen to the eye
- Acts as antioxidant
- Increase prostaglandin E_2 release in stomach mucosa
- Protects liver cells

USES

- Nonspecific, acute diarrhea
- Vascular disorders: varicose veins (supports veins)
- Eye conditions: glaucoma, macular degeneration, improves night vision
- Peptic ulcer: protects gastric mucosa
- Anticancer activity

DOSAGE

- Standardized (25% anthocyanidens) 20 to 40 mg three times a day
- Bilberry extract (25% anthocyanidens) 80 to160 mg three times a day

TOXICITY

- Nontoxic

CONTRAINDICATIONS

- None known

SIDE EFFECTS

- None known

LONG-TERM SAFETY

- Safe
- If diarrhea is present for more than several days, see a health care provider.

PREGNANT/LACTATING/CHILDREN

- Unknown

DRUG INTERACTIONS

- None known

Bibliography

Bomser, J., Madhavi, D. L., Singletary, K., & Smith, M. A. (1996). In vitro anticancer activity of fruit extracts from Vaccinium species. Planta Medica. 62, (3), 212–216.

Colantuoni, A., et al. (1991). Effects of Vaccinium Myrtillus Anthocyanosides on arterial vasomotion. Arzneimittelforschung. 41, (9), 905–909.

Lawrence Review. (1994). The Review of Natural Products. St. Louis, MO: Facts and Comparisons.

Lietti, A., et al. (1976). Studies on Vaccinium Myrtillus Anthocyanosides: I., vasoprotective and antiinflammatory activity. Arzneimittelforschung. 26, 829–832.

Black Cohosh
(Cimicifuga racemosa)

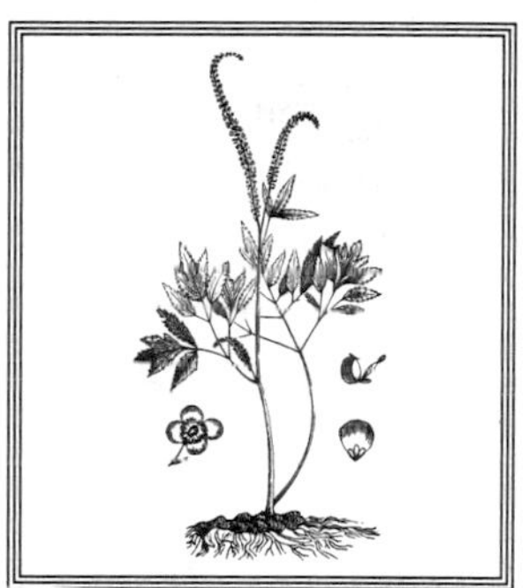

DESCRIPTION

- A striking plant grows in hardwood forests in the United States and Europe
- Grows at edges of woods
- 3 to 9 feet tall
- A member of the buttercup family
- Small white flowers in from July to September

PART OF PLANT USED FOR MEDICINAL PURPOSES

- Rhizome: dig in fall

FOLK USE

Native Americans used it to treat arthritic joints/inflammation, respiratory congestion, relaxing nervine, and reproductive conditions, including menopausal symptoms. Since 1988, black cohosh tinctures has been found to be as effective as estrogen replacement therapy (ERT) in menopausal women in Germany. (Note: as a "folk" remedy (unproven by double-blind trials) it has been used for some menopausal women from early 19th Century through today, not just in Germany, but in the United States, Canada, Australia, and others.)

ACTIVE INGREDIENTS

- Triperpenes glycosides and other glycosides

- Isoflavones
- Alkaloids
- Tannins
- Resins
- Methanol

ACTION

- Estrogen mimetic
- Suppresses LH, therefore helps control hormone surges that cause symptoms in menopause
- Anti-inflammatory

USES

- Helps control signs and changes of menopause or those related to surgical removal of ovaries (will make cycles further apart); 50 to 60% of women have reduction in symptoms in 6 to 8 weeks.
- Hot flashes
- Depression
- Irritability
- Fatigue
- Headache
- Reduces water retention
- Irregular menses
- Vaginal dryness
- Alleviates insomnia and promotes sleep
- Anti-inflammatory for arthritis
- Antipyretic
- During labor when irritated or woman is very tired (small doses under tongue)
- Regular/painful menses/with heavy flow in any age woman
- Decreases symptoms of endometriosis—stops spasm of uterus
- Research has demonstrated that black cohosh can block estrogen's ability to promote tumor growth (this effect is increased with concurrent tamoxifen) (see contraindications.)**

DOSAGE

- Tincture* 10 to 60 drops/day
- Root/rhizome infusion: a swallow at a time up to 250 mL/day
- Powdered root* or as tea: 1 to 2 grams

---

*Estrogen effect greater in dried powder or root, less in tincture.
**Conflicting information at this time.

- Remifemin, a commercial formula: 2 tablespoons twice daily, or 1 tablet two times a day

TOXICITY

- May increase menstrual flow
- Do not use if pregnant
- May increase heart rate
- Possible stomach upset
- Can be used even during menses

CONTRAINDICATIONS

- Has phytoestrogens ability, so do not use with estrogen positive cancer; however, some studies suggest it may be helpful because it blocks ER II receptor sites in cancer.

SIDE EFFECTS

- Headaches (frontal) (mostly with doses higher than 2 mL/day or with standardized extracts)
- Hypotension, usually from overdose
- Visual disturbances
- Can increase or start bleeding again during menopause by stimulating normal function of ovary that isn't "done" yet—not always a dangerous sign. Perimenopausal bleeding must be diagnosed to rule out disease.

PREGNANCY/LACTATING/CHILDREN

- Do not administer to children.

DRUG INTERACTIONS

- None known
- Research is mixed, standardized extracts may or may not be safe used with estrogen

LONG-TERM SAFETY

- Probably safe for several years

Bibliography

Hobbs, C. (1998). Black Cohosh—A woman's herb comes of age. Herbs for Health. March/April, 38–41.

Lieberman, S. (1998). A review of the effectiveness of Cimicifuga racemosa (black cohosh) for the symptoms of menopause. Journal of Womens Health. 7, (5), 525–529.

Snow, J. (1996). Black Cohosh. Protocol Journal of Botanical Medicine. Vol 1, (4), 17–19.

Dong Quai *(Dong gui, Dong gway, Angelica sinensis and several other species)*

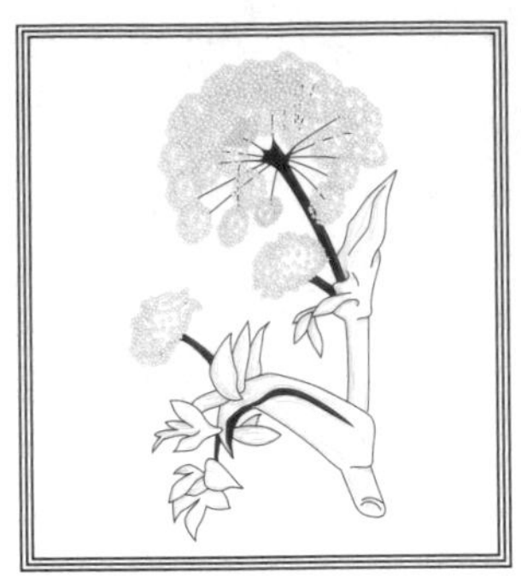

DESCRIPTION

- An aromatic root plant grown throughout the Orient
- Dong quai is yin (see Oriental Medicine for more information)

PART OF PLANT USED FOR MEDICINAL PURPOSES

- Root and rhizomes

FOLK USE

- Dong quai is one of the most frequently used women's herbs in the world
- Has been used by the Chinese for thousands of years as a blood tonic

ACTIVE INGREDIENTS

- Six coumarin derivatives
- Lactones
- Essential oils
- Many others

ACTION

- Peripheral vasodilator
- Antispasmodic, particularly coronary arteries
- Immunosuppressive
- Anti-inflammatory (decreases prostaglandin E_2, not histamine)
- Ca^{++} channel blocking activity: smooth muscle relaxers
- Acts as phytoestrogen, but may suppress estradiol; thus, may be safe in estrogen positive cancers
- Pain relievers
- Potent uterine vasodilation

USES

- Relieves hot flashes (but if you feel hot all the time, don't use because it may increase flashes)

- No. 1 menopausal tonic* to:
  - restore thin, dry vaginal tissues
  - relieve water retention
  - reduce headaches
  - reduce high blood pressure but not enough to eliminate medications
  - ease menopausal insomnia
  - restore emotional calm
  - improve digestion: increases pancreatic function
- Warming herb

DOSAGE

- Tincture of fresh or dried roots, 10 to 40 drops, 1 to 3 times a day
- Dried roots as infusion, up to 250 mL/day
- Root, chew 1/8 to 1/4″ 2 to 3 times/day

(Caution: may increase menstrual flow).

TOXICITY

- relatively nontoxic

CONTRAINDICATIONS

- Do not use if menses is heavy (may increase bleeding), if fibroids or diarrhea are present, of if feeling bloated. If breast tenderness or soreness occurs, discontinue use.

SIDE EFFECTS

- Photosensitizing

LONG-TERM SAFETY

- Unknown

PREGNANCY/LACTATING/CHILDREN

- Unknown

DRUG INTERACTION

- Active ingredients: coumarins, thus do not use with coumadin products
- Careful use with ASA

---

*1997 research has indicated that dong quai is ineffective in stopping menopausal symptoms and does not produce estrogen-like responses, but other studies refute these findings.

Bibliography

Bates, B. (1997). Dong quai shown not effect for menopause. Internal Medicine News. Aug, 1, 46.

Hirata, J.D., Swiersz, L. M., et al. (1997). Does dong quai have estrogenic effects in postmenopausal women? A double-blind, placebo-controlled trial. Fertility and Sterility. 68, (6), 981–986.

Echinacea (*Echinacea augustifolia* and related species)

(*Echinacea purpurea*)

(*Echinacea pallida*)—(purple cone flower)

DESCRIPTION

- Perennial herb, part of the daisy family, native to Midwest North America from Saskatchewan to Texas.
- Height 1.5 to 3 feet
- Purple flowers
- When the flower is chewed, it causes tingling of lips and tongue

PART OF PLANT USED FOR MEDICINAL PURPOSES

- The aerial portion (purpurea) and the root (pallida)

FOLK USE

- Native Americans used echinacea to treat wounds, burns, abscesses, insect bites, toothaches, joint pains, and as an antidote for snake bites.
- In Europe, it was used to treat injuries in horses.
- In 1870 it was introduced as "Meyer's blood purifier" for all matter of ills.
- Germany has officially approved echinacea for use in treating colds, flu, and URI.

ACTIVE INGREDIENTS*

- 0.1% echinacoside
- Complex isobutylamide (echinacein)
- Alkamides

*No single agent appears to be responsible for plant's activity. (Many of the active ingredients are destroyed during processing. Freeze drying is the most effective way to preserve the healing properties.)

ACTION

- Immunomodulators (Several clinical trials say yes; others say no. More research is necessary. It may stimulate lymphokines.)
- Cytotoxic activity against tumor cells
- Stimulates bone marrow macrophages
- Stimulates white blood cell (WBC) production
- Antioxidant
- Decreases cytokine production (IL-6)
- Reduces inflammation (inhibits both enzymes cyclooxygenase and five; lipoxygenase ultimately reducing leukotrienes and prostaglandins, both mediators of inflammation.)
- Turns on T-lymphocytes and NK cells
- Little or no effect on normal immune response in healthy patients
- Elevates neutrophils count and increases their activity
- Shortens duration of URI
- Stimulates production of interferon, which in turn, increases NK cells

USES

- To treat infections, particularly candida (does not treat source of infection)
- The common cold (may decrease the chances of getting a cold, decreases its severity)
- Enhances wound healing
- Relieves arthritis pain
- May enhance WBCs in persons undergoing chemotherapy
- Helps prevent skin photodamage from UV sunlight when used topically
- Used in Germany along with chemotherapy in the treatment of cancer

DOSAGE*

- Research needs to be done to determine the proper form and dose, the best species and part of the plant to use, and the best solvents. Take at first sign of infection. (May need to take 1 gram three times a day.) Do not take continuously for more than 6 to 8 weeks.
- Dried root (or as tea), 1 to 2 grams/day
- Freeze-dried plant, 325 to 650 mg three times a day

  Juice of aerial portion of E. purpurea stabilized in 22% ethanol (preferably standardized to contain a minimum of 2.4% β-1,2-fructofuranosides): 2 to 3 mL (½ to ¾ teaspoon) three times a day

---

*The most research has been conducted in Germany with a product now produced in the United States under the brand name Echinaguard (Nature's Way).

- Tincture (1:5): 3 to 4 mL (¾ to 1 teaspoon) three times a day
- Fluid extract (1:1): 1 to 2 mL (¼ to ½ teaspoon) three times a day
- Solid (dry powdered) extract (6.5:1 or 3/5% echinacoside): 300 mg three times a day

TOXICITY

- Nontoxic at recommended doses.
- Severely allergic people, or people with atopy, may develop a full anaphylactic reaction.

CONTRAINDICATIONS

- Autoimmune diseases such as multiple sclerosis (MS) and HIV (based on the speculation that stimulating an overactive immune system will worsen symptoms, but there is no research to confirm this).
- Diabetes
- Allergy to daisy family (i.e., chrysanthemums) of plants

SIDE EFFECTS

- Minimal
- Nausea

LONG-TERM SAFETY

- Not to be used for more than 8 weeks continuously

PREGNANT/LACTATING/CHILDREN

- Do not take during pregnancy and lactation.
- Do not administer to children younger than 6.

DRUG INTERACTIONS

- May cause liver toxicity with other liver toxic drugs

Bibliography

Bauer, R. & Wagner, H. (1991). *Echinacea* species as potential immunostimulatory drugs. Econ Med Plant Res. 5, 253–321.

Braunig, B., et al. (1992). *Echinacea purpurea* radix for strengthening the immune response in flu-like infections. Z Phytother. 13, 7–13.

Burger, R. A., Torres, A. R., Warren, R. P., Caldwell, V. D., & Hughes, B. G. (1997). Echinacea-induced cytokine production by human macrophages. International Journal of Immunopharmacology. 19, (7), 371–379.

Dorn, M., Knick, E., & Lewith, G. (1997). Placebo-controlled, double-blind study of Echinaceae pallidae radix in upper respiratory tract infections. Complementary Therapeutic Medicine. 3, 40–42.

Facino, R. (1995). Echinacea in preventing skin damage. Planta Medica. 61, 510–514.

Lantz, G. (1997). Cone flower's popularity: prescription for trouble? National Wildlife. 35, (4), 12.

The Lawrence Review. The Review of Natural Products. St. Louis, MO: Facts and Comparisons. 1997–1998.

Mack, R.B. (1998). "A bunch of the boys were whooping it up." Echinacea for what ails ya. North Carolina Medical Journal. 59, (4), 236–237.

Melchart, D., Linde, K., et al. (1994). Immunomodulation with *Echinacea:* a systematic review of controlled clinical trials. Phytomedicine. 1, 245–254.

Myers, S. P. & Wohlmuth, H. (1998). Echinacea-associated anaphylaxis. Medical Journal of Australia. 168, (11), 583–584.

Mullins, R. J. (1998). Echinacea-associated anaphylaxis. Medical Journal of Australia. 16, 168, (4), 170–171.

Parnham, M. J. (1996). Benefit-risk assessment of the squeezed sap of the purple coneflower (Echinacea purpurea) for long-term oral immunostimulation. Phytomedicine. 3, (1), 95–102.

Schoneberger, D. (1992). The influence of immune stimulating effects of pressed juice from Echinacea purpurea on the course and severity of colds. Forum Immunologie. 8, 2–12.

Feverfew *(Tanacetum parthenium)*

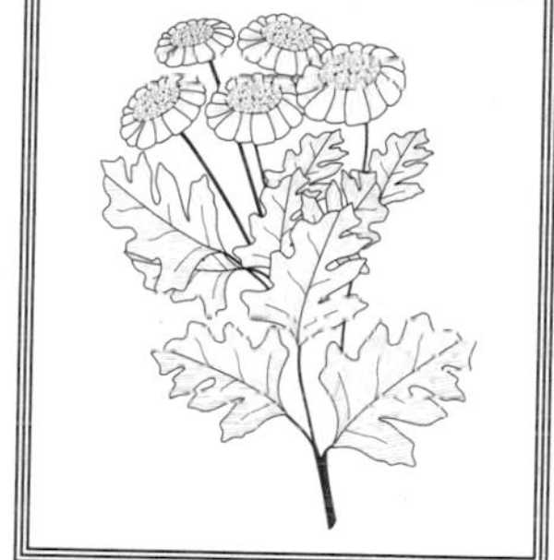

Description

- Member of the sunflower family, which grows throughout the United States and Europe
- Short bushy perennial that grows 15 to 60 cm tall
- Flowers are daisy-like with a yellow center and 10 to 20 white rays; blooms July to October.

Part of Plant Used for Medicinal Purposes

- The leaves (fresh or dried)

Folk Use

- Use dates back hundreds of years (Greeks and early Europeans) for the treatment of fever, migraines, and arthritis.

Active Ingredients

- Sesquiterpene lactones (parthenolide [85%], canin, others)
- Flavonoid glycosides (luteolin, apigenin)
- Monoterpenes

ACTION

- Acts like aspirin, to inhibit the products (prostaglandins, leukotienes, and thromboxanes) that cause inflammation.
- Inhibits platelet activity
- Inhibits inflammatory mediators such as histamine and serotonin
- Relaxes smooth muscles
- Acts as a serotonin antagonist (possibly similar to methysergide [Sansert])
- Antipyretic
- Spasmolytic activity, perhaps through inhibition of extracellular Ca^{++} into smooth muscle cells
- Inhibits release of enzymes from WBCs found in inflamed joints and skin
- Antibiotic activity

USES

- Beneficial in migraine headaches (reduces severity and frequency)
- Reduces inflammation in arthritis
- Is approved in Canada for migraine prevention if it contains 0.2% parthenolide
- Relieves menstrual pain
- Planted around houses to purify the air
- Insect repellent
- Balm for insect bites

DOSAGE

- Fresh plant tincture
- Capsule with 25 mg of freeze dried leaves (product should contain at least 0.2% to 250 μg) parthenolide
- Take 125 mg/day
- Keep in refrigerator to prevent deterioration

TOXICITY

- Mild upset stomach

CONTRAINDICATIONS

- Hypersensitivity

SIDE EFFECTS

- Rebound migraine headaches and joint stiffness may occur after stopping
- Loss of taste
- Lip swelling
- Dermatitis associated with plant
- Allergic reaction (like Echinacea allergy to chrysanthemums)

LONG-TERM SAFETY

- Safe

PREGNANT/LACTATING/CHILDREN

- Do not use if pregnant or lactating (may cause uterine contractions)
- Do not use for children younger than 2

DRUG INTERACTIONS

- Possibly with anticoagulants, may increase bleeding
- Decreases effectiveness of ASA, Tylenol, NSAIDs, and Imitrex

Bibliography

Anonymous. (1996). Efficacy of feverfew as prophylactic treatment of migraine. British Medical Journal. 291, 569–573.

Awang, D. V. C. (1993). Feverfew fever. HerbalGram. 29, 34.

Barsby, R. W. J., et al. (1993). Feverfew and vascular smooth muscle: extracts from fresh and dried plants show opposing pharmacological profiles, dependent upon sesquiterpene lactone content. Planta Medica. 59, 20–25.

deWeerdt, C. J., Bootsma, H. P. R., & Hendricks, H. (1996). Randomized double-blind placebo controlled trial of a feverfew preparation. Phytomedicine. 3, (3), 225.

Hobbs, C. (1990). Feverfew. National Headache Foundation Newsletter. Winter, 10.

Johnson, S. (1984). Feverfew: A traditional herbal remedy for migraine and arthritis. London: Sheldon Press, 19.

Johnson, E. S., et al. (1985). Efficacy of feverfew as prophylactic treatment of migraine. British Medical Journal. 291, 569.

The Lawrence Review of Natural Products. St. Louis, MO: Facts and Comparisons. 1994.

Murphy, J. J., Heptinstall, S., & Mitchell, J. R. A. (1988). Randomized double-blind placebo-controlled trial of feverfew in migraine prevention. Lancet. 8, (601), 189–192.

Palevitch, D., Earon, G., & Carasso, R. (1997). Feverfew (Tanacetum parthenium) as a prophylactic treatment for migraine: a double-blind placebo-controlled study. Phytotherapy Research. 11, 508–511.

Garlic *(Allium sativum)*

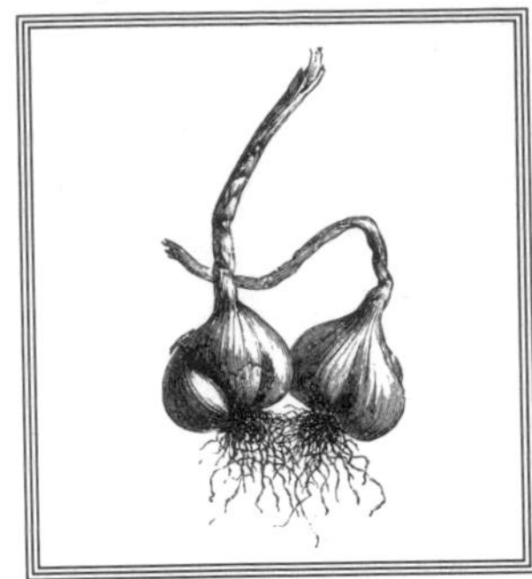

DESCRIPTION

- A member of the lily family that grows worldwide
- The bulb is used as a medicinal or culinary herb
- Contains volatile oil composed of sulfur-containing compounds

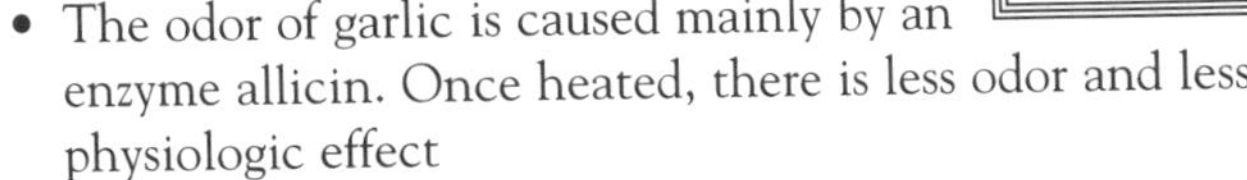

- The odor of garlic is caused mainly by an enzyme allicin. Once heated, there is less odor and less physiologic effect

FOLK USE

- Sanskrit records document the use of garlic 5,000 years ago. The Chinese have used it for at least 3,000 years.
- Hippocrates and Aristotle wrote about garlic to treat many medical conditions
- In ancient Egypt, 15 lb of garlic would buy one able-bodied slave.
- Reportedly cured scurvy in the 1800s
- Relieves wasp and bee stings
- Valued as an aphrodisiac
- Traditional garlic has been and is still used in Chinese, Ayurvedic, and Naturopathic Medicine.

ACTIVE INGREDIENTS

- More than 100 sulphur-containing amino acids, the main one being alliin. It is odorless and makes up a quarter of 1% of the weight of garlic. Allinase is an enzyme that, when the garlic clove is cut or crushed, interacts with alliin and forms allicin. Allicin gives garlic its odor and bitey taste and is responsible for most of the medicinal effects of garlic. It is highly unstable.
- At room temperature it degrades in 3 hours
- During cooking, it degrades in 20 minutes
- Ajoene (antithrombotic activity)
- Dithiins

ACTION

- Has anti-inflammatory properties
- Decreases platelet aggregation

- Antioxidant
- Antimicrobial agent against bacteria, virus, worms, and fungus (It is effective against many bacteria and may be just as effective as penicillin, streptomycin, erythromycin, and tetracycline.)
- Antiyeast properties
- Bacteriostatic to *Helicobacter pylori,* a major cause of gastric ulcers and possibly an increased cancer risk
- Enhances the function of the immune system, increases activity of helper T cells
- Has antitumor properties and decreases the formation of powerful cancer-causing compounds (the allium compound diallyl sulfide may increase levels of glutathione S-transferase, which contributes to detoxification of carcinogens).
- Possibly mediates nitric oxide synthase activation, which helps restore endothelial function, which in turn, improves elasticity of blood vessels and reduces ASHD
- Acts on prostaglandins

USES

- Stimulant
- Diuretic
- Expectorant
- Anti-infective
- Lowers high blood pressure
- Reduces ASHD
- Possible prevention of blood clots
- Decreases LDL (garlic is approved in Europe for its cardiovascular effect to lower blood lipids and decrease atherosclerotic heart disease changes in the blood vessels)

DOSAGE

- One clove of fresh garlic/day. (Fresh is best; if tablets must be taken, buy those standardized for allicin.) As for garlic constituents, the whole is greater than any of the parts. They all work together and have overlapping functions.
- Do not use the odorless variety.
- Chop clove of garlic small and swallow at bedtime. Do not chew.
- Dried garlic does not contain allicin and ajoene. Fresh garlic releases its active ingredients in the mouth because allicin is formed by enzymatic activity.

TOXICITY

- In average doses, no toxicity.

CONTRAINDICATIONS

- Large quantities or long-term use is contraindicated in: acute inflammation, brittle diabetes, hypoglycemia, dehydration, and insomnia.

SIDE EFFECTS

- Heartburn, nausea, flatulence, GI disturbances
- Allergic reactions
- Body and breath odor
- Diarrhea
- Headache
- Insomnia
- Topically, may cause skin irritation, though as an ointment or cream is used for burns, infections, and fungus.

LONG-TERM SAFETY

- Safe

PREGNANCY/LACTATING/CHILDREN

- Safe in moderate doses

DRUG INTERACTIONS

- ASA and coumarin may have increased bleeding tendencies.

Bibliography

Abdullah, T., Kandil, O., et al. (1988). Garlic revisited: therapeutic for the major diseases of our times? Journal of the American Medical Association. 80, 439–445.

Anonymous. (1998). Garlic pills don't lower cholesterol. Health News. 4, (9), 5.

Bergner, P. (1996). The healing power of garlic. Rocklin, CA: Prima Publishing.

Block, E. (1985). The chemistry of garlic and onions. Science America. March, 114–118.

Breithaupt-Grogler, K., Ling, M., Boudoulas, H., & Belz, G. G. (1997). Protective effect of chronic garlic intake on elastic properties of aorta in the elderly. Circulation. 98, (8), 2649–2655.

Dirsch, V. M., Kiemer, A. K., Wagner, H., & Vollmar, A. M. (1998). Effect of allicin and ajoene, two compounds of garlic, on inducible nitric oxide synthase. Atherosclerosis. 139, (2), 333–339.

Dorant, E., van den Brandt, P. A., Goldbohm, R. A., & Sturmans, F. (1996). Consumption of onions and a reduced risk of stomach carcinoma. Gastroenterology. 110, (1), 12–20.

Ernst, E. (1997). Can Allium vegetables prevent cancer? Phytomedicine. 4, (1), 79–83.

Heinrick, L. (1996). Garlic. Baltimore, MD: Williams & Wilkins.

Ho, C., Huang, M., (Eds). (1995). Food phytochemicals for cancer prevention II: teas, spices, and herbs. (ACS Symposium Series 547). Trends Food Science Technology. 6, 216–217.

Koch, H. P. (1993). Garlic—fact or fiction? Phytotherapeutic Research. 7, 278–280.

Simons, L. A., Balasubramanium, S., Konigsmark, M., Parfitt, A., Simons, J., & Peters, W. (1995). On the effects of garlic on plasma lipids and lipoproteins in mild hypercholesterolemia. Atherosclerosis. 113, 219–225.

Steinmetz, K. A., Kushi, L. H., Bostick, R. M., Folsom, A. R., & Potter, J. D. (1994). Vegetables, fruits, and colon cancer in the Iowa Women's Health Study. American Journal of Epidemiology. 139, 1–15.

Ginger *(Zinqiberis rhizoma)*

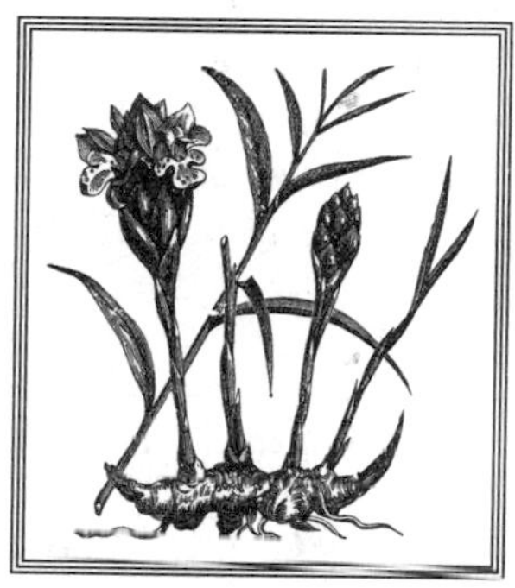

Description

- An erect perennial herb with thick tuberous rhizomes underground and stems that grow to 2 to 4 feet. Grass-like leaves are 6 to 12 in long.
- Grows in the tropics with the major producer being Jamaica.
- Green purple flowers similar to orchids

Part of Plant Used for Medicinal Purposes

- Root or rhizome, is aromatic

Folk Use

- It has been used for thousands of years in China to treat stomach ache, diarrhea, nausea, hemorrhage, arthritis, and toothache.
- It has been used as a spice for cooking in Asia and India.
- Has been used for years in ginger ale, candy, liquors, and cosmetics.
- In China, ginger root and stem are used as pesticides against aphids and fungal spores.

Active Ingredients

- Volatile oil (1–3%) provides the characteristic aroma
- Gingerols (provide pungent qualities)
  - (6) shogaol
  - (6) and (10) dehydrogingerdione
  - (6) and (10) gingendione
  - zingerone
- Zerumbone

ACTION

- Positive inotropic action (dose dependent)
- Inhibits GI motility, antiemetic activity
- Inhibits prostaglandin biosynthesis
- May inhibit growth of bacteria (because of shogaol and gingerols)
- Immune stimulating activity
- Prevents motion sickness (possibly by increasing gastric motility and blocking GI reactions and the subsequent nausea feedback)
- Antioxidant
- Antipyretic
- Analgesis
- Antitussive
- Possible antitumor activity

USES

- Treats arthritis and migraine headaches
- Lowers fevers
- Prevents colds and decreases their severity
- Decreases motion sickness and nausea during pregnancy
- May protect against ulcers caused by stress, alcohol, or aspirin
- Relieves dizziness and vestibular disorders

DOSAGE

- Capsules usually contain 500 mg of ginger
- 1 to 2 grams dry ginger root a day, but may need 8 to 10 grams to obtain results.
- 2 capsules at beginning of migraine to decrease nausea
- Motion sickness: take 0.5 grams of powdered ginger or 0.5 teaspoon of fresh ginger every 15 minutes for an hour before you travel; continue this dosage during the trip if you have any signs of illness.
- Nausea from chemotherapy or surgery: A week before chemotherapy, take 2 grams powdered ginger daily. If you're already undergoing chemotherapy, your digestive tract will be sensitive, so start with 250 mg powdered ginger daily, gradually increasing to a level that is comfortable and effective.
- Digestion: as a digestive tonic, you can take 1 gram powdered ginger before or after a meal. You can also make a digestive tea. Simmer approximately 1 teaspoon of fresh grated ginger in one cup of water for 15 minutes, then strain.

- Ulcers, heart disease and inflammatory ailments: For these serious conditions, it is best to seek the counsel of a trained herbalist or a medical practitioner schooled in the use of botanicals. Dramatic benefits can require high doses; research found that the greatest relief of arthritis pain, for example, occurred with a daily intake of up to 7 grams of powdered ginger and 50 grams of fresh rhizome.
- Colds and flu: take 0.5 to 1 gram/hour of powdered ginger in capsules for 2 to 3 days.

TOXICITY

- Does not appear to be toxic at normal levels
- Overdose may cause central nervous system (CNS) depression and cardiac arrhythmias

CONTRAINDICATIONS

- None known

SIDE EFFECTS

- GI discomfort if taken on an empty stomach

LONG-TERM SAFETY

- Safe

PREGNANCY/LACTATING/CHILDREN

- Safe

DRUG INTERACTIONS

- None known

Bibliography

Fulder, S. (1996). Ginger & pregnancy. Herbalgram. 38, (Fall), 47–50.

Kiuchi, F., et al. (1992). Inhibition of prostaglandin and leukotriene biosynthesis by gingerols and diarylheptanoids. Chemical and Pharmaceutical Bulletin. 40, 387–391.

The Lawrence Review of Natural Products. Facts and Comparisons. St. Louis, MO. 1998.

Reddy, A. C. & Lokesh, B. R. (1992). Studies on spice principles as antioxidants in the inhibition of lipid peroxidation of rat liver microsomes. Molecular Cellular Biochemistry. 111, 117–124.

Schulick, P. (1996). Ginger. Vegetarian Times. May, 80–82.

Surh, Y. J., Lee, E., & Lee, J. M. (1998). Chemoprotective properties of some pungent ingredients present in red pepper and ginger. Mutation Research. 402, (1-2), 259–267.

Visalyaputra, S., Petchpaisit, N., et al. (1998). The efficacy of ginger root in the prevention of postoperative nausea and vomiting after outpatient gynaecological laparoscopy. Anaesthesia. 53, (5), 506–510.

Ginkgo* *(Maidenhair tree)* *(Ginkgo biloba)*

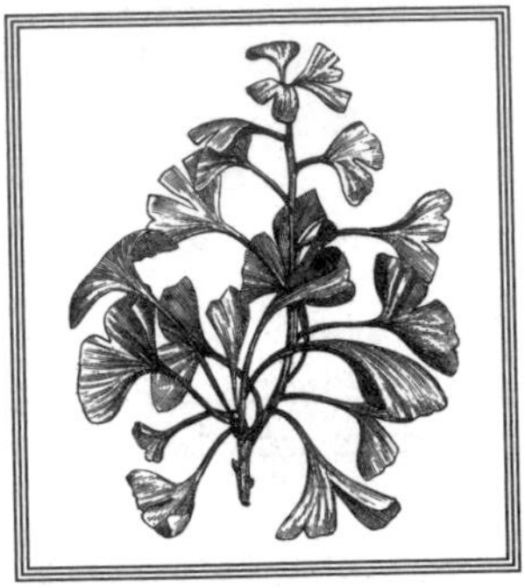

DESCRIPTION

- Deciduous tree that grows 125 feet, 3 to 4 inches in diameter, can live up to 1,000 years, and produces a flower and a fruit.
- Male and female trees look slightly different and bear different flowers
- Male: upright flowers develop on leaf axis
- Female: wider shape and wider crown, flowers have 2 terminal "naked" ovules on stalk
- Fruit is circular, yellow to orange with thick fleshy layers that give off a foul odor when mature (male is less odiferous); female fruit "hides" highly prized inner seed; male does not "fruit"
- Slow growing

PART OF PLANT USED FOR MEDICINAL PURPOSES

- leaf: with highest concentration of active compounds possibly present in autumn (this is debated now, but it is thought when chlorophyll fades, flavonoids are more available)

FOLK USE

- The tree was first cultivated in the Orient, then introduced into Europe in the early 1700s and brought to the United States in the 1780s.
- Use for medicinal purposes, antitussive and antiasthmatic, began 2800 BC
- Written about in Germany in 1771

ACTIVE INGREDIENTS

- Flavonoids (quercetin and 40 others)
- Terpenoids (ginkgolide B)

---

*Standardized ginkgo extracts are regulated as drugs in Germany. In China, ginkgo is available in tablet and injectable forms.

- Benzoids
- Sesquiterpenes
- Diterpenes
- Organic acids (vanilla, ascorbic, p-coumaric)
- Steroids

ACTION

- Antioxidant, nitric oxide, free radical scavenger (from activity of flavonoids and terpenoids)
- Platelet activating factor antagonist
- Vasoregulating effects, relaxes blood vessels
- Inhibits lipid peroxidation of membranes
- Moderates cerebral energy metabolism
- Improves cerebral blood flow and improves membrane integrity—protects neurons and astrocytes
- Antihypotic
- Increases activity of brain waves (different gingko products act in different parts of brain)
- Decreases tumor growth
- Possibly reduces muscle damage in patients with chronic disease, such as Parkinson's and MS

USES

- Cerebral insufficiency (difficulty in concentration and memory, absent mindedness, confusion, lack of energy, depression, dizziness)
- Peripheral vascular insufficiency (intermittent claudication [increases walking distance], Raynaud's disease)
- Alzheimer's disease/dementia
- Impotence
- Antioxidant/neuroprotective effects
- Tinnitis
- Asthma

PHARMACOKINETICS

Onset: readily
Peak: 2 to 3 hours
Duration: unknown
Half-life: 5 hours
Excreted: exhaled air, urine, feces

TOXICITY

- Safe

DOSAGE

- Gingko 1:2 tincture, dose 0.5 to 1 teaspoon three times a day
- Standardized extract of 24% glycosides, 6% terpene lactones
- 40 mg three times a day (80 mg three times a day has been studied in some research)

SIDE EFFECTS

- Minimal and transient
- GI
- Headache
- Dizziness
- Allergic reactions

(The fruit pulp and raw seeds are toxic, but are not used in medicinal preparation. Fruit causes allergic reaction similar to poison ivy when touched.)

CONTRAINDICATIONS

- Do not use if menses is very heavy

PREGNANCY/LACTATION/CHILDREN

- No trials available, so avoid

DRUG INTERACTION

- ASA and coumarin products may increase bleeding tendencies

Bibliography

Eisenburg, D. (1993). Herbal and magical medicine: Traditional healing today. New England Journal of Medicine. 328, 215–216.

Hofferberth, B. (1994). The efficacy of EGb 761 in patients with senile dementia of the Alzheimer type, a double blind placebo-controlled study on different levels of investigation. Human Psychopharmacology. 9, 215–222.

Holgers, K. M., et al. (1994). *Ginkgo biloba* extract for the treatment of tinnitus. Audiology. 33, 85–92.

Hoyer, S. (1995). Possibilities and limits of therapy of cognition disorders in the elderly. Zeitschrift Fur Gerontologie und Geriatrie. 28, (6), 457–462.

Huguet, F. (1994). Decreased cerebral 5-HTIA receptors during aging: reversal by ginkgo biloba extract (EGb 761). Journal of Pharmacy and Pharmacology. 46, 316–318.

Itil, T. (1995). Natural substances in psychiatry (ginkgo biloba in dementia). Psychopharmacology Bulletin. 31, 147–158.

Itil, T. (1996). Early diagnosis and treatment of memory disturbances. American Journal of Electromedicine. June, 81–85.

Kanowski, S. (1996). Proof of efficacy of the ginkgo biloba special extract EGb 761 in outpatients suffering from mild to moderate primary degenerative dementia. Pharmacopsychiatry. 29, (2), 47–56.

Kim, Y. S., Pyo, M. K., et al. (1998). Antiplatelet and antithrombotic effects of a combination of ticlopidine and Ginkgo biloba ext. Thrombosis Research. 91, (1), 33–38.

Kleijnen, J. & Knipschild, P. (1992). *Ginkgo biloba*. Lancet. 340, 1136–1139.

LeBars, P. L., Schatzberg, A. F., et al. (1997). A placebo-controlled, double-blind randomized trial of an extract of Ginkgo biloba for dementia. Journal of the American Medical Association. 278, (16), 1327–1332.

Li, C. L. & Wong, Y. Y. (1997). The bioavailability of ginkgolides in Ginkgo biloba extracts. Planta Medica. 63, (6), 563–565.

Maurer, K., Ihl, R., Dierks, T., & Frolich, L. (1997). Clinical efficacy of *Ginkgo biloba* special extract EGb 761 in dementia of the Alzheimer type. Journal of Psychiatric Research. 31, (6), 645–655.

Oyama, Y., et al. (1996). Ginkgo biloba extract protects brain neurons against oxidative stress. Brain Research. 712, (2), 349–352.

Peters, H., Kieser, M., & Holscher, U. (1998). Demonstration of the efficacy of ginkgo biloba special extract EGb 761 on intermittent claudication—a placebo-controlled, double-blind multicenter trial. Vasa. 27, (2), 106–110.

Sastre, J., Millan, A., Garcia de la Asuncion, J., et al. (1998). A *Ginkgo biloba* extract (EGb 761) prevents mitochondrial aging by protecting against oxidative stress. Free Radical Biology and Medicine. 24, (2), 298–304.

Schatzberg, A. M. (1998). Ginkgo biloba for dementia. The Journal of Family Practice. 46, (1), 20.

Schubert, H. & Halama, P. (1993). Depressive episode primarily unresponsive to therapy in elderly patients: Efficacy of *Ginkgo biloba* extract (EGb 761) in combination with antidepressants. Geriatr Forsch 3, 45–53.

Snow, J. M. (1997). *Ginkgo biloba* L. (Ginkogaceae). Protocol Journal of Botanical Medicine. 2, (1), 9–15.

Snowden, D. A. (1997). Brain infarction and the clinical expression of Alzheimer disease. Journal of the American Medical Association. 277, 813–817.

Wesnes, K. A., Faleni, R. A., et al. (1997). The cognitive, subjective, and physical effects of a *Ginkgo biloba/Panax ginseng* combination in healthy volunteers with neurasthenic complaints. Psychopharmacology Bulletin. 33, (4), 677–683.

Vester, J. (1994). Efficacy of ginkgo biloba in 90 outpatients with cerebral insufficiency caused by old age. Phytomedicine. 1, 9–16.

Ginseng,* Asian, Chinese, Korean *(Panax* ginseng*)*, American *(P. quinquefolius)*

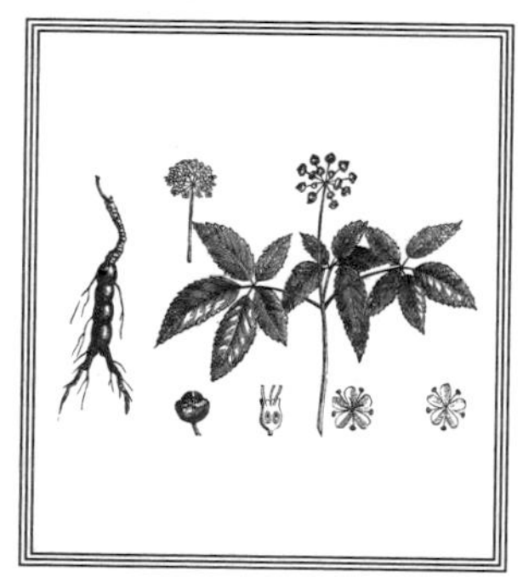

DESCRIPTION

- Ginseng is a shrub approximately 3 to 4 feet tall with erect spiny shoots covered with light grey or brownish bark. Grows abundantly in Asia above the 38th latitude

*(Siberian *Eleutherococcus senticosus* is not a true ginseng.)

- American ginseng grows from Canada to Georgia. It is considered an endangered species, thus ginseng is cultivated. It is slow growing and takes 6 years to produce a marketable root.
- Asian ginseng is considered the strongest. Builds "chi" (energy) said to be "hot"
- American ginseng is milder and less stimulating. Works more systemically, said to be "cold"

PART OF PLANT USED FOR MEDICINAL PURPOSES

- The root is most widely used and is gathered in the fall just before defoliation.
- The leaves may also be used and are gathered in July

FOLK USE

- The Chinese have used ginseng for 4,000 years to increase longevity, improve general health, improve appetite, and restore memory
- Name means "cure-all"
- Russians have used ginseng since 1855
- "Ginseng" is Chinese for "man root" because plant resembles the human form
- As an aphrodisiac

ACTIVE INGREDIENTS

- Many triperpenoid saponin gensenosides (Japanese) are the same as panaxosides (Russian) (often the active ingredients are named differently by different countries using the herb)
- Sterols B_1, B_2, B_{12}
- Amino acids
- Coumarins

QUALITY CONTROL

- Quality root is expensive. The best grades of Korean Red may sell for \$50/oz. Studies have been done on many ginseng products and as many as 25% had no ginseng and 60% did not have enough to create an effect.

ACTION

- Stimulate immune system
- Affect secretion of hormones

- Enhances body metabolism
- Antioxidant
- Decreases platelet aggregation
- May act as hormone regulator in menopause
- Increase NK cell activity (Scaglione, 1996, found that NK levels at 8 and 12 weeks were almost double the controls)
- Ca^{++} antagonists in vascular tissue
- Influences hypothalamus/pituitary/adrenal axis
- Improves glucose homeostasis and insulin sensitivity in the diabetic patient (36 patients, Stooniemi, 1995)
- Increases memory, concentration, and coordination, particularly in the elderly by increasing uptake of ACH

USES

- Not intended to treat specific disease but rather to support health
- Adaptogen or tonic—helps to adapt to physical and mental stress, thus it:
  - improves stamina (not verified by research)
  - increases concentration
  - combats fatigue
  - aids resistance to disease, such as cancer, diabetes, infection
  - may protect from flu and common cold
  - increases energy and physical performance (not verified by research)

DOSAGE**

- Use standardized extracts with 4 to 7% ginsenosides
- Available in many forms usually taken 1 to 3 times a day
- Tablets: 100 to 300 mg/day/divided
- Dried roots: 2 to 4 grams
- Tincture (1:5) 10 to 20 mL
- Fluid extract (1:1) 2 to 4 mL

  } often contain as much as 34 to 45% alcohol*
- Solid (dry powdered) extract (20:1), containing more than 1% eleutheroside E: 100 to 200 mg)

TOXICITY

- Nontoxic

*Products do not have to identify alcohol content.

**Takes 6 to 8 weeks to work. Dose for 1 to 2 months, herb holiday 1 to 2 weeks, then dose 1 to 2 more months.

CONTRAINDICATIONS

- Concurrently with caffeine
- Avoid during menses and an acute illness
- Hypertension
- Schizophrenia, manic
- Brittle diabetics
- In healthy persons younger than 40 years age

SIDE EFFECTS

When given to someone without indications (professional herbalists do not give it out to anyone who is "tired")

- Insomnia
- Diarrhea
- Skin rash
- Sleep quality worsens
- May increase bleeding in postmenopausal women
- Breast tenderness in men

LONG-TERM SAFETY

- Safe

PREGNANCY/LACTATING/CHILDREN

- No studies, probably no
- Inappropriate except in rare cases of older children with chronic disease, not for self-treatment

DRUG INTERACTIONS

- Do not take concurrently with steroids, antipsychotics, MAOI
- Side effects of drugs are increased
- Stop all caffeine
- Interferes with effectiveness of oral birth control pills
- May cause digitalis toxicity
- Do not take concurrently with anticoagulants, may increase bleeding

Bibliography

Anonymous. (1998). Ginseng: many forms, many questions, not enough answers. Environmental Nutrition. June.

Cui, J., et al. (1994). What do commercial ginseng preparations contain? Lancet. 344, 134.

D'Angelo, L., et al. (1986). A double-blind, placebo-controlled clinical study on the effect of a standardized ginseng extract on psychomotor performance in healthy volunteers. Journal of Ethnopharmacology. 16, 15–22.

Dowling, E. A., et al. (1995). Effect of *Eleutherococcus senticosus* on submaximal and maximal exercise performance. Medicine and Science in Sports and Exercise. May, 482–489.

Engels, H.J., et al. (1996). Failure of chronic ginseng supplementation to affect work performance and energy metabolism in healthy adult females. Nutrition Research. 16, 1295–1305.

Farnsworth, N. R., et al. (1985). Siberian ginseng *(Eleutherococcus senticosus)*: current status as an adaptogen. Economic Medical Planning and Research. 1, 156–215.

Hallstrom, C., et al. (1982). Effects of Ginseng on the performance of nurses on night duty. Comparative Medicine East and West. Vol IV, (4), 277–282.

Hermann, J., et al. (1997). No ergogenic effects of ginseng *(Panax ginseng* C.A. Meyer) during graded maximal aerobic exercise. Journal of the American Dietetic Association. 97, (10), 1110–1115.

Kwan, C. Y. (1995). Vascular effects of selected antihypertensive drugs derived from traditional medicinal herbs. Clinical and Experimental Pharmacology and Physiology. (Suppl 1), s297–s299.

Loggia, R., et al. (1991). Anti-stress activity of a ginseng extract: a subchronic study in mice. Planta Medicine. 57, (Suppl 2), A6–A7.

Loi, S. (1996). Ginseng. Australian Journal of Emergency Care. 3, (3), 28–29.

Scaglione, F., et al. (1996). Efficacy and safety of the standardized ginseng extract G115 for potentiating vaccination against common cold and/or influenza syndrome. Drugs Experimental Clinical Research. 22, (2), 65–72.

Sotaniemi, E. A., et al. (1995). Ginseng therapy in non-sinsulin-dependent diabetic patients. Diabetes Care. 18, (10), 1373–1375.

Vigano, C. & Ceppi, E. (1994). What is Ginseng? Lancet. 344, 619.

Green Tea*
(Camellia sinensis)

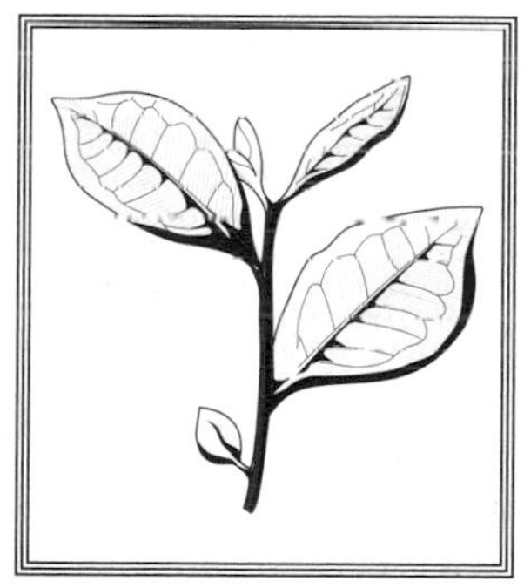

DESCRIPTION

- Tea plants are cultivated in China.
- It is an evergreen shrub, usually kept pruned to 2 to 3 feet tall.
- Parts used include the leaf bud and the two adjacent young leaves together with the stem. Older leaves are inferior.

PART OF PLANT USED FOR MEDICINAL PURPOSES

- Leaves

*Green tea is prepared from steamed and dried leaves.
Black tea leaves are withered, rolled, fermented, and then dried.
Oolong tea is considered half fermented, approximately halfway between green and black

FOLK USE

- Used for more than 3,000 years as a beverage.
- Chinese believe green tea is a cure for cancer.
- Used as a diuretic.
- The word tea can be traced back to 1655 when the Dutch introduced the word and beverage to England.

ACTIVE INGREDIENTS

- Polyphenols
- Tannins
- Protein
- Fiber
- Sugar
- Fluoride
- Methylxanthines
- Caffeine 1 to 4% (6 oz C = 10 to 50 mg)
- Flavonoids

ACTION

- Caffeine is a CNS stimulant, thus it:
  increases nervousness
  insomnia
  tachycardia
  increases blood sugar
  increases cholesterol (9c/da)
  increases stomach acid
- Tannins decrease development of colon polyps
- Protects from fatal diseases, increases longevity
- Antioxidant (effect decreased by milk)
- May directly bind to certain carcinogens
- May mediate apoptosis (cancer cell destruction)

USES

- As a drink
- Diuretic
- Cancer prevention (cancer onset in tea drinkers is delayed by years)

DOSAGE

- 1 cup or more/day; steep tea in hot water for 1 to 2 minutes

TOXICITY

- With great intake, may lead to esophageal cancer

CONTRAINDICATIONS

- In infants, may impair iron metabolism

SIDE EFFECTS

- Fluoride stains teeth
- Hyperactivity in children
- May remove calcium from the bone
- Insomnia
- Jitteriness
- Increased urination

LONG-TERM SAFETY

- Safe

PREGNANCY/LACTATION/CHILDREN

- Avoid in pregnancy, lactation, and children (yet to be proven in humans)

DRUG INTERACTIONS

- Methylxanthine component decreases the absorption of Ca^{++}. Separate by at least 2 hours.

Bibliography

Ali, M., Afzal, M., Gubler, C.J., et al. (1990). A potent thomboxane formation inhibitor in green tea leaves. Prostaglandins Leukot Essent Fatty Acids. 40, 281–283.

Canfielf, L. M., Forage, J. W., & Valenzuela, J. G. (1992). Carotenoids as cellular antioxidants. *Proceedings of the Society for Experimental Biology and Medicine*. 200, 260–265.

Chen, Z. P., Schell, J. B., Ho, C. T., & Chen, K. Y. (1998). Green tea epigallocatechin gallate shows a pronounced growth inhibitory effect on cancerous cells but not on their normal counterparts. Cancer Letters. 129, (2), 173–179.

Fujiki, H., Suganuma, M., et al. (1998). Cancer inhibition by green tea. Mutation Research. 402, (1-2), 307–310.

Gutman, R. (1996). Discovering tea. Herbalgram. Summer, No. 37, 33–41.

Hibasami, H., Komiya, T., et al. (1998). Induction of apoptosis in human stomach cancer cells by green tea catechins. Oncology Report. 5, (2), 527–529.

Keli, S. O., Hertog, M. G. L., Feskens, E. J. M., et al. (1996). Dietary flavonoids, antioxidant vitamins and incidence of stroke. Archives of Internal Medicine. 154, 637–642.

The Lawrence Review of Natural Products. Facts and Comparisons. St. Louis, MO. 1998.

Middleton, E., & Kandaswami, C. (1994). Potential health-promoting properties of citrus flavonoids. Food Technology. November, 115–119.
Murray, M. (1995). The healing power of herbs. Prima Publishing, San Francisco, CA. p. 162.
Yang, G. Y., Liao, J., Kim, K., et al. (1998). Inhibition of growth and induction of apoptosis in human cancer cell lines by tea polyphenols. Carcinogenesis. 19, (4), 611–616.

Hawthorn *(Crataegus oxyacantha)*

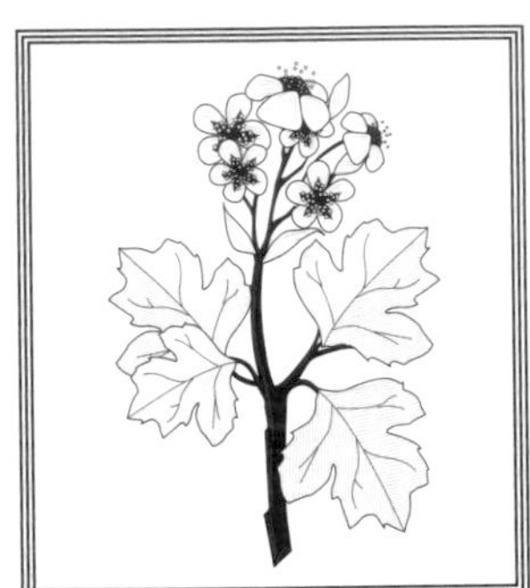

DESCRIPTION

- Spiny tree, native to Europe
- May be grown as a hedge but can grow to 15 to 18 feet.
- Produces white, strong-smelling flowers in large bunches from April to June.
- Spherical bright red fruit, contains 1 to 3 nuts.

PART OF PLANT USED FOR MEDICINAL PURPOSES

- Blossoms, flowers, leaves, and fruit

FOLK USE

- Dates back to Dioscorides
- Used since the 1700s for sore throats and heart problems such as heart failure, angina, and hypertension.

ACTIVE INGREDIENTS

- Flavonoids
  - quercetin
  - hyperoside
  - vitex inrhamnoside
  - lactones
- Anthocyanidins
- Proanthocyanidins
- Cardiotonic amines
  - tyramine
  - phenylethylamine and others

ACTION

- Strong cardiac activity
- Dilates blood vessels (particularly the coronary arteries)

- Increases force of contraction
- Inhibits angiotensin-converting enzyme
- Lowers blood pressure
- Increases cAMP by lowering enzyme phosophodiasterase
- Reduces triglycerides, cholesterol, and blood sugar
- Stabilizes vitamin C by lowering its oxidation, which lowers capillary permeability and fragility
- Stabilizes collagen, which strengthens connective tissue
- Antioxidant and free radical scavenger
- Decreases inflammation
- Decreases release of prostaglandins, histamines, and leukotrienes.

USES

- Reduces inflammation and pain in arthritis
- Reduces congestive heart failure*
- Reduces abnormal cardiac rhythms*
- Lowers blood pressure*

DOSAGE**

- Berries or flowers (dried): 3 to 5 grams or as an infusion
- Blossoms: harvest in May (Shake branch in paper bag and use 1 to 5 teaspoons in 1 C boiling water, infuse for 10 minutes.)
- Tincture (1:5): 4 to 5 mL (alcohol may elicit pressor response in some individuals)
- Fluid extract (1:1): 1 to 2 mL
- Freeze-dried berries: 160 mg
- Flower extract (standardized to contain 1.8% vitexin 04'-rhamnoside or 20% procyanidins): 100 to 250 mg

TOXICITY

- Low toxicity in appropriate doses
- High doses may induce hypotension, sedation, and arrhythmia

CONTRAINDICATIONS

- In persons trying to self-medicate for potentially serious heart disease

---

*Should not be used alone to treat these conditions. See an experienced herb practitioner and advise your physician if using Hawthorn for these conditions.

**To be effective, hawthorn may need to be administered for 2 weeks or more. In Germany, only flowers and leaves are approved, not berries. Occasional dosing is of no value; take regularly.

SIDE EFFECTS

- Rare

LONG-TERM SAFETY

- Safe for lifetime use

PREGNANCY/LACTATION/CHILDREN

- Safe

DRUG INTERACTIONS

- Digitalis products may potentiate hawthorn

Bibliography

Anonymous. (1998). Crataegus oxycantha. Common name: hawthorn. Alternative Medicine Review. 3, (2), 138–139.

Nasa, Y., et al. (1993). Protective effect of crataegus extract on the cardiac mechanical dysfunction in isolated perfused working heart. Arzneim Forsch/Drug Research. 43, (9), 945–949.

Schmidt, U., et al. (1994). Efficacy of Hawthorn (Crataegus) preparation of LI 132 in 78 patients with chronic congestive heart failure. Defined as NYHA Functional Class II. Phytomedicine. 1, 17–24.

Schussler, M., et al. 91995). Myocaridal effects of flavonoids from Crataegus species. Arzneimittelforschung. 45, (8), 842–845.

Kava Kava *(Piper methysticum)*

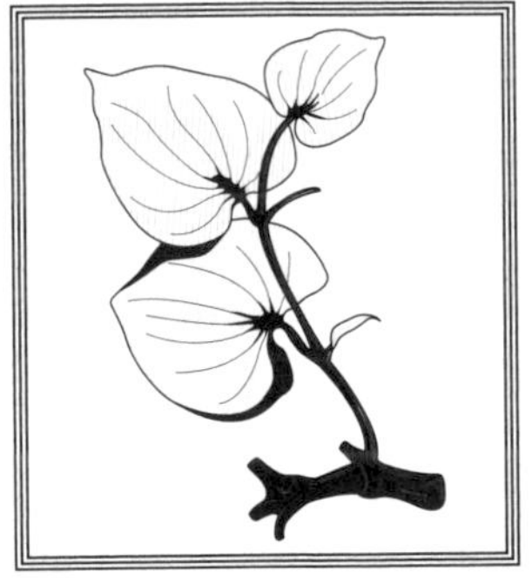

DESCRIPTION

- More than 20 varieties have been identified
- Member of the black pepper family

PART OF PLANT USED FOR MEDICINAL PURPOSES

- Root

Research demonstrates that kava may be an alternative to benzodiazepines in anxiety disorders.

FOLK USE

- Used for hundreds of years by natives of the South Pacific Islands as a ceremonial and celebratory, nonalcoholic, calming drink
- Used by South Pacific Islands to treat gonorrhea, bronchitis, rheumatism, headaches, colds, and to enhance wound healing
- In Europe, widely used as a sedative
- Enhances relaxing and a social atmosphere
- Polynesian cultures (usually young men or women) would prepare root by mastication and then spitting the chewed material into a bowl and then adding water

ACTIVE INGREDIENTS

- Several arylethylene pyrones
- Dihydropyrones (which possess CNS activity)
- Kava lactones and 5,6-dihydro kava lactones

ACTION

- Local anesthetic activity comparable to cocaine
- Analgesia through nonopiate pathways (naloxone does not reverse kava), acts like lidocaine
- Reduces nonpsychotic anxiety
- May act directly on the limbic system
- Poorly soluble in water
- Promotes sleep in the absence of sedation
- Produces mild euphoric changes, such as happiness and fluent and lively speech
- Modifies GAMA receptors in brain
- May have dopamine antagonistic properties

USES

- Relieves anxiety without affecting alertness
- Relieves tension headaches and muscle spasm
- Relieves insomnia
- Enhances REM sleep without the hangover effect in morning
- Anti-inflammatory
- Improves memory
- Possibly controls pain
- Possibly relieves anxiety and sleep disorder during menopause

DOSAGE

- Use standardized extracts in 30% to 50% concentration

TOXICITY

- Skin discoloration
- Chronic ingestion may lead to kavaism, dry, flaking, discolored skin, blood count abnormalities (increased RBC, decreased platelets, decreased lymphocytes), some pulmonary hypertension, and reddened eyes (possibly related to interference with cholesterol metabolism. All symptoms are reversible when kava intake is stopped.
- Ethanol increases toxicity

CONTRAINDICATIONS

- Parkinson's disease

SIDE EFFECTS

- Yellowing of skin, hair, nails
- Signs of drunkenness with excess, not with usual dosing
- Drowsiness

LONG-TERM EFFECTS

- Safe in moderate doses
- Kava abuse is a possibility but it is not addicting
- No withdrawal symptoms have occurred when discontinued

PREGNANCY/LACTATING/CHILDREN

- Do not use during pregnancy and when lactating
- Safety unknown for children

DRUG INTERACTIONS

Potentiates:
- Alcohol
- Tranquilizers
- Antidepressants
- Benzodiazepines
- Botanical herbs: St. John's wort, valerian root
- Do not use concurrently

Bibliography

Bone, K. (1993–1994). Kava—a safe herbal treatment for anxiety. British Journal of Phytotherapy. 3, (4), 147–153.

Cantor, C. (1997). Kava and alcohol. Medical Journal of Australia. 167, 560.

The Review of Natural Products. Kava-kava. St. Louis, MO: Facts & Comparisons. November, 1996.

Gebner, B. (1994). Extract of kava-kava rhizome in comparison with diazepam and placebo. Zeitschrift fur Phytotherapie. 15, 30–37.

Herberg, K. W. (1993). Effect of kava-special extract WS 1490 combined with ethyl alcohol on safety relevant performance parameters. Blutalkohol. 30, 96–105.

Lehmann, E. (1996). Efficacy of a special kava extract (Piper methysticum) in patients with states of anxiety, tension and excitedness of non-mental origin-a double blind placebo-controlled study of four weeks treatment. Phytomedicine. 3, 113–119.

Lindenburg, D. L. (1990). Kavain in comparison with oxazepam in anxiety disorders. A double-blind study of clinical effectiveness. Fortschritte der Medizin. 108, 49–50.

Munte, T. F. (1993). Effects of oxazepam and an extract of kava roots on event-related potentials in a word recognition task. Neuropsychobiology. 27, 46–53.

Norton, S. & Ruze, P. (1994). Kava dermopathy. Journal of the American Academy of Dermatology. 31, (1), 89–97.

Singh, Y. N. (1992). Kava: an overview. Journal of Ethnopharmacology. 2, (37), 13–45.

Singh, N.N., et al. (1998). A double-blind, placebo controlled study of the effects of kava (Kavatrol) on daily stress and anxiety in adults. Alternative Therapies. 4, (2), 97–98.

Spillane, P. K., et al. (1997). Neurological manifestations of kava intoxication. Medical Journal of Australia. 167, 172–173.

Voltz, H.P. & Kieser, M. (1997). Kava-kava extract WS 1490 versus placebo in anxiety disorders—a randomized placebo-controlled 25-week outpatient trial. Pharmacopsychiatry. 30, 1–5.

Warnecke, G. (1991). Psychosomatic dysfunctions in the female climacteric. Fortschitte der Medizine. 109, 119–122.

Licorice (*Gylcyrrhiza glabra*)

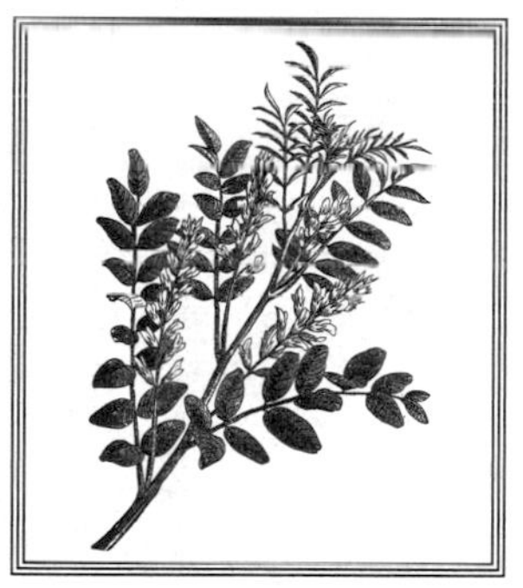

Description

- 4- to 5-foot shrub, grows in subtropical climates in rich soil.
- Gylcyrrhiza means "sweet root"
- Spanish licorice has blue flowers
- Russian licorice has violet flowers
- Licorice is 50 times sweeter than sugar

Part of Plant Used for Medicinal Purposes

- Root

Folk Use

- Roman empire used licorice
- Hippocrites and Pliny the Elder (23 AD) used licorice as expectorant and carminative

- In China, licorice was thought to lengthen life

ACTIVE INGREDIENTS

- Ammonia
- Cleanane triterpenoids
- Glycoside glycyrrhizin (7–10%) (active ingredients are flavonoids)
- Starches, sugars
- Isoflavonoids
- Coumarins
- Lignins
- Amino acids
- phytosterols
- Volatile acids

ACTION

- Inhibition of renin/aldosterone/angiotensin axis
- Weak antibacterial and antiviral agent
- Inhibits prostaglandin E_2
- May help clear immune complexes
- Inhibits histamine release
- May reduce plaque formation in persons with ASHD
- Estrogen adaptation (if estrogen too low, increase levels; if estrogen too high, decrease levels)

USE

- Chiefly as a flavoring agent that masks bitter agents
- Expectorant
- Anti-inflammatory
- Lung infections, sore throats
- Antitussive
- May help to reduce symptoms of PMS because it possesses antiestrogenic properties and suppresses the breakdown of progesterone (administer 2 weeks before menses)

DOSAGE

Three times a day
- Powdered root: 1 to 2 grams
- Fluid extract (1:1): 2 to 4 mL
- Solid (dry powder) extract (4:1): 250 to 500 mg (adverse effects may occur with 100 mg/day)

TOXICITY

May begin to develop after one month of usage

- Facial weakness
- Dulled reflexes
- Hypertensive encephalopathy

CONTRAINDICATIONS

- Hypersensitivity to licorice
- Preexisting renal, hepatitic, and cardiovascular (CV) disease because of risk of side effects
- Hypertension
- Low potassium
- Pregnancy

SIDE EFFECTS*

- Hyperaldosteronism
- Hypertension
- Edema
- Hypokalemia
- Sodium retention

LONG-TERM SAFETY

- Unknown

PREGNANCY/LACTATION/CHILDREN

- Cautious use is advised.
- Use only low dose in children.
- Avoid for more than 2 weeks during pregnancy

DRUG INTERACTIONS

- Diuretics inhibits fluid loss
- Antihypertensives inhibits activity
- Digitalis decreases effectiveness and increases side effects related to K^+ and Na^+

Bibliography

The Lawrence Review of Natural Products. St. Louis, MO: Facts and Comparisons. 1998.

*All side effects more pronounced in elderly.

Milk Thistle *(Silybum marianum/or Cardui marianum)*

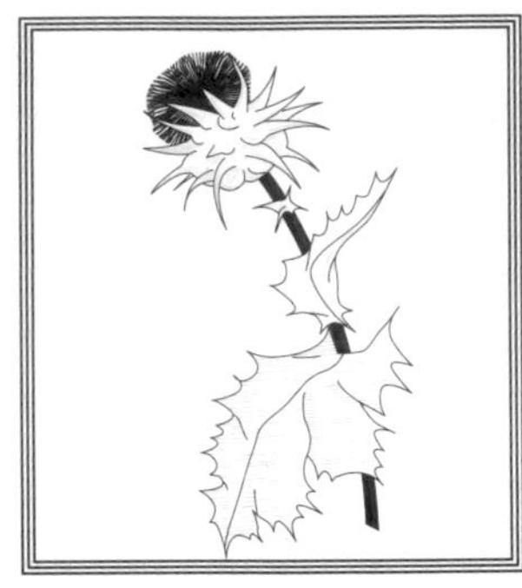

DESCRIPTION

- Annual/biennial plant found in rocky soils in South and West Europe and some parts of the United States
- Grows 5 to 10 feet high, has dark shiny green leaves with white veins
- Has solitary flower heads that are reddish-purple with spines from June to August
- Has milky white veins on its green leaves

PART OF PLANT USED FOR MEDICINAL PURPOSES

- Seeds, fruits, and leaves are all used for medicinal products.

FOLK USE

- Used for more than 2,000 years as a liver protectant
- Used in England to remove obstructions of liver and spleen and for treatment of jaundice
- In the 19th and 20th Century, used to treat varicose veins, menstrual difficulties, and congestion of liver and spleen
- Once grown in Europe as a vegetable. The de-spined leaves were used as a spinach substitute and the flower eaten "artichoke style." The roasted seeds were used as a coffee substitute.
- Homeopathic remedy includes seeds and is used to treat jaundice, peritonitis, bronchitis, and varicose veins
- Used for many years to stimulate milk production in lactating women

ACTIVE INGREDIENTS

- Silymarin, which consists of several flavonolignans
    - Silybin (antioxidant and hepatoprotection)
    - Silychristin
    - Silidianin
    - Silibinin
- Apigenin
- Silybonol (fixed oil)
- Palmitic and stearic acids

- Betaine hydrochloride
- Triamine
- Histamine

ACTION

- Antioxidant
- Hepatoprotectant (undergoes extensive enterohepatic circulation; moves from plasma to bile and concentrates in liver cells)
- Stimulates DNA and RNA synthesis within hepatocyte activating regeneration of liver cells
- Prevents toxins from entering liver cells by preventing binding (may prevent liver damage from tetracycline, tylenol, thallium, erthromycin, amitriptyline, and long-term phenothiazines. More research needs to be done to clarify and verify this information.)
- Blocks peroxidation of fatty acids and damage to lipid membranes
- May have anti-inflammatory activity
- May enhance immune function (PMNNs, T-lymphocytes)
- May lower cholesterol production
- Increases bile secretion
- May decrease diabetic complications and protect from outside insults such as alcohol
- Increases glutathione in liver (enzyme responsible for detoxifying a wide range of toxins, hormones, and drugs)
- Free radical scavenger
- Decreases prostaglandin synthesis

USES

- Improves survival in patients with cirrhosis, may reverse liver damage (patient must stop drinking alcohol to maximize effectiveness)
- Improves immune function in patients with cirrhosis
- Improves acute and chronic hepatitis (B and C types)
- Improves quality of life
- May prevent or treat gallstones
- In certain occupations (farmers, chemical workers) to protect liver from toxins
- In Europe for Amanita mushroom poisoning (poison deathcap or toadstool mushroom)
- Improves appetite and reduces nausea in patients with cirrhosis

DOSAGE*

- Standardized extracts with 35 to 70 mg or 70% to 80% of silymarin (the active component) three times a day. Average dose is 280 to 420 mg/day.
- Alcohol-based extracts are contraindicated because of the need to administer relatively high amounts of alcohol to obtain an adequate dose of silymarin.

PHARMACOKINETICS

- Absorbs readily
- Peak: 1 hour
- Onset 5 to 8 days
- Reversal of damage: 1 to 2 months
- Remission in chronic hepatitis: 6 months to 1 year

TOXICITY

- No toxicity, considered safe

CONTRAINDICATIONS

- In severe liver disease

SIDE EFFECTS

- Mild laxative effect
- GI symptoms
- Mild allergic reactions
- Hepatitic disease conditions

LONG-TERM SAFETY

- Safe and nontoxic

PREGNANCY/LACTATION/CHILDREN

- Safe

DRUG INTERACTIONS

- None known

---

*The product researched most widely and available in Europe is Legalon. Another product, Thisilyn, also widely researched in Europe, is available in the United States through Nature's Way.

Bibliography

Albrecht, M. (1992). Therapy of toxic liver pathologies with Legalon. Zeitschrift fur Klin Medizine. 47, (2), 87–92.

Awang, D. (1993). Milk thistle. Canadian Pharmaceutical Journal. 422, 403–404.

Bisset, N. (1994). Herbal drugs and phytopharmaceuticals. London: CRC Press. 121–123.

Buzzelli, G. (1993). A pilot study on the liver protective effect of silybin-phosphatidylcholine complex (IdB1016) in chronic active hepatitis. International Journal of Clinical Pharmacology Therapeutic Toxicology. 31, 456–460.

Flora, K., Hahn, M., Rosen, H., & Benner, K. (1998). Milk thistle (Silybum marianum) for the therapy of liver disease. American Journal of Gastroenterology. 93, (2), 139–143.

Foster, S. (1991). Milk thistle-Silybum marianum. Botanical Series #305. Austin, TX: American Botanical Council. 3–7.

Grossman, M. (1995). Spontaneous regression of hepatocellular carcinoma. American Journal of Gastroenterology. 90, (9), 1500–1503.

Hobbs, C. (1992). Milk thistle: the liver herb. 2nd Ed. Capitola, CA: Botanica Press. 1–32.

The Lawrence Review of Natural Products. St. Louis, MO: Facts and Comparisons. 1998.

Mascarella, S. (1993). Therapeutic and antilipoperoxidant effects of silybin-phosphatidycholine complex in chronic liver disease: preliminary result. Current Therapeutic Research. 53, (1), 98–102.

Palasciancio, G. (1994). Milk thistle. Current Therapeutic Research. 55, (5), 537–545.

Skottova, N. & Kreeman, V. (1998). Silymarin as a potential hypocholesterolaemic drug. Physiological Research. 47, (1), 1–7.

von Schonfeld, J., Weisbrod, B., & Muller, M. K. (1997). Silibinin, a plant extract with antioxidant and membrane stabilizing properties, protects exocrine pancreas from cyclosporin A toxicity. Cellular Molecular Life Sciences. 53, (11–12), 917–920.

Saw Palmetto (Serenoa repens)

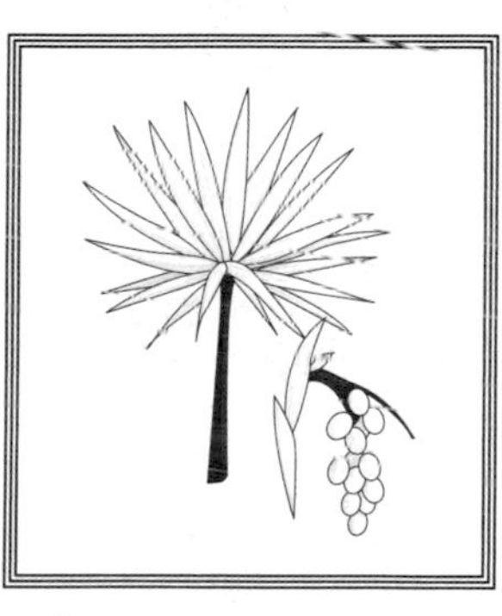

Description

- Small palm tree native to West Indies and Atlantic coast of North America from South Carolina to Florida.
- Grows 6 to10 feet high, with 2- to 4-foot spiny-toothed leaves that form a circular, fan-shaped outline
- Fruit is blue black, shriveled and somewhat oily
- Seed in fruit are hard, flat, and reddish brown

Part of Plant Used

- Berries

Folk Uses

North American herb doctors used the berries for treatment of genitourinary disturbances, prostate problems in men, and breast problems in women.

ACTIVE INGREDIENTS

- Fatty acids (caproic, oleic, linoleic, linolenic)
- Steroids
- Diterpenes
- Triterpenes
- Sesquiterpene
- Alcohols

ACTION

- Antiandrogenic
- Inhibits 5 reductase (enzyme responsible for catalazation of testosterone to 5-DHT).
- Promotes fertility in both genders

USES

- Reduces symptoms of benign prostatic hypertrophy
- Urinary antiseptic
- Diuretic activity
- Stimulates appetite
- May enhance sexual functioning and desire
- Increases testicular function
- Reduces cystic acne
- Reduces cysts in breasts

DOSAGE

- 160 mg twice daily

TOXICITY

- Safe

CONTRAINDICATIONS

- None known

SIDE EFFECTS

- Minimal
- GI

LONG-TERM SAFETY

- Safe, but when used for more than 3 months, patient should be observed by a health care provider
- Not for self-diagnosis and treatment

PREGNANCY/LACTATING/CHILDREN

- Contraindicated in pregnancy. By reducing 5 reductase, it can affect unborn male fetus.

DRUG INTERACTION

- None known

Bibliography

Anonymous. (1998). Herbal supplements. Is saw palmetto good for the prostate? Harv Health Letters. 23, (7), 6.

Braeckman, J. (1994). The extract of *Serenoa repens* in the treatment of benign prostatic hyperplasia. Current Therapeutic Research. 55, 776–785.

Champault, A. (1984). Double-blind trial of an extract of the plant Serenoa repens in benign prostate hyperplasia. British Journal of Clinical Pharmacology. 18, 461–462.

Gerber, G. S., Zagaja, G. P., Bates, G. T., et al. (1998). Saw palmetto in men with lower urinary tract symptoms: effects on urodynamic parameters and voiding symptoms. Urology. 51, 1003–1007.

Murray, M. (1994). Saw palmetto extract vs. Proscar. The American Journal of Natural Medicine. 1, (1), 8–9.

Powers, J. E. (1997). That pesky prostate and the saw palmetto. South Dakota Journal of Medicine. 50, (12), 453–454.

St. John's Wort (*Hypericum perforatum*)

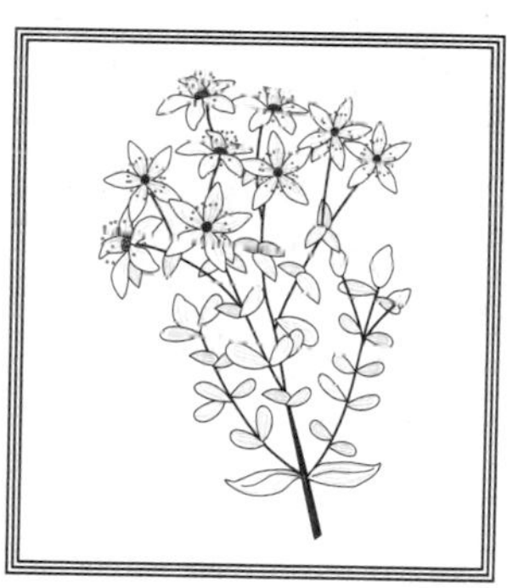

DESCRIPTION

- Shrubby perennial plant with bright yellow flowers. Some say they are at their brightest coincidental with the birthday of John the Baptist (June 24).
- Native to Europe but now grows in many parts of the world in dry, gravelly soils and sunny places
- Grows 1 to 2 feet, considered an aggressive weed

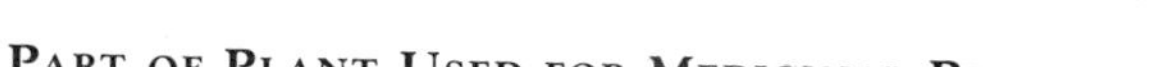

PART OF PLANT USED FOR MEDICINAL PURPOSES

- Flowering tops

FOLK USE

- Dioscorides used St. John's wort in the 1st Century for sciatica, burns, and fever

- Hippocrates used St. John's wort to treat many diseases
- Greeks and other Europeans from Middle Ages thought St. John's wort to have magical powers
- Folk remedy to treat wounds, kidney and lung disease, and depression
- In Europe it was used internally for diarrhea, dysentery, worms, jaundice, and nervous disorders
- The early church said the red dots on the yellow flower was the blood of St. John the Baptist

ACTIVE INGREDIENTS

- Quinoids (Hypericin, pseudohypericin, protohypericin, protopseudohypericin)
- Phenol (p-coumaric acid and others)
- Flavonoids (Quercitin, and others)
- Hyperforin (potent uptake inhibitor of serotonin 5-HT, norepinephrine, GABA, and L-glutamate)
- Xanthones
- Polypropanoids
- Alicyclic acid
- Alkanes
- Monoterpenes
- Essential oils and tannins (10%)
- Carotenoids
- Pectin

ACTION

- Antidepressant
- Antiviral
- Anti-inflammatory
- Antimicrobial
- Astringent (because of 10% tannins)
- Previously thought to act as MAOI but recent research indicates this is not true
- Acts as selective serotonin reuptake inhibitor (SSRIs) (keeps serotonin active in the brain)
- Suppresses interleukin 6, release probably affecting mood through neurohormonal pathways
- May increase number of neurotransmitters in brain (under investigation)
- May inhibit catechol-o-transferase
- Normalizes regular sleep patterns

USES

- Mild to moderate depression (inappropriate for severe depression or bipolar disorders)
- Antiviral activity against herpes type 1 and 2, mononucleosis, influenza (take at first sign of herpes infection)
- Antibacterial activating against gm^+ and gm^- bacteria
- Eases pain of sciatica and arthritis
- Eases menopausal symptoms
- Anti-inflammatory
- As a lotion, speeds healing of wounds, burns, and sunburn
- May decrease signs of dementia
- Helps heal damaged nerve tissue after CVA or neurologic trauma

DOSAGE

- 300 mg three times daily with meals; standardized extract of 0.3% hypericin
- Available as tea, powder, oil, liquid, capsules, tablets
- Oil infusion of fresh flowers (1 tsp two to three times daily)
- With food to prevent GI upset (only necessary for side effects or high dose tincture)
- Tincture 1:2, 2 to 4 mL three times a day for 8 weeks

The following are recommended doses:

- As an antidepressant, take 300 mg three times daily, but for no more than 8 weeks without physician supervision. Some trials have shown that 300 mg three times daily has less of an antidepressant effect than amitriptyline (Elavil) at a dose of 25 mg three times daily, but more of an effect than placebo.
- As a tea, steep 2 to 4 grams (1 to 2 teaspoons) of leaves and flowers 5 to 10 minutes in one cup of boiling water. The dose is one to two cups twice daily for 4 to 6 weeks.
- As an anti-inflammatory or for wound epithelization, use a tincture, and cover wound with gauze or bandage until healing is established.
- For children 6 to 12 years of age, the dose should be half to two thirds of the adult dose.

PHARMACOKINETICS

Onset: absorption: 2 to 2.6 hours
Peak: 5 hours

Dosing varies between preparations, but the equivalent dose should be 2 to 4 grams of dried herb a day.

Duration: takes 4 to 6 weeks to be effective
Steady state: (with long-term use) 4 days
Half-life: 24 to 48 hours
Met/Ex: unknown

TOXICITY

- Photosensitivity may occur, so be careful of sun exposure

CONTRAINDICATIONS

- Fair skin people who must have prolonged sun exposure
- Severe depression
- Seizures because there have been isolated anecdotal reports of seizures occurring with St. John's wort
- Migraines because duration and intensity may increase

SIDE EFFECTS*

- Headache
- Nervousness
- Itching
- Fatigue
- GI irritation
- Restlessness

LONG-TERM SAFETY

- Safe, but not for self-diagnosis and treatment for more than 3 to 4 months

PREGNANCY/LACTATING/CHILDREN

- Avoid during pregnancy; may be administered during pregnancy, but should be supervised by an herbalist
- Decrease production of milk by inhibiting secretion of prolactin
- Not in children younger than 6 years

DRUG INTERACTION

- Caffeine, theophylline, beta $_2$ agonists with St. John's wort increases anxiety, nervousness, and worsens panic disorder
- Concurrent disulfiram (Antabuse) and metronidazole (Flagyl)

---

*Usually subside with long-term use. If side effects occur, decrease dose and then gradually increase again. Side effects usually subside.

- Increased likelihood of severe antabuse reaction. Allow 48 to 72 hours between dosing of these products
- Serotonin syndrome with SSRIs (sweating, agitation, tremor)
- MAOIs
- Tricyclic antidepressants
- Some atypical antipsychotics such as olanzapine (Zyprexa) or risperidone (Risperdal)
- Amphetamine-like drugs
- Dopamine agonists
- Over-the-counter drugs, especially cough and cold remedies, diet drugs with dextromethorphan, ephedrine, pseudoephedrine, or phenylpropanolamine
- Other herbal agents such as cocaine, 1-tryptophan, yohimbe, ma huang, ginseng, feverfew
- Does not potentiate alcohol
- Do not combine with any sleep aids—have difficulty waking and wake up groggy

Bibliography

To date there have been at least 25 well-controlled, placebo trials that confirmed efficacy of St. John's wort for depression. Most trials have been short-term, 6 to 8 weeks, thus long-term efficacy needs to be studied fully. Research was funded by the National Institutes of Health in early 1998. The FDA has sanctioned hypericin as an investigative new drug that is in clinical trials with the name VIMRXYN

Chatterjee, S. S., Bhattacharya, S. K., et al. (1998). Hyperforin as a possible antidepressant component of hypericum extracts. Life Sciences. 63, (6) 499–510

Ciordia, R. (1998). Beware "St John's Wort," potential herbal danger. Journal of Clinical Monitoring and Computing. 14, (3), 215.

Cott, J. M. & Fugh-Berman, A. (1998). Is St John's wort (Hypericum perforatum) an effective antidepressant? Journal of Nervous and Mental Disease. 186, (8), 500–501.

Degar, S., et al. (1992). Inactivation of the human immunodeficiency virus by hypericin: evidence of photochemical alterations of p24 and a block in uncoating. AIDS Research and Human Retroviruses. 8, 1929–1936.

DeSmet, P. A. G. M., et al. (1993). Adverse effects of herbal drugs, vol. 2. Berlin: Springer-Verlag, pp. 9, 10, 49, 50

Evans, M. (1997). St. John's wort: an herbal remedy for depression? Canadian Family Physician. Oct 43, 1735–1736.

Gordon JB: SSRIs and St John's Wort: possible toxicity? Am Fam Physician. 1998 Mar 1;57(5)950.

Hansgen, K. D., et al. (1994). Multicenter double-blind study examining the antidepressant effectiveness of the Hypericum extract LI 160. Journal of Geriatric Psychiatry and Neurology. 7, (Suppl 1), s15–s18.

Harrer, G: (1995). Effectiveness and tolerance of the hypericum extract LI 160 compared to maprotiline: a multicenter double-blind study. Journal of Geriatric Psychiatry and Neurology. 7, (Suppl 1):s24–s28.

Heiligenstein, E. & Guenther, G. (1998). Over the counter psychotropics: a review of melatonin, St John's wort, valerian and kava-kava. Journal of the American College of Health. 46, (6), 271–276.

Hudson, J. B., et al. (1991). Antiviral activities of hypericin. Antiviral Research. 15, 101–112.

Lavie, G., et al. (1990). Hypericin as an antiretroviral agent—mode of action and related ana-

logues. Annals New York Academy of Sciences. 556–562.
Linde, K., et al. (1996). St. John's wort for depression—an overview and meta-analysis of randomised clinical trials. British Medical Journal. 313, 253–258.
Martinez, B., et al. (1993). Hypericum in the treatment of seasonal effective disorders. Journal of Geriatric Psychiatry and Neurology. 7, (Suppl 1), s29–s33.
Miller, A. L. (1998). St John's Wort (Hypericum perforatum): clinical effects on depression and other conditions. Alternative Medicine Review. 3, (1), 18–26.
Muller, W. E. G. & Russul, R. (1994). Effects of Hypericum extract on the expression of serotonin receptors. Journal of Geriatric Psychiatry and Neurology. 7, (Suppl 1), s63–s64.
Perovic, S. (1995). Pharmacological profile of hypericum extract. Effect on serotonin uptake by postsynaptic receptors. Arzneimittelforschung 45, (11), 1145–1148.
Ramirez, L. K., et al. (1996). St. John's wort for depression—an overview. British Medical Journal. 313, (7052), 253–258.
Snow, J. M. (1997). *Hypericum perforatum* L. (Hyperiaceae). The Protocol Journal of Botanical Medicine. 2, (1), 16–21.
Sommer, H. (1994). Placebo-controlled double-blind study examining the effectiveness of a hypericum preparation in 105 mildly depressed patients. Journal of Geriatric Psychiatry and Neurology. 7, (Suppl 1), s9–s11.
Stix, G. (1998). Plant matters. Scientific American. 278, (2), 30–32.
Volz, H. P. (1997). Controlled clinical trials of Hypericum extracts in depressed patients—an overview. Pharmacopsychiatry. 30, (Suppl), 72–76.
Vorbach, E. V., et al. (1994). Effectiveness and tolerance of the Hypericum extract LI 160 in comparison with imipramine: randomized double-blind study with 135 outpatients. Journal of Geriatric Psychiatry and Neurology. 7, (Suppl 1), s19–s23.
Vorbach, E. V., et al. (1997). Efficacy and tolerability of St. John's wort extract LI 160 versus imipramine in patients with severe depressive episodes according to ICD-10. Pharmacopsychiatry. 30, (Suppl), 81–85.
Wheatley, D. (1997). LI 160, an extract of St. John's wort, versus Amitriptyline in mildly to moderately depressed outpatients—a controlled 6-week clinical trial. Pharmacopsychiatry. 30 (Suppl), 77–80.
Woelk, H. (1994). Benefits and risks of the hypericum extract LI 160: drug monitoring study with 3250 patients. Journal of Geriatric Psychiatry and Neurology. 7 (Suppl 1), s34–s38.

INTERNET

www.hypericum.com
(800) 543-3101

Tea Tree Oil *(Melaleuca alternifolia)*

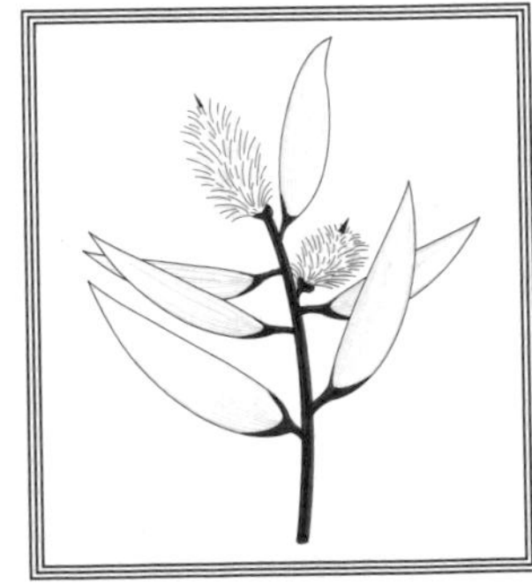

DESCRIPTION

There are many plants known as "Tea Trees," but the species *Melaleuca alternifolia* is responsible for tea tree oil.

- Small tree, native only to the northeast coastal region of New South Wales, Australia.

- Evergreen shrub, grows 8 feet tall
- Fruits grow in clusters and white flowers bloom in summer

PART OF PLANT USED FOR MEDICINAL PURPOSES

- Leaves, the source of the oils, are steam distilled to produce the oil

FOLK USE

- Used by the Aborigines of Australia as a treatment for cuts, abrasions, burns, and insect bites
- Referred to by Captain Cook in 1777
- During World War II, used by soldiers as a disinfectant
- In the 1920s, it was used in surgery and dentistry

ACTIVE INGREDIENTS

- Volatile oil (2%)
- Terpin: 4-01 (40%)
- Terpene hydrocarbons
  - pinene
  - terpinene
  - cymene
- Oxygenated terpenes
- Sesquiterpene hydrocarbons
- Eucalyptol
- Nerolidol
- Viridiflorol

ACTION

- Antimicrobial, against:
  - *Candida*
  - *E. coli*
  - *S. aureus*
  - *P. aeruginosa*
  - fungus, yeast
  - possibly MRSA
- Parasitic agent
- May remove transient skin flora without removing resident flora

USES

- Acne
- Burns

- Herpes
- Cosmetics
- Impetigo
- Insect bites
- Lice, ring worm
- Psoriasis
- Infections
- Nail fungus (onychomycosis)

DOSAGE

- Oil applied topically 1 to 2 times daily

TOXICITY

- With ingestion, ataxia and drowsiness have been reported
- Topically, rare

CONTRAINDICATIONS

- Hypersensitivity

SIDE EFFECTS

- Contact dermatitis
- Allergic contact eczema

LONG-TERM SAFETY

- Safe with topical use

PREGNANCY/LACTATION/CHILDREN

- Safe if used topically

DRUG INTERACTIONS

- None known

Bibliography

Bassett, I. B., et al. (1990). A comparative study of tea-tree benzoylperoxide oil versus in the treatment of acne. Medical Journal of Australia. 153, (8), 455–458.

Buck, D. S., Nidorf, D. M., & Addino, J. G. (1994). Comparison of two topical preparations for the treatment of onychomycosis: Melaleuca alternifolia (tea tree) oil and clotrimazole. Journal of Family Practice. 38, 601–605.

Chan, C. H. & Loudon, K. W. (1998). Activity of tea tree oil on methicillin-resistant *Staphylococcus aureus*. Journal of Hospital Infections. 39 (3), 244–245.

Cox, S., et al. (1998). Tea tree oil causes K^+ leakage and inhibits respiration in *E. coli*. Letters in Applied Microbiology. 26, 355–358.

Gustafson, J., et al. (1998). Effects of Tea tree oil on *E. coli*. Letters in Applied Microbiology. 26, 194–198.

Hammer, K. A., et al. (1996). Susceptibility of transient and commensal skin flora to the essential oil of Melaleuca alternifolia. American Journal of Infection Control. 24(3), 186–189.

Raman, A., et al. (1995). Antimicrobial effects of tea-tree oil and its major components on *Staphylococcus aureus*, Staph. Epidermidis and Propionibacterium Acnes. Letters of Applied Microbiology, 21(4), 242–245.

Valerian *(Valeriance officinalis)*

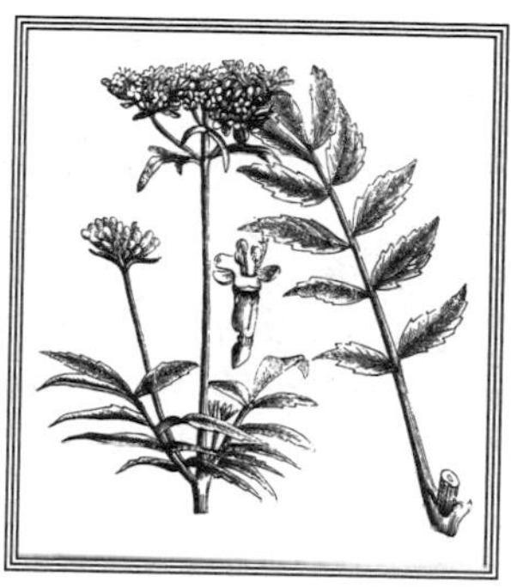

DESCRIPTION

- Perennial plant native to North America and Europe
- Tuberous root produces a flowering stem 2 to 4 feet high
- White to cream-colored flowers bloom June to September

PART OF PLANT USED FOR MEDICINAL PURPOSES

- Rhizome

FOLK USES

- Used for hundreds of years in Europe as a sedative to relieve insomnia, anxiety, and conditions associated with pain
- American Indians boiled the roots into a tea for calming the nerves

ACTIVE INGREDIENTS

- Valepotriates
- Valeric acid
- Volatile oils
- Flavonoids
- Steroids
- Alkaloids

ACTION

- Acts on CNS as sedative, binds to same brain receptors as Valium and other benzodiazepines
- Lowers blood pressure
- Anti-inflammatory (increases Omega 3s)

USES

- Improves sleep
- Relieves insomnia
- Lowers blood pressure
- Relaxes intestinal muscles
- Possibly for antitumor activity
- Acts as a sedative

DOSAGES*

- Dried root (or as tea): 1 to 2 grams
- Tincture (1:5): 4 to 6 mL (1 to 1.5 teaspoons)
- Fluid extract (1:1): 1 to 2 mL (0.5 to 1 teaspoon)
- Valerian extract (0.8% valeric acid): 150 to 300 mg
- For sleep: 300 to 500 mg before bedtime
- For anxiety: 150 to 500 mg a day, divided

TOXICITY

- Safe and approved for food use by the FDA

CONTRAINDICATIONS

- Schizophrenia, bipolar disorders

SIDE EFFECTS

- Rare, but hypersensitivity with overdoses

LONG-TERM USE

- Safe

PREGNANCY/LACTATING/CHILDREN

- Safe

DRUG INTERACTION

- May intensify the effects of sedatives
- Has no effect with alcohol
- Increases seizure activity while taking anticonvulsants

---

*For sleep, take 1 hour before bedtime.

Bibliography

Blumenthal, M. (1998).USP publishes information monographs on ginger and valerian. HerbalGram #43. 3, 12.

Leuschner, J., Muller, J., & Radioman, M. (1993). Characterization of the central nervous depressant activity of a commercially valuable valerian root extract. Arzneimittelforschung. 43 (6), 638–643.

Lindahl, O. & Lindwall, L. (1989). Double blind study of a valerian preparation. Pharmacology. Biochemistry, and Behavior. 32, (4), 1065–1066.

Pinco, R. G. & Israelsen, L. D. (1998). European-American Phytomedicines Coalition Citizen Petition to amend FDA's monograph on nighttime sleep-aid drug products for over-the-counter ("OTC") human use to include Valerian. USP Publishes Information Monographs on Ginger and Valerian. 12 (3).

Sakamoto, T., et al. (1992). Psychotropic effects of Japanese valerian root extract. Pharmaceutical Society of Japan. 40 (3), 758–761.

Schultz, V., Hubner, W. D., & Ploch, M. (1997). Clinical trials with phyto-psychopharmacological agents. Phytomedicine. 4 (4)., 379–387.

Tatsuya, S., Yoko, M., & Dazu, N. (1992). Psychotropic effects of Japanese valerian root extract. Chemical and Pharmaceutical Bulletin. 40 (3), 758–761.

USP. (1998). Valerian (*Valeriana officinalis*). Information Monographs on Ginger and Valerian. 12(3).

Wagner, J., Wagner, M. L., & Hening, W. A. (1998). Beyond benzodiazepines: alternative pharmacologic agents for the treatment of insomnia. American Pharmacotherapy. 32 (6), 680–691.

Willey, L. B. Valerian overdose: a case report. Veterinary and Human Toxicology. 37 (4), 364–365, 1995.

Vitex (*Agnus castus*) (Chaste tree, Monk's pepper)

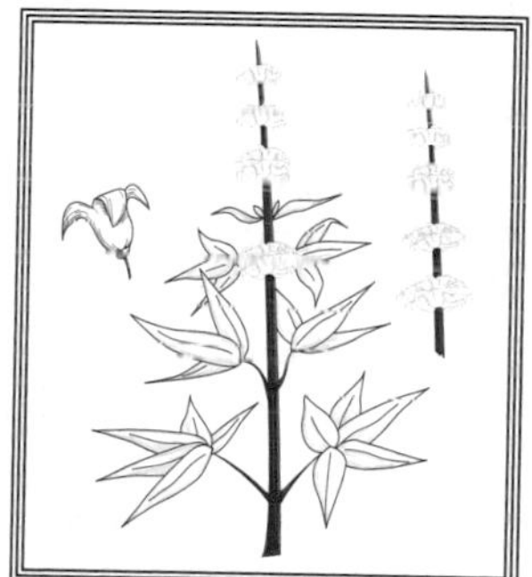

DESCRIPTION

- Grows abundantly in Southern Europe and the Mediterranean
- Grows 22 in tall
- Has purple flowers in summer, black fruit in autumn

PART OF PLANT USED FOR MEDICINAL PURPOSES

- The dried fruit

FOLK USE

- Vitex has been used for more than 2,000 years as a treatment for female problems, such as menstrual cramps, irregular cycles, and abnormal bleeding. Legend has it that it was an "anti-aphrodisiac" for men and has been called "monk's pepper."
- Used by Hippocrates

- Symbol of chastity by medieval European church; where it is native (Mediterranean, Greek Islands) in pre-Christian times its use was sacred to Hera, protectress of women.

ACTIVE INGREDIENTS

- Iridosides
- Flavonoids (luteolin 6-C, luteolin 7-0, luteolin, artemetin, and others)
- Progestins
- Essential oils
- Steroids
- Monoterpenoids
- Sesquiterpenoids

ACTION

- Antiandrogen lowers male hormones
- Balances progesterone and estrogens, therefore regulates female cycle
- Decreases breast pain
- Increases LH

USES

- To treat perimenopause
- Hot flashes
- Relieve anxiety
- Relieve pain in breasts
- Treat vaginal dryness
- Irregular menstrual cycles
- May treat annovulatory cycles
- May increase ovulation and thus increase likelihood of becoming pregnant
- Increases milk production during lactation

DOSAGE

- Tincture (1:5): 24 mL, 1 to 2 times a day
- For menstrual cramps, 1 teaspoon every 2 hours until cramps are gone
- Tea: 1 to 3 cups of freshly powdered berries

TOXICITY

- Nontoxic

CONTRAINDICATIONS

- Unknown

SIDE EFFECTS

- Nausea, vomiting
- Allergic reaction: itch, rash
- Headache
- Increased menstrual flow

LONG-TERM SAFETY

- Safe

PREGNANT/LACTATION/CHILDREN

- Safe in pregnant and lactating women
- Safety in children not until after menarche

DRUG INTERACTION

- Unknown

Bibliography

Hirobe, C., Qiao, Z. S., Takeya, K., & Itokawa, H. (1997). Cytotoxic flavonoids from Vitex agnus-castus. Phytochemistry. 46 (3), 521–524.

Lauritzen, D., et al. (1997). Treatment of premenstrual tension syndrome with *Vitex agnus-castus*. Controlled, double-blind study versus pyridoxine. Phytomedicine. 4 (3), 183–189.

Snow, J. (1996). Vitex. Protocol Journal of Botanical Medicine. 1, (4), 20–23.

INTERNET

Associations

AANP
http://infinity.dorsai.org/Naturopathic.Physician/Welcome.html

American Herbalists Guild
http://www.healthy.net/pan/pa/herbalmedicine/ahg/index.html

Phytonet
http://www.exeter.ac.uk./phytonet/welcome.html

National Cancer Institute
http://web.fie.com/htdoc/fed/nih/nci/any/menu/any/nciindex.htm

WH Traditional Med. Program
http://www.who.ch/programmes/dap/trm0.html

American Society Of Pharmacognosy
http://www.temple.edu/ASP/

Centers for Disease Control and Prevention
http://www.cdc.gov/

Office of Alternative Medicine
http://altmed.od.nih.gov/

Internet for Medicinal Plant Research

Alta Vista	http://altavista.digital.com/
Deja News - Internet Newsgroups	http://www.dejanews.com/
HealthWorld Online	http://www.healthy.net/
Phytopharmacognosy	http://www.mdx.ac.uk./www/pharm/
Medline via PubMed	http://www.ncbi.nlm.nih.gov/PubMed/medline.html
Browse the MeSH Hierarchy	http://muscat.gdb.org/repos/medl/browse/nest.html
ChemFinder Searching	http://chemfinder.camsoft.com/
Phytochemical & Ethnobotanical Database	http://www.ars-grin.gov/cgi-bin/duke/farmacy1.pl
Phytochemical & Natural Products Links	http://uchii1.ch.umist.ac.uk/group/subtopics/phyto.html
Journals/Books	
Modern Herbal Home Page	http://www.botanical.com/botanical/mgmh/mgmh.html
Eclectic Materia Medica (Felter)	http://chili.rt66.com/hrbmoore/FelterMM/Felters.html
Ellingwood's Therapeutist	http://chili.rt66.com/hrbmoore/Journals/Ellingwood.html
Culbreth's Materia Medica	http://chili.rt66.com/hrbmoore/ManualsOther/Culbreth.html
Classic Texts	http://chili.rt66.com/hrbmoore/ManualsOther/ManOther.html
Journal of Natural Products	http://pubs.acs.org/journals/jnprdf/index.html
Journal of Ethnopharmacology	http://www.elsevier.nl/estoc/publications/store/1/03788741/
Journal of Pharmacognosy	http://www.swets.nl/sps/journals/ijp.html
Botanical Research Bulletin	http://www.herbsinfo.com/pages/botan-r1.htm
RSC Natural Product Reports	http://chemistry.rsc.org/rsc/nprpub.htm
Planta Medica	http://www.thieme.com/aec.htm
Herbal Gram	http://www.healthworld.com/library/periodicals/journals/HerbalGram/index.html
Journal of Naturopathic Medicine	http://www.healthy.net/library/journals/naturopathic/index.html

Gesellschaft fuer Arzneipflanzenforschung- Society for Medicinal Plant Research	http://www.rz.uni-duesseldorf.de/WWW/GA/english/ewelcome.htm
Protocol Journal of Botanical Medicine	http://www.herbalresearch.com/botjrn.htm
Quarterly Review of Natural Medicine	http://www.healthy.net/library/journals/quarterlyreview/index.html
Databases	
NIH Web Search	http://search.info.nih.gov/
Directory for Economic Botany	http://www.helsinki.fi/kmus/botecon.html
Subject-Oriented Internet Resource Guides	http://www.lib.umich.edu/chhome.html
Libary of Congress	http://marvel.loc.gov/
WWW Virtual Library	http://www.w3.org/pub/DataSources/bySubject/Overview.html
Resources of Scholarly Societies	http://www.lib.uwaterloo.ca/society/subjects_soc.html
Biological, Agricultural & Medical INFOMINE	http://lib-www.ucr.edu/bioag/
Starting Points: Scientific Resources	http://library.niehs.nih.gov/start.htm
Intro to Using WWW Databases	http://www.inform.umd.edu/PBIO/MEDICAL_BOTANY/internet.htm
NAPRALERT	http://pcog8.pmmp.uic.edu/mcp/nap1.html
American Indian Ethnobotany DB	http://www.umd.umich.edu/cgi-bin/herb/
PLANTS National DB	http://plants.usda.gov/plants/
Medicinal & Poisonous Plant DB	http://www.inform.umd.edu/PBIO/Medicinals/medicinals.html
Smell Database	http://hydrogen.cchem.berkeley.edu:8080/Smells/
Natural Products	http://lib.upm.edu.my/iisnp.html
National Center for Development of Natural Products	http://www.olemiss.edu/depts/ncdnp/

CHAPTER 4

Nutrition As a Way to Health

The human body is a complex organism with the ability to heal itself. Each cell can be thought of as a complex engine. Some work alone, others work in unison, but they all work 24 hours a day and they all require fuel. The fuel comes directly from the things we eat. The nutrients in food provide our cells with the materials needed to carry on daily activity. If our nutrition is inadequate, bodily function is impaired. This impairment may lead to organ dysfunction, often years after the nutritional imbalance, deficiency, or excess began.

The past 20 years have brought to light new knowledge about nutrition and its effects on the body. *Phytochemicals* (chemicals present in plants), which give the plant color, flavor, and protection, have been identified. *Nutraceuticals* (the newest type of dietary supplement), which enhance normal and regular food with herbs, vitamins, and antioxidants, have been born. Through understanding of the concepts of holistic nutrition, health can be promoted and disease can be prevented.

WHAT WE EAT

The National Cancer Institute reported that 45% of Americans consume no fruit in a day, and 22% do not eat vegetables. On average, the typical American consumes only three servings of fruit and vegetables a day. Our new food pyramid calls for the consumption of eight fruits (three) and vegetables (five) a day. Many people do not consume 60 mg of vitamin C each day, let alone the minimum daily requirement of 200 mg. Just about everyone could spend more time in the produce section of their local grocery store. Fresh is best. Organically grown is possibly even better.

Look for crisp, plump, firm, and unbruised produce. Smell the fruit at room temperature. If it smells how you want it to taste, then it is the one to buy.

If fresh is unavailable, frozen is next best. Do not buy frozen fruit and vegetables if the bag has frozen ice crystals inside. Do not allow the product to come to room temperature before you refreeze. Canned produce is the last resort. If you buy canned, buy products canned in their own juice.

Be careful with barbecuing. While grilled food is great for low fat diet, heavily charred meats can contain high levels of carcinogens called *heterocylic aromatic* amines. It is wise not to indulge in grilled meat too often. When you want to grill, try fish instead of red meat.

Our food pyramid suggests a healthy daily eating plan (Fig. 4-1).

Fruits and Vegetables

One serving of fruits and vegetables is equal to:

1 cup of raw leafy vegetables
1/2 cup of other vegetables (cooked or chopped raw)
3/4 cup vegetable or fruit juice
1 medium apple, banana, or orange
1/2 cup fruit (chopped, cooked, frozen, or canned)
2 tablespoons dried fruit

How to Count Fiber

Fiber intake should be 25 to 30 grams/day. Here are some guidelines for counting fiber:

5 grams each
- 1/2 cup cooked, dried beans, peas, or lentils
- 1 serving of high-fiber, wheat-bran cereal

2 grams each
- 1 serving of fruit or vegetable (not counting juice)
- 1 serving of any whole-grain food; for example:
  - 1 slice whole-wheat bread
  - 1/2 cup whole-wheat pasta
  - 1/2 whole-wheat bagel
  - 1 slice rye crisp bread

1 gram each
- 1 serving of a refined grain food

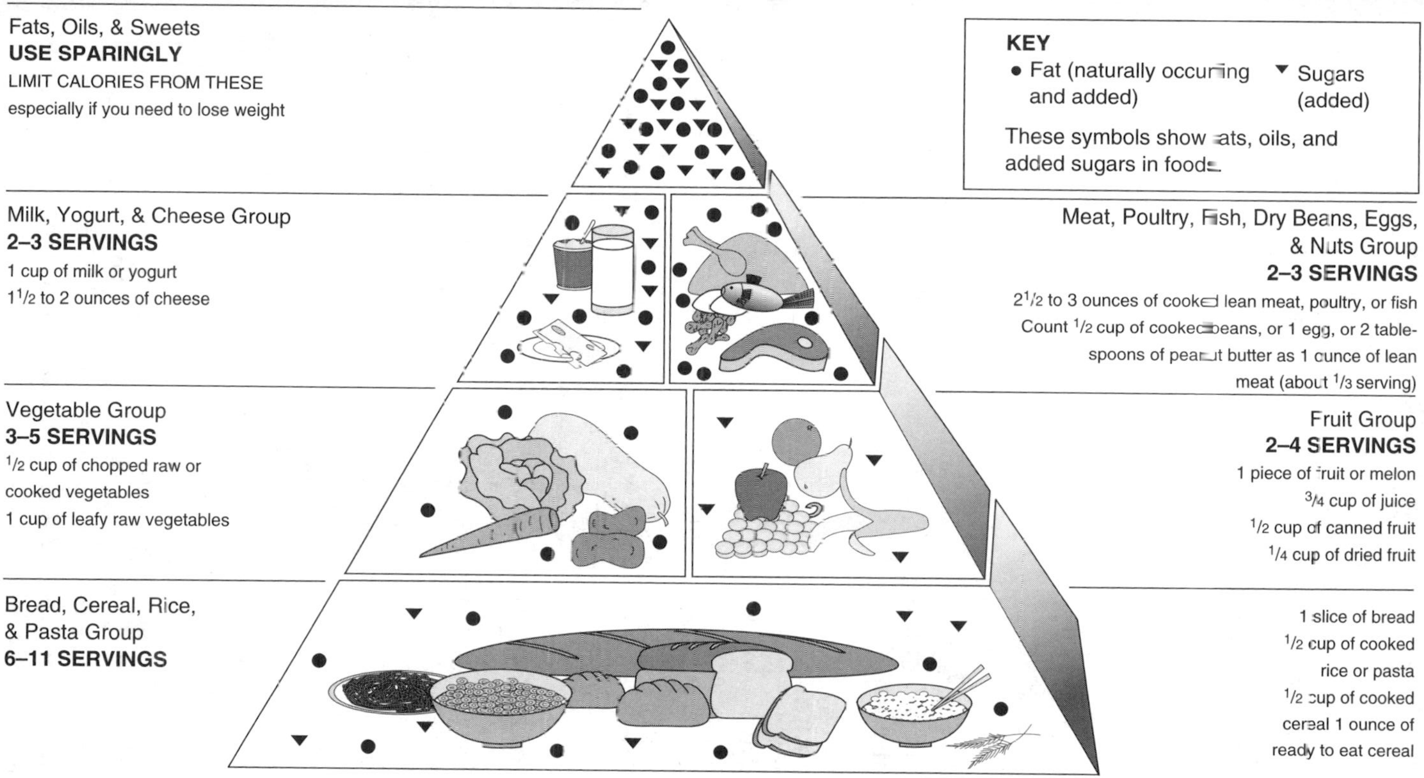

Fats, Oils, & Sweets
USE SPARINGLY
LIMIT CALORIES FROM THESE
especially if you need to lose weight

KEY
- ● Fat (naturally occurring and added)
- ▼ Sugars (added)

These symbols show fats, oils, and added sugars in foods.

Milk, Yogurt, & Cheese Group
2–3 SERVINGS
1 cup of milk or yogurt
$1\frac{1}{2}$ to 2 ounces of cheese

Meat, Poultry, Fish, Dry Beans, Eggs, & Nuts Group
2–3 SERVINGS
$2\frac{1}{2}$ to 3 ounces of cooked lean meat, poultry, or fish
Count $\frac{1}{2}$ cup of cooked beans, or 1 egg, or 2 tablespoons of peanut butter as 1 ounce of lean meat (about $\frac{1}{3}$ serving)

Vegetable Group
3–5 SERVINGS
$\frac{1}{2}$ cup of chopped raw or cooked vegetables
1 cup of leafy raw vegetables

Fruit Group
2–4 SERVINGS
1 piece of fruit or melon
$\frac{3}{4}$ cup of juice
$\frac{1}{2}$ cup of canned fruit
$\frac{1}{4}$ cup of dried fruit

Bread, Cereal, Rice, & Pasta Group
6–11 SERVINGS
1 slice of bread
$\frac{1}{2}$ cup of cooked rice or pasta
$\frac{1}{2}$ cup of cooked cereal 1 ounce of ready to eat cereal

FIGURE 4-1
The Food-Guide Pyramid.

Along with this eating plan, we should include 5- to 8-oz glasses of water a day. Water has been demonstrated to prevent constipation and decrease the risk of colon cancer.

In the 1990s, Dr. C. Everett Koope, then surgeon general of the United States, identified six dietary-related diseases:

Heart disease
Cancer
Obesity
Arthritis
Osteoporosis
Diabetes

Many dietary modifications and special diets have been developed to prevent and treat these diseases, some of which are valuable; some of which are not.

Enzymes

The late Dr. Edward Howell, a physician and pioneer in enzyme research, called enzymes the "sparks of life." Enzymes are responsible for nearly every facet of life and health. Each body cell has an excess of 100,000 enzyme particles necessary for normal metabolic processes. All metabolic processes at every level of the cell depend on the life-sustaining action of enzymes. An enzyme is a large protein molecule containing vitamins, amino acids, and trace minerals such as zinc, selenium, manganese, and copper. Enzymes cannot function properly without the presence of co-enzymes—vitamins, minerals, and proteins.

Demineralization of the soil, as a result of poor crop rotation and fertilization schedules and the application of pesticides, have left most crop land deficient in trace minerals needed to manufacture enzymes in plants and the higher species (man included) that consume them. Natural farming methods (see Pesticide section) help revitalize the soil.

Enzymes are divided into two groups: digestive and metabolic enzymes. Digestive enzymes (amylase breaks down carbohydrates; protease breaks down protein; lipase breaks down fat) break down foods along the gastrointestinal (GI) tract, enabling the nutrients to be absorbed into the blood stream. Metabolic enzymes catalyze various chemical reactions in the cell, such as energy production and detoxification. Two metabolic enzymes are important: superoxide dismutase (SOD) protect the cells by acting as an antioxidant and O_2 free radical scavenger and catalase that breaks down hydrogen peroxide, a metabolic waste product, and liberates O_2 for body use.

The body manufactures many enzymes, but it is also important to obtain enzymes from food. Enzymes are sensitive to heat, and temperatures above 116° F destroy most food enzymes, so cooked food is dead food. To obtain an adequate supply of food enzymes, raw food must be consumed or enzyme supplements can be taken.

Enzymes can be found in many different foods, from plant and animal sources. Avocados, papayas, pineapples, bananas, and mangos are all high in enzymes. Sprouts are the richest source of enzymes, so SOD occurs naturally in a variety of food sources, including barley grass, broccoli, Brussels sprouts, cabbage, wheat grass, and most green plants.

Supporters of enzyme supplementation suggest that enzyme therapy can eliminate heartburn, gas, headaches, bloating, constipation, diarrhea, stress, fatigue, food allergies and hay fever, and overweight and underweight problems. It is suggested by authors writing popular books regarding enzyme therapy that enzymes are as justified as a dietary substance as minerals and vitamins (D. Morrison, *Body Electronics Fundamentals*; E. Howell, *Enzyme Nutrition*; E. Howell, *Food Enzymes for Health and Longevity*; M. Wolf and K. Ransbager, *Enzyme Therapy*; H. Santillo, *Food Enzymes, The Missing Link to Radiant Health*).

Most commercially available enzymes are digestive enzymes extracted from various sources. Enzymes cannot be manufactured synthetically. Some companies produce enzymes from animal products (pancreatin and pepsin). Other companies produce their enzyme extracts from aspergillus, a type of fungus. SOD and catalase enzymes should be contained in an enteric-coated product that allows the SOD to pass intact through the stomach acid and be absorbed in the small intestine. All forms of enzymes should be kept in a reasonably cool place to insure potency.

WHAT TO LOOK FOR WHEN PURCHASING FOOD ENZYMES

- Food enzymes made from a plant source are superior in their effectiveness to animal-derived digestive enzymes such as pepsin, pancreatin, and oxbile.
- Food enzymes should be labeled in "units of activity," not by weight. The units of activity are based on the "Food Chemical Codex," set forth by the National Academy of Sciences.
- Beware of double and triple strength enzymes. High levels of protease initiate the breaking down of the other enzymes, which results in less activity, not more.
- Many enzymes require specific vitamins and minerals (cofactors) for optimal functioning in the digestive process.

NUTRITIONAL DISEASES

Heart Disease

Heart disease is the number one killer of men and women older than 65 in the United States. Diet modification should begin in the 20s in persons with family histories of coronary problems. General guidelines include:

- Reduce saturated fat and cholesterol intake
- Reduce transfatty acids such as margarine
- Substitute monounsaturated fats such as olive oil for butter or other vegetable oils
- Increase fiber
- Do not smoke
- Control homocysteine levels (more later)
- Exercise regularly
- Maintain normal body weight
- Increase omega 3 in diet (high in fatty fish such as salmon, tuna, mackerel)
- Reduce sodium intake

Several dietary programs have been developed and have proven beneficial to persons in reducing ASHD deposits. However, these programs are restricting and take much dedication to follow. Both are approved by the American Heart Association, and both have much research that supports their use.

PRITIKIN PROGRAM

- Developed by Dr. N. Pritikin in the 1960s
- Regular exercise: 45-minute walk/day
- Diet should be less than 10% fats, low in cholesterol (three 1/2 oz animal protein and 2 glasses skim milk/day), and high in complex CHO
- Multivitamins daily

Con:

- Possible deficiency in iron and other nutrients

ORNISH PROGRAM

- Developed by Dr. D. Ornish in the 1970s
- Plan reverses ASHD deposits
- Exercise: 1 hour/day
- Meditation: 20 minutes/day

- No smoking
- Improved communication with others
- Diet should be 1800 calories/day, 10% fats, no animal protein, caffeine, nuts, seeds, egg yolk, or dairy except for 1 cup nonfat milk or yogurt daily
- 75% CHO, 2 oz alcohol/day
- Supplemental vitamins

Con:

- Too low in fat and protein; may lead to deficiencies
- Possible deficiency in iron and vitamins

HOMOCYSTEINE

Homocysteine, a sulfur-containing amino acid, is produced by the breakdown of the essential amino acid methionine and is found in complete dietary proteins. Evidence is mounting that suggests that as homocysteine levels increase, so does the incidence of arterial disease. Nygard, et al (1997) found that when studying 587 patients, total homocysteine levels are a strong predictor of mortality. The higher the homocysteine level, the greater the likelihood of death.

The cardiovascular danger zone appears to begin at homocysteine concentrations that surpass 15(μmol/L), though levels as low as 10 μmol/L are also suspect. An unpublished University of Washington study reported that, among 465 women age 18 to 44 (79 of whom had been diagnosed with myocardial infarction), those whose blood homocysteine levels were 15.6 μmol/L or greater had 2.3 times the risk of heart attack as women with less than 10 μmol/L. This finding was after adjusting for cardiovascular risk factors.

Laboratory studies indicate that high homocysteine possibly contributes to atherosclerosis in three ways: by damaging the inner lining of blood vessels, promoting plaque buildup, or altering blood's clotting mechanism to make clots more likely in the heart or brain. Early evidence suggests that homocysteine, together with glycine, may also destroy brain cells as a result of stroke or head trauma.

Research suggests that boosting the intake of the B vitamin folate (folic acid 400 μg) or combinations of folate, B_6 (pyridoxine 3 mg), or B_{12} (cobalamin 2 mcg) helps decrease homocysteine levels. These B vitamins help regulate homocysteine metabolism. In the Washington study, the women whose folate levels were 8.39 nmol/L or greater had approximately 50% less risk of heart attack than those whole folate measured below 5.27 nmol/L. The scientists found little association between

B_{12} levels and heart attack risk. Folate and B_{12} help recycle homocysteine back into methionine, while B_6 helps break it down into harmless subunits. Five servings of fresh fruits and leafy greens per day are also a rich source. As of January 1, 1998, manufacturers are required by the U.S. Food and Drug Administration (FDA) to add folate to certain grain products, including enriched breads, cereals, noodles, flours, and cornmeal. Some experts predict that this step, by increasing folate intake, will decrease homocysteine levels nationally.

Cancer and Cancer Development

One of three Americans will develop cancer during his or her lifetime. Second only to heart disease, cancer deaths account for 23% of all U.S. deaths. The four organs most affected are lungs, colon, rectum, and prostate. For most cancers, the death rate has remained approximately the same since the 1930s, which indicates that little or no real progress has been made in survival of cancer. Thus, this information would indicate there is no effective treatment for most cancers.

There is a strong correlation between diet or nutrition and many cancers. Chemical and environmental factors, including diet and lifestyle, may be responsible for causing 80% to 90% of all cancers. The older one gets, the greater the risk for developing cancer and the shorter the survival rate than the average 5 years.

Researchers suggest that cancer is a four stage process:

- ***Initiation*** begins after a single application/exposure to a subcarcinogenic substance (e.g., smoke, pesticides, drugs, electromagnetic waves, radiation). Initiation can permanently damage genetic material within the cell.
- ***Promotion*** occurs after a second or repeated exposure of the same or different subcarcinogenic substance. Promotion involves cellular proliferation. During early stages, cellular proliferation is reversible but later becomes irreversible.
- ***Progression*** is the actual division and multiplication of the tumor over the next 10 to 15 years. At first, most tumors are slow growing. As they become bigger, their division speeds.
- ***Metastasis*** is the final step when the tumor spreads diffusely throughout the body.

VEGETABLES

Vegetables block the initiation phase and inhibit or reverse the promotion phase. Some research suggests that vegetarian diets as a whole protect against cancer by their lack of the enzyme 6-desaturase. This enzyme is necessary for cell metabolism, and although normal human cells have it, cancer cells generally do not and require an exogenous supply. By depriving cancer cells of 6-desaturase, vegetarian diets decrease the cells' viability. A vegetarian diet with no added vegetable oil maximizes the amount of protective nutrients while minimizing the amount of carcinogenic nutrients and therefore may be the most effective diet for preventing cancer and for improving the prognosis of those who have disease.

GERSON THERAPY

- Known as metabolic therapy
- Developed by Dr. M. Gerson (1881 to 1959)
- Combines vigorous detoxification with nutrition to restore immunity and healing
- Diet: organic fresh fruits and vegetables
  - 13 glasses fresh squeezed juices/day (diet is high in antioxidants, vitamin C, beta-carotene)
  - Supplements such as thyroid extract, potassium iodide, liver extract, pancreatic enzymes, and niacin
  - No meat or animal protein for first 6 to 12 weeks, then minimal after that
  - Fat free, but some dairy is allowed (Gerson believes all fats promote tumor growth)
  - Linseed oil, a rich source of omega 3
  - Coffee enemas several times daily (caffeine stimulates action of liver, increases bile flow, and opens bile ducts so liver can rid the body of toxic wastes)
- Numerous research articles indicate that there are remissions and cures using this therapy

RESOURCES

Gerson Institute
P.O. Box 430
Bonita, CA 91908
(619) 472-7450

KELLEY'S NUTRITIONAL METABOLIC THERAPY

- Developed by Dr. W. Kelley, a dentist at Centro Hospitalrio Internationale del Pacifico, S.A., Playas, Tijuana, Mexico

- Combines nutrition, detoxification, and supplements of pancreatic enzymes
- Diet tailored to the person's metabolic make-up
- Supplements of vitamins, minerals, pancreatic enzymes (150 tablets/day) (the enzymes help digest the tumor)
- Detoxification: 1 coffee enema/day, and a supplement holiday periodically to allow the body time to "catch up" with ridding itself of toxins
- Chiropractic or osteopathic adjustments to stimulate nerves
- Spiritual component: encourage patient to reestablish a faith in a higher power

Numerous research studies have verified remissions and cures using this technique.

RESOURCES

Nicholas Gonzalez, MD
737 Park Avenue
New York, NY 10021
(212) 535-3993

LIVINGSTON TREATMENT

- Developed by Dr. V. Livingston during the 1940s
- Primary aim: restore the body's natural defenses by strengthening the immune system
- Vaccination: one vaccine prepared from a culture of the patient's own bacteria and Bacillus Calmete Guérin (BCG) vaccine. (Vaccines were needed because she thought that cancer is caused by a pleomorphic organism, progenitor cryptocides. Progenitor cryptocides are present in all of us at birth and normally remain dormant. When the immune system is weakened, the microbe causes cancer.)
- Largely vegetarian raw food high in abscesic acid (carrots, mango, avocados, tomatoes, lima beans, and green leafy vegetables)
- No coffee, alcohol, refined sugar, flour, and all processed foods
- As recovery occurs, fish is allowed

The University of Pennsylvania Oncology link suggests that there is no evidence of progenitor cryptocides and the organism that Dr. Livingston identified as staphylococcus epidermides. They further suggest that there is no evidence to support the treatment.

RESOURCES

Livingston Foundation Medical Center
3232 Duke Street
San Diego, CA 92110
(619) 224-3515

WHEAT GRASS THERAPY

- Developed by Dr. A. Wigmore
- Wheat grass, grown from wheat berries, is rich in chlorophyll, a substance nearly identical to hemoglobin
- Wheat grass has 60 times more vitamin C than citrus fruit
- Wheat grass contains more than 100 vitamins, minerals, and nutrients, all eight essential amino acids, and many bioflavonoids
- Wheat grass contains anticancer substances—abscises acid and laetrile
- Attempts to rebuild the body, detoxifies, and enhances the function of the immune system
- Wheat therapy preceeded by a 3-day juice cleansing fast along with enemas. The juice is wheat grass juice, green drinks, vegetables, and naturally sweetened lemon water and Rejuvelac (a fermented wheat berry drink). The enemas are with water and wheat grass.
- Raw foods, nothing cooked
- No supplements are necessary
- Research exists that verifies remissions and cures. The promoters of the diet say the diet cures nothing, but allows the body to cure itself.

RESOURCES

Ann Wigmore Foundation
196 Commonwealth Avenue
Boston, MA 02116
(617) 267-9424

Ann Wigmore Research and Educational Institute
P.O. Box 429
Rincon, Puerto Rico 00677
(809) 868-6307

Hippocrites Health Institute
1443 Palmdale Court
West Palm Beach, FL 33411
(407) 471-8876

New Hippocrites Health Institute
One Shipyard Way
Medford Square, MA 02155
(617) 395-1608

Health Institute of San Diego
6970 Central Avenue
Lemon Grove, CA 91945
(619) 464-3346

Creative Health Institute
918 Union City Road
Union City, MI 49094
(517) 278-6260

Obesity

Obesity is an excess of body fat, 20% higher than normal body weight. The U.S. population is becoming more obese each year with more than 60% of adults today being overweight. New books are constantly appearing on the best seller list on "new" ways to lose weight. And, although many of these diets may cause weight loss, the weight loss usually is not sustained. The basic, and probably oversimplified, principles of weight loss are:

- Eat fewer calories/day than you require
- Drink 5 to 8 (8 oz) glasses of water/day
- Exercise 4 to 6 times/week for at least 30 to 60 minutes
- Change your eating habits
- Do not chew gum (activates digestive juices, which provokes hunger)

Arthritis

Arthritis, the inflammation of the joints, is suffered by more than 50 million people in the United States. Diet modification has been demonstrated to reduce the symptoms in some people. Dietary modifications include:

- Eat more sulfur-containing foods, such as asparagus, eggs, garlic, and onions. Sulfur is needed for the repair and rebuilding of bone, cartilage, and connective tissue, and helps the body absorb calcium. Other good foods include green leafy vegetables (which supply vitamin K), fresh vegetables, nonacidic fresh fruits, whole grains, oatmeal, brown rice, and fish.

- Eat fresh pineapple frequently. Bromelain, an enzyme found in pineapple, is excellent for reducing inflammation. (To be effective, the pineapple must be fresh because freezing and canning destroy enzymes.)
- Eat some form of fiber, such as ground flaxseeds, oat bran, or rice bran daily.
- Avoid the nightshade vegetables (peppers, eggplant, tomatoes, white potatoes). These foods contain solanine, to which some people, particularly those suffering from arthritis, are highly sensitive. Solanine interferes with enzymes in the muscles and may cause pain and discomfort.
- Do not take iron supplements or a multivitamin containing iron. (Iron is suspected of being involved in pain, swelling, and joint destruction. Consume iron in foods instead. Good sources include blackstrap molasses, broccoli, Brussels sprouts, cauliflower, fish, lima beans, and peas.)
- Check for possible food allergies. Many sufferers of neck and shoulder pain have found relief when they eliminate certain foods.
- Spend time outdoors for fresh air and sunshine. Exposure to the sun prompts the synthesis of vitamin D, which is needed for proper bone formation.
- Get regular moderate exercise.
- If you are overweight, lose the excess pounds. Being overweight can cause and aggravate arthritis.
- Eating deep-sea fish, which are rich in eicosapentaenoic acid (EPA) and docoshahexaenoic acid (DHA), was found to help relieve the symptoms of rheumatoid arthritis in an unpublished study conducted by Charles Dinarello, MD, of the Tufts University School of Medicine.
- Chlamydia, the organism responsible for many cases of urethritis, has been linked to a form of arthritis that affects young women. In nearly half of the women with unexplained arthritis tested in one study, chlamydia was found in the joints. Seventy-five percent had elevated levels of antibodies to chlamydia in their blood.
- Decrease acid ash foods, which increase pain (grains, red meat, peas, citrus)
- Increase alkaline ash foods (vegetables and fruit). Vegetarian diets may lessen symptoms of rheumatoid arthritis.
- Increase antioxidant nutrients such as vitamin E, C, and beta carotene. Vitamin E may reduce inflammation, vitamin C may slow the progression of osteoarthritis (particularly of the knee), and a beta carotene deficiency may be linked to the development of rheumatoid arthritis. Until more research is performed, it is best to increase antioxidant foods rather than taking antioxidant supplements.

Osteoporosis

Osteoporosis is a progressive disease in which the bones gradually become weaker causing changes in posture and making the individual more prone to fractures. Osteoporosis is found in women more than men. The death rate from osteoporosis and its complications is greater than from breast cancer. Dietary and life style habits are important in preventing and managing osteoporosis.

- Eat plenty of foods rich in calcium (dairy products, soy products such as tofu, oily sea fish, parsley, alfalfa, and green vegetables such as kale), 1000 to 2000 mg/day.
- If calcium supplements are taken, use calcium citrate/calcium colanate because they are more absorbable, and stay away from calcium from oyster shells or dolomite because they contain higher levels of toxic substances such as lead or mercury. Do not take calcium products within 2 hours of coffee, tea, soft drinks, spinach, broccoli, bran,
  protein foods, and alcohol because they bind to calcium, decreasing its absorbability. Calcium is best absorbed with meals (see earlier exclusions). Many health practitioners suggest taking Ca^{++} at bedtime to avoid drug and food interactions.
- Eat less meat and include more completely vegetarian meals (meat leaches calcium from bones).
- Limit caffeine in all forms, including coffee, tea, soft drinks (caffeine leaches calcium from bones).
- Limit sugar (decreases calcium absorption).
- Exercise 4 to 6 times/week with weight-bearing exercises
- Increase phosphate, boron, and magnesium in the diet (all needed for inner and outer bone strength).
- Postmenopausal women may want to consider hormone replacement therapy until approximately age 75 (bone loss slows at approximately that age).
- Avoid yeast products (yeast leaches calcium from bones).
- Avoid, if at all possible, thyroid drugs, steroids, diuretics, and dilantin (they leach calcium from the bones).

ORTHOMOLECULAR THERAPY

What Is Orthomolecular Therapy?

The term orthomolecular therapy was coined in 1968 by the Nobel Prize winner, Linus Pauling, PhD, to describe an approach to treating disease with naturally occurring substances found in the body. "Orthos" means correct. Pauling continued his research and in 1970, published numerous papers on the use of mega doses of vitamin C to prevent or minimize symptoms of the common cold and flu, and to cause tumor regression. His studies are still being refused today.

R. J. Williams, PhD, in the 1970s and 1980s, began to realize that each individual is unique nutritionally. The government has developed our recommended daily allowances (RDA), for nutrients that prevent severe deficiency states. Orthomolecular medicine says that these levels do not provide for optimal health, and people may need many times more than the RDA levels.

In 1987, R. Kunin, MD, of San Francisco, CA, summarized the principles of orthomolecular therapy.

- Nutrition comes first in medical diagnosis and treatment, and nutrient-related disorders are usually curable once nutritional balance is achieved.
- Biochemical individuality is the norm in medical practice; therefore, universal RDA values are unreliable nutrient guides. Many people require an intake of certain nutrients beyond the RDA suggested range (often called a megadose) because of their genetic disposition or the environment in which they live.
- Drug treatment is used only for specific indications and is always mindful of the potential dangers and adverse effects.
- Environmental pollution and food adulteration are a fact of modern life and are a medical priority.
- Blood tests do not necessarily reflect tissue levels of nutrients.
- Hope is the indispensable ally of the physician and the absolute right of the patient. Basically, orthomolecular therapy attempts to create a healthier diet by eating nutritious, whole food, high in fiber and low in fat, and by eliminating junk foods, refined sugars, and food additives. In addition, additives of vitamins and minerals are included daily or several times daily. This therapy is referred to as "Megadose Therapy" because the dosages of vitamins and minerals are far above the RDA's.

One of the major criticisms of orthomolecular medicine is that megadosing can cause toxicity. Orthomolecular medicine physicians closely monitor patient's progress with blood and urine tests and monitor nutrient levels so toxicity does not occur. Persons participating in megadose therapy without a doctor's supervision can get into trouble. For example, daily vitamin C intake can be determined by bowel tolerance. Every several days, increase the vitamin C dosage by 500 to 1000 mg until diarrhea occurs, then drop back 1000 mg. That dose will then be the ideal megadose for optimal health.

What Is the History of Orthomolecular Therapy?

The basis of orthomolecular therapy dates to the 1920s when vitamins and minerals were first used to treat diseases that were unrelated to nutritional deficiencies. Several concepts were discovered:

- Vitamin A could prevent childhood deaths from infectious illness
- Magnesium could stop cardiac arrhythmias

In 1950, additional discoveries were made:

- Vitamin B_3 (niacin) in high doses, along with traditional psychotropic drugs of the day, doubled the number of recoveries from schizophrenics (this therapy was later rejected by the American Psychiatric Association).
- Malnutrition and improper nutrition places a person at risk for the development of disease and psychiatric disorders.
- Health can be impaired as a result of the consumption of refined, empty calorie foods (white bread, pastries, sugar).
- Mental illness may be related to decreases in fiber, minerals, and complex carbohydrates.

What Research, Reviews, and Comments Exist?

PRO

Research has verified that many conditions are improved by administering larger than usual doses of vitamins and minerals. Megadosing of niacin has become an accepted therapy to reduce cholesterol levels. Vitamin E, up to 2000 IU/day is used to control hot flashes associated with menopause to reduce the incidence of a second MI, and to improve memory and decrease the decline in patients with Alzheimers. In the 1980s, intravenous magnesium became an accepted treatment for arrhythmia control after an MI. Magnesium has also been accepted therapy in preventing and controlling symptoms of pregnancy-induced hypertention.

Research in orthomolecular medicine needs to be continued as a way of contributing to the overall health of the person, and in prevention of chronic disease. Possibly, we need optimal daily requirements instead of minimal RDAs.

CON

Not found in a literature search.

What Is Orthomolecular Therapy Used to Treat or Improve?

Research is ongoing, but some conditions may be improved or prevented by megadosing. See Table 4-1.

What Happens During Orthomolecular Therapy?

Orthomolecular therapy physicians will obtain a health history, appropriate diagnostic tests, and proceed to develop a plan of supplements appropriate for the individual. Progress is monitored and adjustments are made as needed.

TABLE 4-1

Cancer prevention	Beta carotene (precursor to vitamin A) Selenium Vitamin C
Pregnant mothers to prevent neural tube defects	Folic acid
Birth control use	Folic acid
Myocardial infarction and arrhythmias	Magnesium (IV)
Hypercholesterol	Niacin
Diabetes to enhance insulin utilization	Chromium
Heart disease, Psoriasis	Omega 3 oils
Rheumatoid arthritis	Omega 6 oils
Effects of aging	Beta carotene, vitamin E, selenium, vitamin C
Depression or anxiety	Amino acids or GABA supplements
Asthma	Magnesium
Alzheimer's	Vitamin E
Hot flashes	Beta carotene, vitamin E

Are There Any Risks Involved With Orthomolecular Therapy?

When properly monitored by a physician, no risk exists; but when attempted by an individual, risk of organ toxicity exists.

What Training Is Required of the Practitioner?

Orthomolecular Therapy physicians are traditionally educated physicians with additional training in nutrition.

Further Reading

Hoffer, A. & Walker, M. (1978). Orthomolecular nutrition, revised edition. New Canaan, CT: Keats Publishing, Inc.

Huemer, R. (1986). The roots of molecular medicine: a tribute to Linus Pauling. New York: W.H. Freeman and Co.

Lieberman, S. & Bruning, N. (1990). The real vitamin and mineral book. Garden City Park, NY: Avery Publishing Group, Inc.

Werbach, M. (1992). Nutritional influences on illness. 2nd ed. Tarzana, CA: Third Line Press.

Wright, J. (1990). Dr. Wright's guide to healing with nutrition. New Canaan, CT: Keats Publishing, Inc.

RESOURCES

International Academy of Nutrition & Preventive Medicine
P.O. Box 18433
Asheville, NC 28814
(704) 258-3243

INTERNET

Council for Responsible Nutrition
www.crnusa.org

American Society for Clinical Nutrition
www.faseb.org/ascn

Food Zone
http://birdsong.cudenver.edu

Tufts University - Nutrition Navigator
http://navigator.tufts.edu

People crave laughter as if it were an essential amino acid.
— PATCH ADAMS, MD

TABLE 4-2 DRUGS THAT DEPLETE NUTRIENTS

Products	Depleted Nutrients
Acetaminophen	C
Alcohol	Mg, B complex, C, D, E, K^+, Zinc
Allopurinol	Iron
Accupril	Ca^{++}, Phosphate, A, B, D
Antacids	A, B_1, Folic acid, Ca^{++}, Copper, Iron, Phosphorous
Antibiotics	B, K^+
Antihistamines	C
Aspirin	Ca^{++}, Folic acid, K^+, A, B, C, Iron, Zinc
Barbiturates	C
Caffeine	K^+, B, Zinc, Biotin
Chlorothiazines	Mg, K^+
Clonidine (Aldomet)	Ca^{++}, Vitamin E
Corticosteroid	Ca^{++}, A, B_6, C, D, Zinc, K^+
Digoxin	Thiamine, B_1, B_6, Zinc, Ca^{++}, Mg^{++}
Dilantin	Ca^{++}, Mg^{++}, D, Vitamin K, B_6, B_{12}, Folic acid
Diuretics	Ca^{++}, Iodine, Mg^{++}, K+, B_2, C, Zinc
Estrogen	Folic acid, B_6
Ismelin (Methyldopa)	B_{12}, Folic acid
Indocin	Vitamin C, Iron
INH	Iron
H_2 inhibitors	B_{12}
Laxatives	B_6, Niacin
Nadolol	Choline, Chromium, B_5
Nitrates	Niacin, Selenium, Vitamin E, B_{15}
Birth control pills	B complex, C, Zinc, Ca^{++}, Mg^{++}
Penicillin	B_2, Niacin, B_6, C, D, Ca^{++}, Iron, Mg^{++}, K^+, Zinc
Phenobarb	Folic acid, B_{12}, D, B_6, Vitamin K, Ca^{++}, Mg^{++}
Prednisone	K^+, B_6, C, Zinc
Premarin	B_2, B_6, B_{12}, Folic acid, Mg^{++}, Zinc
Propanolol	Chromium, B_5, choline
Reserpine	K+, B_2, B_6
Sulfa	PABA
Thiazides	Mg^{++}, K^+, B_2, Zinc

NUTRACEUTICALS

Nutraceuticals, functional foods, pharmafoods, or designer foods are the new "healthy foods." These foods include antioxidant (fortified juices, botanical teas), herb (spray snacks), and vitamin-fortified candy. Old foods (orange juice, cranberry juice, fast food snacks, teas) now have added nutrients and phytochemicals (see Phytochemical section). These products are more like medicine or supplements masquerading as food.

Not all products provide the benefits they promise. How about Ginkgo Biloba Rings, Kava Kava Corn Chips, Echinacea Shells? Herbs hold promise, but what part of the herb are we really getting and what happens to it after it has been processed with the food?

Before you buy these products, keep the following in mind:

- Maintain a healthy degree of skepticism. Call the manufacturer if you have a specific question about a product's claim or check with a health professional.
- Check the price and nutrition label of a products before buying it. Ask yourself if there is a better, less expensive way to get the nutrients and health benefits from whole foods instead.
- Remember that nutraceuticals alone cannot guarantee good health. Health benefits are best realized when you eat a variety of whole foods, including fruits, vegetables, grains, and legumes.

ORGANIC VERSUS CONVENTIONAL FOODS

Agricultural chemicals came into widespread use in the 1920s. Since that time, there has been concern about the safety of food grown with pesticides. Organic produce is becoming widely available, so which should you buy—organic or conventional produce?

In a recent study, organic, or green, produce had 25% residual pesticides, but they were less toxic than conventional produce. Organic means grown without pesticides, not pesticide free. Pesticides may arrive on the produce from the air or water. Pesticides enhance soil quality, which should ultimately enhance the quality of the food.

Worthington (1998) evaluated 34 studies that compared organic with conventional management in relation to nutrient content. Although the studies were different in their techniques, a clear trend supporting the notion that organic produce is more nutritious emerges, but is inconclusive. An overall trend shows higher nutrient content in organic produce, possibly caused by lower water content in the organic crops. Consistently higher levels of vitamin C and lower levels of nitrates are found in organically grown food.

National standards are long overdue. The U.S. Department of Agriculture is in the process of developing standards, which include:

- Food must be grown on land to which no prohibited fertilizers or pesticides have been applied in the previous 3 years.
- Organic growers must use sustainable farming methods, including crop rotation, composting, and natural pest controls.
- Foods meeting the regulations (verified by USDA-approved

certifiers) may carry a USDA organic seal. States, such as California, that have additional requirements can display their own seal instead. Labeling noncertified products as organic will be a federal offense.

- Products that have detectable pesticide residues exceeding certain unavoidable levels cannot be sold as organic.
- Farm animals for organic dairy and meat products must be raised under conditions that enhance health and minimize stress. Growth hormones and the routine use of antibiotics are not allowed.
- Packaged foods labeled organic must contain at least 95% organic ingredients by weight. Products with 50% to 95% organic ingredients may state only that they "contain" organic ingredients. Products with less than 50% organic ingredients may include the word organic only in the ingredient listing.

FOOD ADDITIVES

Additives are placed in foods for several reasons, to:

- lengthen shelf life
- enhance color
- enhance texture
- enhance taste
- make product more marketable

Additives include sugars (natural or synthetic, such as aspartame, sucratose, and monosodium glutamate [MSG]) and other chemicals and colors. To decrease exposure to food additives, strive for freshly picked and prepared foods.

Aspartame

Aspartame, or NutraSweet, has soared in popularity because of America's obsession with dieting. Aspartame is found in diet foods, but also in many other processed foods. Aspartame consists of three components: the amino acid, phenylalanine, aspartic acid, and methanol or wood alcohol. Persons have reported headaches, bloating, gas, mood swings, changes in vision, nausea, diarrhea, sleep disorders, confusion, and asthma after ingestion. The cumulative effects of high doses of aspartame are unknown. Aspartame has been found to be reasonably safe in all persons with the exception of persons with phenylketonuria (PKU), a rare genetic condition in which the body cannot properly metabolize the amino acid phenylalanine (a component of aspartame). Aspartame has not been allowed as a sweetener in Europe for more than 10 years.

Saccharin

Although saccharin has been used since the 1970s in more than 100 countries, safety issues have not been resolved. Studies have demonstrated that saccharin can cause bladder cancer in rats. In 1997, a panel of experts narrowly voted to recommend saccharin remain on the government's list of "likely" carcinogens.

Acesulfame K

Acesulfame K (Sunett) was first approved in 1988, but was only recently approved for use in soft drinks. Research has not demonstrated that acesulfame K poses any cancer risk. Acesulfame K is even sweeter when used in combination with aspartame.

Sucralose

Sucralose (Splenda) is a water-soluble, noncaloric powder with 320 to 1000 times the sweetness of table sugar. Plasma half-life is 2 to 5 hours and unabsorbed sucralose and metabolites are excreted in urine. It tastes like sugar and has no after taste. It is not destroyed at usual temperatures and pH reached during cooking and baking. Its long-term safety is unknown.

Monosodium Glutamate

Monosodium glutamate (MSG) is used without warning as a flavor enhancer. MSG is a concentrated form of sodium usually extracted from grains or beets. MSG can be disguised by many different names:

hydrolyzed plant protein	hydrolyzed food protein
hydrolyzed food starch	natural flavors
monosodium glutamate	vegetable protein

Many packaged, frozen, processed, dried, or canned foods may contain MSG, but those foods that most consistently contain MSG include:

Bouillons	Consommés	Dips
Fish and shellfish (canned, jarred)	Meats (canned)	Hot dogs
Luncheon meats	Salad dressings	Miso (soybean paste)
Poultry (canned)	Soups	Sauces
Soybeans (roasted or boiled)	Teriyaki sauce	Stocks
	Soy sauce	Stews
	Tempeh	

In addition to those above, look out for following restaurant foods that most consistently contain MSG:

Cheese sauces	Sauces (on meats and poultry, in particular)	Hot dogs
Luncheon meats	Stews	Asian dishes
Soups		

In children, MSG has been associated with asthma, hyperactivity and learning disabilities. When an attempt is made to eliminate MSG from the diet, it takes approximately 10 to 14 days to clear the body. The only way you are completely safe from MSG is to have the label say MSG free.

Olestra

Olean or Olestra (the trade name) is a fat substitute made from sugar and soybean oil, approved in 1996 for use in snack foods. It has the taste and texture of fat, but the molecules are too large for the body to digest, so olestra passes through the digestive system unabsorbed. Sounds like a "snacker's" dream come true, but when eaten in large quantities (maybe a half bag of chips or more) a laxative effect may occur. Olestra also inhibits the absorption of carotenoids (antioxidants) and fat-soluble vitamins (A, D, E, and K). Olestra in foods encourages people to snack on low-quality foods that are highly processed in favor of other more nutritious foods such as fresh fruits and vegetables.

PLASTIC AND FOOD SAFETY

Are plastics safe in the microwave? Some plastic containers such as margarine tubs and some plastic wraps may soften and melt. This is not caused by the microwaves, but by the heat of the food. Any contact between hot food and plastic can be a problem. And the hotter the food, the bigger the problem. Fatty foods such as ground beef, gravies, or cheese, and sugary foods such as peach cobbler or a jelly doughnut get particularly hot in the microwave.

Plastic particles melting into food is a concern because some byproducts of plastics are thought to be *endocrine disrupters* (hormone disrupters, or pseudohormones)—substances that mimic and may interfere with the body's natural hormones. Plasticizers (compounds that add flexibility to plastic food wraps) are particularly suspect.

In a recent Consumers Union test, plasticizers were found in only two of seven national and store brands of plastic wraps analyzed. But the two—*Saran Wrap* and *Reynolds Plastic Wrap*—are well-known, big-selling brands. Hamburgers wrapped in either of these wraps, then reheated in a microwave, showed evidence that the plastic compounds had migrated into the burgers wherever the wrap made contact with them.

It is difficult to say if ingesting trace amounts of plasticizers is harmful. The theory that the chemicals in plastic may be harmful is suggested by animal research but has not yet been convincingly demonstrated in humans. Experts take both sides.

Because there are more questions than answers surrounding this issue, it pays to be cautious and choose materials least likely to react should they come in contact with hot foods—especially since that is not difficult to do. Here are *Environmental Nutrition's* guidelines on what to use:

Green Light (does not react with hot food)

- Glass, including tempered glass, such as Pyrex
- Ceramic glass, such as Corningware

Yellow Light (some scientists express concern)

- Rigid plastic labeled for microwave use, such as Rubbermaid's Intellivent, Tupperware's CrystalWave, TupperWave, and Rock 'N Serve
- Plastic wraps made from polyethylene, such as Glad Cling Wrap Crystal Clear Polythylene

Red Light (most scientists recommend avoiding)

- Food containers such as margarine tubs and take-out containers
- Plastic containers not labeled microwave-safe
- Shrink wraps and cling-type plastic wraps that contain plasticizers, such as Reynolds Plastic Wrap and Saran Wrap

(From: Environmental Nutrition: 7, 1998.)

PESTICIDES

Did you ever read the label on a pesticide? Most say something like this:

"Extreme caution, Do not inhale. Use in well-ventilated areas. Do not allow any contact with skin or hair. Do not dispose of near water. Keep away from livestock and feed. May cause blindness or death if taken internally. Read all instructions carefully. Federal law requires application in accordance with label data."

And now, we will apply this to our growing food. Crop loss from insect damage has doubled since World War II. Insecticide use is up more than 10 times in that same period. DDT, a primary insecticide for all plants used to kill mosquitoes, became ineffective in the 1950s to 1960s. The

TABLE 4-3 THE "DIRTY DOZEN"

Strawberries (1 cup)	Cherries, U.S. (1 cup)
Apples (1)	Cantaloupe, Mexican ($^1/_4$)
Apricots (4)	Grapes, Chilean ($1^1/_2$ cup)
Blackberries (1 cup)	Pears (1)
Raspberries (1 cup)	Nectarines (1)
Spinach ($^1/_2$ cup)	Peaches (1)

National Cancer Institute confirmed in 1988 what environmentalists have been saying for years. After years of testing, the main ingredient in DDT is a cause of cancer in humans.

Research has shown a connection between pesticide exposure and spontaneous abortion, testicular cancer, and low sperm counts. Recently, researchers at Mount Sinai School of Medicine at New York University found that women who had high levels of DDE, a breakdown product of DDT, had breast cancer. The women with low levels of DDE did not have breast cancer.

Pesticides have estrogenic effects and are stored throughout the body in concentrations proportional to the lipid content of tissues. Therefore, the fatter the individual, the more storage there can be. The breast has a high concentration of fat.

Pesticides are only regulated in the United States. Foods entering the United States from other countries may contain unregulated, illegal, or dangerous pesticides. Limit or avoid these foods if possible.

Researchers at the Environmental Working Group periodically review fruits and vegetables for the pesticide load. Table 4-3 lists the Dirty Dozen from 1996. Whenever possible, use organic varieties of the fruits and vegetables.

To limit your exposure, buy certified organic produce. Organically grown products contain more natural vitamins and minerals. Pesticides are also found in meat and meat products. Removal of fat (pesticides concentrate in fat) reduces your exposure.

Follow these suggestions to reduce your exposure to pesticides:

1. Wash all produce. Add a drop or two of soap to the water to help remove pesticides and rinse thoroughly, or soak produce for 5 to 10 minutes in one to two drops of Clorox bleach, then resoak in water for 10 minutes to rinse.
2. Use a vegetable scrub brush for potatoes, sweet potatoes, carrots, and other hard-surface produce whose skin you plan to eat.
3. Chop spinach, cauliflower, broccoli, and other produce with irregular surfaces before you wash it.

4. Peel nonorganic produce that has been treated with a wax coating, including cucumbers, apples, eggplant, carrots.
5. Discard the outer leaves of iceberg and other lettuce and cabbage. Trim the leaves and top from celery.
6. Purchase organically grown produce (labeled "Certified Organic") or produce grown locally with no pesticides. (Somer, 1995)

Alternatives to pesticides are natural farming methods that quickly remineralize the soil and regenerate microbial life.

1. Seaweed fertilizers and seaweed folier sprays
2. Finely ground rock, called "rock dust"
3. Colloid soft rock phosphate
4. Composted organic matter

SPECIAL DIETS

There are many types of diets, some being made famous by several famous authors: A *Program for Reversing Heart Disease* by Dean Ornish, *The Zone* by Barry Sears, *The Naturopathic Diet* by Michael Murrary, or *The Atkins Diet* by Robert Atkins. All of these diets have their pros and cons. They vary in the philosophy and the intake of carbohydrates (CHO), protein, and fat. All have developed scientific rationales (however, the research is often missing from the book) for their diet. See Table 4-4 for a review of these diets.

Fresh Juice Diets

Fruits and vegetables are an excellent source of a wide range of vitamins, minerals, and nutrients. Proponents of juicing suggest that two glasses of fresh juice are required a day to maintain health, and four glasses a day to speed healing and recovery from illness.

To release the minerals, chemicals, vitamins, enzymes, and hormones from the tiny microscopic cells of the fiber of fruits and vegetables, proper juicers must be used. Hand juicers only partly crush the fibers and because they cannot pulverize, extraction of all the vital elements is impossible. Pulverization is the fundamental principle in reclaiming all of the vital elements. Most commercial juices are heat treated to lengthen shelf-life so many of the important parts of the fruits and vegetables may be lost or damaged. In addition, preservatives or chemicals may be added. Thus, it is best to prepare juices fresh from locally grown organic produce. The fresher the produce, the greater the nutrient value. Three types of juices are most common: vegetable, green, and fruit juices.

VEGETABLE JUICES

Fresh vegetable juice:

- restores and builds tissues
- enhances immune system function
- helps remove toxic acid wastes
- balances metabolism
- reduces caloric intake, thus may enhance weight loss

Garlic is a great addition to any vegetable juice. Before juicing, drop the garlic into vinegar for 1 minute to destroy any bacteria on its surface. To reduce GI discomfort, use a maximum of 1 clove/2 glasses of juice. For the greatest health benefit, combine multiple vegetables.

Carrot juice is probably the most popular, and is packed with beta carotene. Because carrot juice is sweet, it is often mixed with other juices. Strong-flavored vegetables (broccoli, onions, rutabaga, turnips, celery) should be used only in small amounts.

GREEN JUICES

Green juices cleanse the body of pollutants and have a rejuvenating effect. Green juices are rich in chlorophyll, which helps purify the blood, build red blood cells, detoxify the body, and provide energy. Green juices are made from: alfalfa sprouts, cabbage, kale, spinach, wheat grass, and other greens. Wheat grass is particularly beneficial during chemotherapy and radiation to heal and protect the GI system. Barley grass or spiralina may be added to increase nutritional value, and carrot or apple juice may be used to sweeten green juice; 8 to 10 oz/day is recommended.

FRUIT JUICES

Fruit juices help cleanse and nourish the body, particularly with antioxidants. One of the most healthy juices is watermelon (see Phytochemicals for more information). The whole watermelon, rind intact, is used. Other great fruits for juicing include kiwi, melons, bananas, berries, apples, and apricots; 10 to 12 oz/day is recommended.

JUICE SUGGESTIONS AND PRECAUTIONS

- Use only organic fruits and vegetables, but wash thoroughly using a vegetable brush.
- Avoid potatoes with green tint (the green color is solanine, which can result in diarrhea, vomiting, and abdominal pain).
- Kiwi and other tropical fruit skins should not be used. They may contain residues of harmful sprays not used in the United States.

TABLE 4-4 POPULAR DIETS

Diet		Cons	Pros
Low-fat vegetarian Resources: The McDougall Plan (New Win Publishing) by John A. McDougall, MD, and Mary A. McDougall; Dr. Dean Ornish's Program for Reversing Heart Disease (Ballantine) by Dean Ornish, MD	Fat 5–10% Carbohydrates 75–85% Protein 10–15%	Not healthy for people who are carbohydrate/sensitive or allergic to grains. Inappropriate as a maintenance diet for some people because it doesn't contain nuts, so is very low in protein and fat. Low in several micronutrients essential for health such as essential fatty acids, zinc, and vitamin B_{12}.	Teaches creative ways to cook plant foods; emphasizes fresh foods. Can be a short-term therapeutic diet for reversing heart disease for people who have overindulged in fatty meats and refined fats. A good cleansing diet that restores proper elimination because it's rich in fiber.
Naturopathic diet Resources: Encyclopedia of Natural Medicine (Prima) by Michael Murray, ND and Joseph Pizzorno, ND; Heart Disease and High Blood Pressure (Prima) by Michael Murray, ND	Fat 15–25% Carbohydrates 60–75% Protein 10–20%	Emphasizes 6 to 13 servings of grains and starches a day, which isn't appropriate for people who are carbohydrate or grain sensitive. Includes fruit juices that wreak havoc with blood sugar balance. Too low in protein and zinc for immunocompromised individuals and athletes who have high requirements for these nutrients.	Stresses the importance of eating high-quality, organic foods and replacing refined foods with nutrient- and fiber-rich whole food carbohydrates. Emphasizes healthy sources of fat to prevent essential fat deficiencies and encourage better function of hormone-like prostaglandins. Contains a nutrient balance more appropriate for many people than vegetarian and macrobiotic diets.

Zone diet Resources: The Zone (HarperCollins) by Barry Sears, PhD, with Bill Lowren; Mastering the Zone (Harper Collins) by Barry Sears, PhD	Fat 30% Carbohydrates 40% Protein 30%	Difficult to consistently follow for each meal and snack. Contains common food allergens such as dairy products, eggs, and soy products. Sometimes includes processed meats, refined grain products, and foods with unhealthy additives.	Teaches the importance of emphasizing lower-carbohydrate fruits and vegetables over grains, which many people don't tolerate well. Serves as a bridge between the high carbohydrate diets and the low carbohydrate diets. A good maintenance diet because it contains a variety of essential vitamins and minerals, with a macronutrient balance to stabilize blood sugar.
Higher protein, Higher fat diet Resources: Protein Power (Bantam) by Michael R. Eades, MD, and Mary Dan Eades, MD; Dr. Atkins' New Diet Revolution (Avon) by Robert C. Atkins., MD	Fat 30–50% Carbohydrates 15–35% Protein 30–45%	Unhealthy for people who have trouble digesting protein and fat or for those with kidney disorders. Too low in fiber for proper elimination in some people. Overemphasizes common food allergens such as eggs and dairy products, and uses some processed meats and condiments that contain unhealthy additives.	Helpful for preventing cravings and binge-eating for people who have overindulged in sugar and refined carbohydrates. Therapeutic for people who have carbohydrate sensitivity, grain allergies, or insulin-related health problems. Contains better-quality fats and carbohydrates than the typical American diet.

Modified from Smith M. How Popular Diets Stock Up. Delicious, Jan., 1998.

- The skin of citrus fruit is bitter and may contain toxic spray residues. It is best to discard these, but keep the white matter that is below the skin. It contains a large amount of antioxidants.
- When using soft fruits that contain little water, add water or add these to other juices.
- Always remove carrot and rhubarb greens and the seeds of apples because they contain toxic substances.
- Very sweet juices (pear, grape, apple) may cause bloating gas, so it is best to dilute these with pure water and drink on an empty stomach.
- To prevent GI discomfort, consume green juice gradually and in moderation.
- Juices are contraindicated in persons with diabetes and persons with food allergies.
- Juicing is not an alternative to eating whole foods for more than 2 to 3 days.
- Juices are not recommended for long-term use in elderly, infants, and children unless under medical supervision.

Fasting

Fasting has been used for thousands of years as a pathway to spiritual enlightenment and holiness. The devout have used it to heighten their awareness, the ancient pagans to appease their Gods, the Greeks to bring hallucinatory dreams, and the religious to add a depth of meaning to their holy days.

Believers of fasting suggest that this is the only way to rid the body of toxins. While drinking water only, the body is eliminating toxins and no new toxins are being introduced with food. Therefore, the net result of 5 days or more of fasting is a healthier, toxin-free body. Proponents of fasting suggest that it extends life, health, and youthfulness and it promotes mental and spiritual well being. Proponents of fasting suggest that fasting can improve:

asthma	arthritis	multiple sclerosis
hypertension	heart disease	inflammatory bowel disease
ulcers	migraines	hay fever
tumors	nephritis	

and many other chronic diseases.

Some research has been performed that shows a decrease in symptoms after a fast. Although we understand that many diseases may be diet related, there are probably many more that we are unaware of. Pros and cons to fasting are:

Pro	Con
Weight loss	Dehydration, possible
Speeds resolution of minor diseases	May be harmful because of nutrient deprivation
Rests digestive system and eliminates some toxins	Lowers blood sugar, increases muscle breakdown and NH_3 production

THE PROCEDURE

The day leading to a fast is preceded by a day of fresh vegetables seasoned with virgin olive oil and organic vegetable juices and fresh squeezed fruit juices. During the fast, the person may drink only water or a combination of fresh fruit and vegetable juices. When the fast is to be broken, after 2 to 3 days, the first day includes fresh vegetables with vegetable juice and fruit juices. Whole foods are added slowly. Small meals are suggested to give the GI tract time to readjust to food. Highly refined and spicy foods are added after several days. A reduction in physical activity is recommended during and for a short time after the fast.

ADVERSE EFFECTS

During the fast the person may experience bad breath, a bad taste in the mouth, coated tongue, and exhaustion. Promoters of fasting say that these symptoms are the toxins being released from the body. These may all be symptoms of ketosis from lack of proper nutrition. Dehydration is always a concern. The individual will need to drink at least 1 to 2 quarts of liquid/day.

CONTRAINDICATIONS

Pregnant and lactating women

Children

Macrobiotic Diet

The macrobiotic or Zen diet was developed in Japan to enhance spiritual and physical well being ("macro" meaning great, "bios" meaning life; therefore, great view of life). It consists primarily of whole grains with brown rice as being the perfect food. The central concept of this diet is "balance = spiritual health." The balance is not only the selection of the food, but its preparation and combination of color, texture, and flavors.

TABLE 4-5 MACROBIOTICS: FOOD CLASSIFICATION

Yang	Yin	Equal Yang and Yin
meat	alcohol	beans
poultry	tea	grains
fish	coffee	nuts
seafood	sugar	fruit
eggs	milk	vegetables
hard cheese	cream	
salt	yogurt	
	herbs	

TABLE 4-6 STAGES 1 AND 10 OF THE MACROBIOTIC DIET

	Cereal	Fruit/ Salads	Vegetables	Soup	Desserts	Animal foods
Stage 1	10%	15%	30% (2/3 cooked) (1/3 raw)	10%	5%	30% (no meat)
Stage 10	60%	none	30%	10%	none	none

Foods are categorized as yin, yang, and equal yin and yang (Table 4-5). The originator of the macrobiotic diet was G. Ohsawa (1893–1966), who reportedly recovered from a serious disease by changing to this simple diet of brown rice, steamed vegetables, and miso soup (soybean soup). The diet has 10 stages. From least stringent to severely limiting.

Before Stage 1, stop eating meat.

American style of the Macrobiotic Diet is less severe than the traditional Japanese diet. American Macrobiotic Diet includes seafood, beans and legumes, and nuts and seeds, which contain iron and protein. Rare cases of nutritional deficiencies exist with this diet.

PRO

The diet is low in fat.

CON

The diet is too low in calories, fat, and protein. It is also deficient in B_{12}, vitamin D, protein, and iron (anemia is common). Parsons, et al (1997) found that adolescents eating a macrobiotic diet had a reduced bone mineral content (BMC). A reduction in BMC in adolescents may hold important implications for fracture risk in later life. Diet is inappropriate for children and pregnant or nursing women. To be healthy, persons on a macrobiotic diet need supplements to ensure proper nutrition.

After a book published in the 1980s, *The Cancer Prevention Diet* by Kushi, the macrobiotic diet has become highly recommended by some for the treatment of cancer. Little research exists, but the diet is deficient in growth-promoting substances; therefore, if there is no way of treating the cancer, the diet may help.

OTHER HEALTH-ENHANCING SUBSTANCES

Chromium Picolinate (the mineral)

Chromium Glucose Tolerance Factor (the supplement)

Chromium picolinate is involved with the metabolism of glucose and the synthesis of cholesterol, fats, and protein. It helps maintain a stable blood sugar through proper insulin use. In general, the average American diet is deficient in chromium because of a lack of chromium in the soil and water supply and a diet high in refined carbohydrates. The RDA for chromium is 120 μg. This was established in 1996. However, evidence states that if you consume 50 μg (Table 4-7), you will not have a deficiency. Doses up to 200 μg are probably safe. When doses range from 300 to 400 μg, toxicity can develop (toxicity results in renal and liver disease).

TABLE 4-7 CHROMIUM CONTENT OF SELECTED FOODS

Food	Chromium Content (μg/serving)	Serving Size
Cereal, 100% fortified, dry	30.70	1¾ oz
Broccoli	22.00	1 cup
Mushroom, white	16.40	½ cup
Wheat cereal, dry	16.40	1¾ oz
Oatmeal, instant	12.90	1¾ oz
Oyster, raw	12.60	3 oz
Bran cereal, dry	12.60	1¾ oz
Turkey ham	10.40	3 oz
Wine, table	7.60	3½ oz
Grape juice	7.50	1 cup
Waffles	6.70	1 each
Oat cereal, dry	6.20	1¾ oz
English muffin	3.60	1 each
Brewer's yeast	3.30	1 tbsp

Recent research in diabetes has demonstrated a decreased glycosylate hemoglobin after 1 month of 200 μg of chromium/day. In addition, diabetic patients taking chromium have shown an 8 to 10 lb weight loss the first year, most likely as a result of the increased use of insulin.

Chromium has also been advertised to "melt the pounds off," "enhance weight loss," and "lower your percent of body fat." Unfortunately, no research is available to verify these statements. When chromium has been consumed in large doses (300 μg/day), the only loss has been liver or renal dysfunction. There was a small study in 1995 that suggested chromium could cause chromosomal damage, thus precipitating cancer, so more research is needed in this area.

Coenzyme Q10

Also known as ubiquinone and vitamin Q, Coenzyme Q10 (CoQ10) is a nutrient that is made by the body and found in a variety of foods. CoQ10 is fat soluble, so it needs a little oil or fat to be absorbed. CoQ10 acts as a shuttle to move electrons from one molecule to another inside the mitochrondria. Therefore, the mitochrondria can make more energy more efficiently.

Japanese researchers, in the 1970s, found that hearts of people with CHF who died had lower levels of CoQ10 than in those who lived. In the 1980s, after further research, CoQ10 administration became part of normal cardiology practice in Japan. CoQ10 should not replace standard therapy for CHF, but it is used in conjunction with current therapy. Additional studies have shown that the more severe the heart disease, the lower the level of CoQ10. Dr. Langsjoen, a cardiologist in Tyler, TX, after his research, thinks that CoQ10 reduces symptoms and improves longevity, and thus administers 20 mg two times a day to all his patients diagnosed with cardiomyopathy.

CoQ10 is also an antioxidant that some researchers feel protects vitamin E, which in turn protects LDL from oxidation. Research performed at the University of Maryland Medical Center in 1997 also found that CoQ10 hampered the ability of the blood to clot. Ironically, some drugs such as the HMG CoA drugs (including lovastatin) and beta blockers (including propranolol) interfere with the body's production of CoQ10.

It has also been suggested that CoQ10 has a role in cancer therapy; however, the information is conflicting. Some research indicates tumors (breast/prostate) recede; others show no change. CoQ10 may protect cells, particularly in the heart, from injury during chemotherapy. However, there is concern that this action may interfere with the chemotherapy effect, so caution is advised until more research is completed.

Colloidal Minerals

Colloidal minerals are a combination of 60 minerals combined with water and clay, which are supposed to be 98% absorbable. When water is mixed with clay, the minerals of the clay become dispersed in the water and a colloidal mineral is created. When the minerals are dispersed in the mixture, they are still solid in form; they are suspended, but not dissolved, in the liquid.

A leading expert, Dr. R. Wood, chief of the Mineral Bioavailability Lab at Tufts University says he has never seen any research that suggests colloidal minerals are an absorbable source of minerals. Dr. Wood suggests that it is "best to obtain your minerals from real food." The colloidal mineral preparations may also contain other potentially toxic metals, such as arsenic, cadmium, thallium silver, lead, and others, and costs $25 to $50/month.

DHEA

Dehydroepiandrosterone (DHEA) is an adrenal androgen being marketed as a "food supplement" that will:

- prevent aging
- be the fountain of youth
- enhance the immune system
- prevent heart disease
- enhance weight loss

DHEA is a precursor of androgens and estrogens. Plasma levels peak at age 20 and decline with age. There is no convincing evidence that DHEA has any beneficial effect on aging or any other disease. People are well advised not to take it.

SIDE EFFECTS

Side effects associated with DHEA use are:

- androgenic effects such as acne, hair loss, hirsutism, and deepening voice in women (may be irreversible)
- increased growth of prostate, breast, and ovarian cancers

Glucosamine Sulfate/Chondrotin

Glucosamine sulfate is a nutrient found in small amounts in food. Its primary role is to produce long chain sugars (GAGs) to rebuild cartilage.

TABLE 4-8 DOSAGE OF GLUCOSAMINE AND CHONDROITIN BY WEIGHT

Pounds	Glucosamine (mg)	Chrondroitin (mg)
<120		800
120–200	1,500	1,200
>200	2,000	1,600

The media is suggesting that glucosamine sulfate and another major cartilage builder *chondrotin* (made from cow, shark, or whale cartilage) can provide relief and perhaps even reverse the disease process of osteoarthritis. Chondrotin, also present in cartilage, is composed of chains of glucosamine sulfate molecules and may inhibit the enzymes that break down cartilage. Many double-blind, controlled studies were performed in Europe in the 1980s, and most showed impressive results with pain control and symptom relief occurring in several weeks.

It is important to take the proper dosages of glucosamine sulfate and chondrotin to obtain results. Research has demonstrated that dosage is based on body weight (see Table 4-8).

Divide the total dose into 3 to 4 doses/day and take with food. As improvement occurs, the dose should be reduced to the lowest effective dose. European studies suggest that people who are obese or on diuretics may need even higher doses.

The Arthritis Foundation points out that all the research has only evaluated short-term results and that longer, better-controlled clinical trials are necessary. Quality control of available over-the-counter products is a problem. It is also important to manage other contributing factors to arthritis, continue to exercise, make diet modifications (reduction of acid forming foods), and maintain a normal weight.

Melatonin

Melatonin is a hormone produced by the pineal gland during sleep. Melatonin production peaks in early childhood and decreases with age. Melatonin has been linked to:

- enhancing sleep
- stimulating the immune system
- acting as an antioxidant
- preventing cancer
- buffering the effects of stress
- lowering cholesterol levels

Little research is available that supports melatonin use for anything other than sleep problems. For melatonin to be produced, the pineal gland must perceive darkness. People who work swing shifts and must sleep during the day make less melatonin and therefore have difficulty obtaining restful sleep and multiple REM cycles.

Drugs that may deplete melatonin are included in Table 4-9. Foods high in melatonin are included in Table 4-10.

Cautions that are associated with the use of melatonin include:

- pregnancy and lactation
- when attempting to get pregnant
- severe mental illness
- autoimmune disease
- cancer of the immune system
- normal children

TABLE 4-9 DRUGS THAT MAY DEPLETE MELATONIN

- NSAID
- Beta blockers
- Ca^{++} channel blockers
- Antianxiety drugs such as diazepam (Valium) and alprazalan (Xanax)
- antidepressants
- B_{12} in large doses
- caffeine
- steroids
- alcohol and tobacco

TABLE 4-10 FOODS HIGH IN MELATONIN

Food	Melatonin (picograms/gram)
Oats	1,796
Sweet corn	1,366
Rice	1,006
Ginger	583
Tomatoes ("Sweet 100s")	500
Bananas	460
Barley	378
Connoisseurs of Japanese food can add these foods to their list:	
Japanese radish	657
Ashitaba	623
Chungiku	417

Side effects associated with melatonin include:

- vivid dreams

Dosing suggestions:

- For sleep only: up to 1 mg 1 hour before sleep (most sleep research has studied 0.1 to 0.3 mg)
- For jet lag, start a day before travel. Traveling west, take melatonin at waking, traveling east take it mid afternoon. When you arrive, continue on the same pill-taking schedule according to your home town clock.

There are long-term safety issues yet to be researched.

Pycnogenol

A French chemist isolated the first pycnogenol in 1947. The term pycnogenol was christened in 1979. Pycnogenol, derived from the bark of the maritime pine found in France or from grape seeds, is a mixture of antioxidant molecules or proanthocyanidolic oligomers (PCO). Research is conflicting about the best source of pycnogenol. The antioxidant effect of pycnogenol is 50 times greater than vitamin E. Pycnogenol strengthens weakened blood vessels, prevents further fluid loss out of the blood vessel, prevents macula degeneration, reduces bronchospasm in asthma, reduces joint pain in arthritis, reduces symptoms of attention deficit disorder (ADD) in children and adults, reduces inflammation in skin conditions such as psoriasis, and enhances immune function.

Pycnogenol binds to collagen and elastin in the vascular wall, preventing their degradation and encouraging their synthesis and maturation. Pycnogenol also appears to help control two crucial neurotransmitters (dopamine and norepinephrine) that are involved with the excitation response. Therefore, using pycnogenol in ADD seems appropriate. Pycnogenol also assists with moving nutrients to the brain (zinc, manganese, selenium, copper).

Recommended dose is 1 mg of PCO for every 1 lb of body weight, 50 to 100 mg/day of pycnogenol to maintain health, or 150 to 300 mg/day to treat disease. Adverse effects have not been reported.

O_2 FREE RADICALS

Highly reactive substances, O_2 free radicals, are produced in the body during the normal metabolic process. There are several known free radicals:

superoxide, hydroxy radicals, hydrogen peroxide, nitric oxide, and others. O_2 free radicals are also formed by exposure to radiation, toxic chemicals such as those in cigarette smoke, overexposure to the sun's rays, and the breakdown of stored fat molecules for energy. A diet that is high in fat can increase free radical activity because oxidation occurs more readily in fat molecules than in carbohydrate or protein molecules. Cooking fats at high temperatures, particularly frying in oil or grilling, can produce many free radicals. O_2 free radicals are also found in air pollution, radiation, herbicides, and rancid fatty foods. Free radicals are kept in check by the action of free radical scavengers that occur naturally in the body. However, our bodies generally are making more O_2 free radicals than our normal scavengers can eliminate.

Antioxidants, obtained from food sources, assist the body in protecting itself against O_2 free radicals. Several nutrients act as antioxidants: vitamin A, C, and E, beta-carotene, selenium, zinc, and the hormone melatonin. In addition, sprouted grains and fresh fruits and vegetables contain high levels of antioxidants. "Antioxidant scores" have recently been identified (Cao, et al, 1996; Wang, et al, 1996). These scores indicate the ability of each vegetable to neutralize disease-causing radicals. The top nine antioxidant vegetables include: kale, beets, red bell peppers, Brussels sprouts, spinach, potatoes, sweet potatoes, and corn. Remember, antioxidant value is not the only item that counts; there are also fiber and minerals. A high intake of antioxidant nutrients appears to be especially protective against cancer.

Free radicals attack body cells, producing more free radicals, and eventually cause cell damage and death. The free radicals cause damage to the cell walls, thus allowing naturally occurring products within the cell (proteases) to leak out where they cause damage. The damaged cell can no longer transport nutrients, O_2, and water into the cell or regulate the removal of waste products. In addition, free radicals can alter the way in which cells code genetic material. Changes in protein structure can occur as a result of errors in protein synthesis. The body's immune system may then see this altered protein as a foreign substance and try to destroy it. The formation of mutated proteins can eventually damage the immune system and lead to cancer and a host of other diseases. O_2 free radicals can cause the cell to die because its mutated genetic code cannot be duplicated. The power center of the cell, the mitochondria, is vulnerable to attack by free radicals. When damaged, the mitochondira shuts down energy production, ages, and dies.

An analogy may help you to think about O_2 free radical damage. Imagine a bright room lit with many candles. A gentle but persistent breeze begins, one by one, the breeze blows out the lights. As the room dims, it becomes harder and harder to see your way around. Finally, when the last candle is extinguished, you are in total darkness and cannot find your way out of the room—the equivalent of many years of unrestrained O_2 free radical damage. Antioxidants deactivate O_2 free radicals so they cannot attach to membranes or cellular components. Antioxidants block the breeze from blowing out the candles, if you will.

PHYTOCHEMICALS

During the last 10 years, and particularly the last 5 years, there has been a proliferation of research conducted on plants. Can plants have a protective value or even a curative effect on the body? It appears that the best prevention and treatment for cancer may be right in the kitchen. The advice from mother "eat your fruits and vegetables" may be life-saving advice. Chances are that mom did not really mean one vitamin from the white pile, one from the yellow pile, and one from the red pile. It is whole foods that pack the disease-prevention wallop. Until recently, scientists did not know most of these products existed; therefore, these kinds of products are not packed in pills, at least not yet. *Phytochemicals* are active components in fruits and vegetables. *Phytonutrition* is the role of these substances in cultural food practices that support or improve health.

Phytochemicals, are abundant in fruits, vegetables, grains, legumes, and seeds, and in many less common foods including licorice, soy, and green tea. Examples of phytochemicals include indoles (broccoli, cabbage, Brussel sprouts), isothiocyanates (broccoli, watercress, cauliflower), sulforaphane (vegetables such as broccoli), allylic sulfides (onions and garlic), isoflavonoids (soybeans), and carotenoids (kale). There are more than 600 carotenoids and 1,700 bioflavonoids that have been identified. There may be thousands of categories of phytochemicals discovered in the future.

Phytochemicals are inessential to sustain life but most likely are essential for optimal health and the prevention of chronic disease. Phytochemicals may be thought of as secondary metabolites or nonnutritional dietary components. Phytochemicals may be termed *functional* food. Food is defined as any substance taken into the body, enabling growth and maintenance needed to keep the animal alive. A functional food must perform a function above and beyond this. Therefore, that function is to cure, heal, or relieve disease. Phytochemicals are blocking or suppressing agents. Phytochemicals give plants their color and flavor. They also serve as part of a plant's defense system against disease, sunlight, and oxidation from air and pollutants. Best of all, once they are in our bodies, phytochemicals defend us.

Scientists know that phytochemicals increase resistance to disease and boost immunity. What scientists do not know is why phytochemicals seem to lose their disease-fighting powers when they are isolated from the "host" plant. It has become clear that "whole foods" contain the protective power; pills do not. Be wary of manufacturers that offer phytochemicals in a pill or powder format.

The National Cancer Institute (NCI) is so excited about these findings they have launched a multimillion dollar project to find, isolate, and study phytochemicals. Phytochemicals seem to have an ability to block the multiple processes that lead to cancer. There is increasing evidence that these natural products can take tumors, defuse them, and turn off the proliferative process of cancer. For example, cancer can begin when a carcinogenic molecule—from the food consumed or the air breathed—invades the cell. But, if sulforaphane, a phytochemical found in broccoli, also reaches the cell, it activates a group of enzymes that whisk the carcinogen out of the cell before it can cause any harm.

The NCI, with the American Dietetic Association (ADA), is hoping that detailed dietary guidelines designed to achieve specific disease-prevention goals can eventually be established. The idea is to have food tables for phytochemicals, just as we do for vitamins and minerals The ADA notes that the health benefits of phytochemicals are best obtained through the consumption of a varied diet using our normal food supply rather than through the use of supplements (Anonymous, 1995). Recent research indicates that the average American consumes two fruits and vegetables/day; far less than our food pyramid suggests with eight to nine fruits and vegetables/day.

Each member of a plant family contains similar but different phytochemicals. For example, grapefruit contains naringeinin, a major phytochemical. Naringeinin does not occur in major amounts in any other citrus fruit. Naringeinin slows the way the liver detoxifies chemicals and drugs. Recent research has identified that drinking two glasses of grapefruit juice a day while taking cyclosporine (a drug used in transplant patients to decrease episodes of rejection) reduces the rate at which cyclosporine is detoxified and improves its clinical benefits. The question becomes, when does phytonutrition cease and phytotherapy begin?

Several groups of phytochemicals are reviewed as to the food source, cooking effects, and mechanism of action. Selected research studies are listed for further review.

Antioxidants

Antioxidants are a group of vitamins, minerals, enzymes, and others (coenzyme Q10) that act as scavengers, cleaning the body of free radicals and protecting against their destructive power.

The vitamins include A, beta-carotene, C, and E; the minerals are selenium and zinc; and the enzymes are superoxide dismutase, methionine reductase, catalase, and glutathione peroxidase. Another antoxidant is the hormone melatonin. Certain herbs can have antioxidant value (Ginkgo biloba, Bilberry, green tea, pycnogenol).

Antioxidants are obtained from many food sources (see Table 4-11), but are often difficult to obtain in sufficient quantities so supplements are necessary. A high intake of antioxidant nutrients appears to be especially protective against cancer and atherosclerosis and particularily the oxidation of LDL.

Vitamin E reduces the incorporation of cholesterol into arteries and decreases the damage in heart muscle during a myocardial infarction. Vitamin E can also help prevent reperfusion damage caused by the increased generation of free radicals. Selenium also plays a role in the prevention of atherosclerosis. Vitamin E has recently been associated with decreasing the incidence of prostate cancer in smoking men. Cataracts and macular degeneration are slowed with the use of zinc and vitamin E and C. It also appears that antioxidant therapy with vitamin A, E, and C can help decrease the side effects of chemotherapy and radiation and do not affect them negatively. Treatment may potentiate the destruction of cancer cells.

Food Sources: See Table 4-12
Cooking effects: Varied
Mechanism of action:

- decreases O_2 free radical activities in the body
- scavenges O_2 free radicals
- increases longevity
- decreases aging of body
- suppresses rate of brain cell damage
- decreases ASHD deposits
- decreases oxidation of LDL
- decreases incidence of cancer

TABLE 4-11 ANTIOXIDANT-RICH FOODS

	Serving	Amount of Antioxidants
Vitamin C[a]		
• protects other antioxidants such as vitamin E		
• plays role in immunity by increasing synthesis of interferon		
• needed by adrenal gland to synthesize hormones		
• needed for growth and repair of all tissues		
• increases ability to absorb iron		
• increases level of HDL cholesterol		
Green bell pepper	1 large	128 mg
Red bell pepper	1/2 cup diced	95 mg
Orange juice	6 oz glass	90 mg
Grapefruit	1 medium	76 mg
Brussels sprouts	1/2 cup cooked	48 mg
Orange	1 medium	66 mg
Strawberries	1/2 cup	66 mg
Broccoli	1/2 cup cooked	52 mg
Collard greens	1/2 cup cooked	23 mg
Grapefruit juice	6 oz glass	38 mg
Beet greens	1/2 cup cooked	18 mg
Tomato juice	16 oz glass	30 mg
Cabbage	1/2 cup cooked	24 mg
Asparagus	1/2 cup cooked	19 mg
Beta-carotene[b]		
• destroys carcinogins		
• guards against myocardial infarction and stroke		
• lowers cholesterol		
• increases production of CD_4 (helper T cells) so may benefit persons who are HIV positive		
Carrot juice	8 oz glass	11,520 IU
Carrot	1 medium, raw	11,000 IU
Sweet potato	1 small	8,100 IU
Spinach	1/2 cup cooked	7,300 IU
Apricots	8 dried halves	5,500 IU
Collard greens	1/2 cup cooked	5,400 IU
Beet greens	1/2 cup cooked	5,100 IU
Cantaloupe	1/4 melon	3,400 IU
Peach	1 medium	2,170 IU
Romaine lettuce	3 1/2 cup chopped	1,900 IU
Asparagus	5 spears cooked	622 IU
Brussels sprouts	9 cooked	550 IU

[a]*The RDA for vitamin C is 60 mg, but intakes of up to 250 mg or more are safe and possibly beneficial to health.*

[b]*There is no RDA for beta-carotene, but intakes of up to 15,000 IU are safe and possibly beneficial to health.*

Continued

TABLE 4-11 ANTIOXIDANT-RICH FOODS—Continued

	Serving	Amount of Antioxidants
Vitamin E[c]		
• protects lipid coat on all cells		
• improves oxygenation		
• enhances immune response		
• may prevent cataracts		
• reduces risk of cardiovascular disease (CV)		
• improves wound healing and reduces scar formation		
• reduces fibrocystic breasts		
• improves symptoms of premenstrual syndrome		
• reduces hot flashes		
Wheat germ oil	1/4 cup	63.6 IU
Wheat germ	1/2 cup	27 IU
Almonds	1/4 cup	25 IU
Safflower oil, preferably cold pressed	1/4 cup	19.51 IU
Cottonseed oil	1/4 cup	13 IU
100% whole grain cereal	1 cup	0.4 IU
100% whole wheat bread	1 slice	0.39 IU
Selenium[d]		
• reduces cancer growth		
• prevents CV disease		
• improves skin condition (along with vitamin E)		
• improves muscle function		
• improves mental well-being		
• reduces toxicity in heavy metal poisoning		
Brazil nuts	1 nut	150–200 μg
Organ meats	4 oz cooked	149.6 μg
Red snapper	3 oz cooked	42 μg
Salmon (Coho)	3 oz cooked	39 μg
Seafood	4 oz cooked	37.9 μg
Halibut	3 oz cooked	31 μg
Sunflower seeds	1 oz	23 μg
Wheat germ	1/4 cup	23 μg
Lean meat	4 oz cooked	22.7 μg
Chicken without skin	4 oz cooked	22.7 μg
Brown rice	1/2 cup cooked	19 μg
100% whole wheat bread	1 slice	12 μg
100% whole grain cereal	1/2 cup	12 μg
Nonfat milk	1 cup	3.6 μg
Vegetables	1 serving	1.6 μg (average)
Garlic	3 cloves	1.3 μg
Fruits	1 serving	0.9 μg (average)

[c] *The RDA for vitamin E is 12 to 15 IU, but intakes of up to 400 IU are safe and possibly beneficial to health.*

[d] *The RDA for selenium is 130 μg, but intakes of up to 200 μg are safe and possibly beneficial to health.*

TABLE 4-11 ANTIOXIDANT-RICH FOODS—Continued

	Serving	Amount of Antioxidants
Zinc[e]		
• constituent of enzyme superoxide dismutase		
• helps maintain vitamin E levels		
• promotes grandular and reproductive health		
• promotes immune function		
• important for taste		
• enhances function of the iris and retina		
• lowers development of macular degeneration and cataracts		
• improves response to stress		
• may improve anorexia nervosa		
• improves health of prostate		
• shortens the duration of the common cold		
Oyster, Eastern, wild raw	3 oz	76 mg
Oyster, Eastern, farmed, raw	3 oz	32 mg
Oyster, Pacific, raw	3 oz	14 mg
Garden burger	1 each	7.5 mg
Crab, Alaskan King	3 oz	6.7 mg
Ground beef, lean, broiled	3 1/2 oz	5.4 mg
Wheat germ, toasted	1/4 cup	4.8 mg
Baked beas, vegetarian	3 1/2 oz	5.4 mg
Lobster, Northern	3 oz	2.5 mg
Pumpkin seeds	1 oz	2.1 mg
Blackeyed peas, cooked	1/2 cup	1.7 mg
Pecans	1 oz	1.6 mg
Tahini	2 tbsp	1.4 mg
Barley, cooked	1 cup	1.3 mg
Wild rice, cooked	1/2 cup	1.1 mg
Peanut butter, chunky style	2 tbsp	0.9 mg
Rye wafers	1 triple cracker	0.7 mg
Buckwheat pancake	1/4 cup	0.54 mg
Egg yolk	1 yolk	0.5 mg
Refined wheat, cooked	1 cup	0.33 mg

[e]*The RDA for zinc is 15 μg, but intakes of up to 22.5–50 μg are safe and possibly beneficial to health. More than 50 mg can lower HDL.*

(From Somer E. Food and Mood: The complete guide to eating well and feeling your best. NY: Henry Holt, 1995: 184–185.)

TABLE 4-12 FOOD SOURCES OF CAROTENOIDS

Fruit/Vegetable	Alpha-Carotene (mg)	Beta-Carotene (mg)	B-Cryptoxanthin (mg)	Lutein/Zenxanthin (mg)	Lycopene (mg)
Apricot halves, 6 dried	0.00	3.70	0.00	0.00	0.20
Broccoli, 1/2 cup cooked	0.00	1.00	0.00	1.40	0.00
Cantaloupe, 1 cup chunks	0.10	4.80	0.00	0.00	0.00
Carrot, 1 medium raw	2.60	5.70	0.00	0.20	0.00
Collard greens, 1/2 cup cooked	0.00	3.50	0.00	10.40	0.00
Grapefruit, pink, 1/2 medium	0.00	1.60	0.00	0.00	4.10
Kale, 1/2 cup cooked	0.00	3.10	0.00	14.20	0.00
Mango, 1 medium	0.00	2.70	0.10	0.00	0.00
Mustard greens, 1/2 cup cooked	0.00	2.00	0.00	7.40	0.00
Orange, 1 medium	0.00	0.10	0.20	0.00	0.00
Papaya, 1/2 medium	0.00	0.20	1.10	0.00	0.00
Pepper, red, 1/2 raw	0.00	0.80	0.00	2.50	0.00
Pumpkin, 1/2 cup cooked or canned	4.70	3.80	0.00	1.80	0.00
Romaine lettuce, 1 cup	0.00	1.10	0.00	3.20	0.00
Spinach, 1/2 cup cooked	0.00	5.00	0.00	11.30	0.00
Spinach, 1/2 cup raw	0.00	2.30	0.00	5.70	0.00
Sweet potato, 1/2 cup mashed	0.00	14.40	0.00	0.00	0.00
Tangerine, 1 medium	0.00	0.00	0.90	0.00	0.00
Tomato, 1 medium	n/a	0.60	0.00	0.10	3.80
Tomato sauce, 1/2 cup	n/a	1.20	0.00	0.20	7.70
Watermelon, 1 cup, cubed	0.00	0.40	0.00	0.00	6.60

n/a, not available.
Source: U.S. Department of Agriculture/National Cancer Institute carotenoid database.
Strive for 5 servings a day.

Bibliography

Ames, B. N., et al. (1990). Oxidants, antioxidants, and the degenerative diseases of aging. Proceedings of the National Academy of Sciences USA. 90, 7915–7922.

Block, G., Patterson, B., & Subar, A. (1992). Fruit, vegetables and cancer prevention: a review of the epidemiological evidence. Nutrition and Cancer. 18, 1–29.

Canfield, L. M., Forage, J. W., & Valenzuela, J. G. (1992). Cartenoids as cellular antioxidants. Proceedings of the Society of Experimental Biology and Medicine. 200, 260–265.

El-Bayoumy, K., et al. (1995). Ehemoprevention of cancer by organoselenium compounds. Journal of Cellular Biochemistry. 22, (Suppl), 92–100.

Godfrey, J. C., et al. (1996). Zinc for treating the common cold: review of all clinical trials since 1984. Alternative Therapies. 2, (6), 63–72.

Lu, J., et al. (1996). Effect on a aqueous extract of selenium-enriched garlic on in vitro markers and in vivo efficacy in cancer prevention. Carcinogens. 17, 1903–1907.

Luoma, P. V., et al. (1995). High serum alpha-tocopherol, albumin, selenium and cholesterol, and low mortality from coronary heart disease in Northern Finland. Journal of Internal Medicine. 237, 49–54.

Patterson, B. H. & Levander, O. A. (1997). Naturally occurring selenium compounds in cancer chemoprevention trials: a workshop summary. Cancer Epidemiology, Biomarkers and Prevention. 6, 63–69.

Plotnick, G. D., et al. (1997). Effect of antioxidant vitamins on the transient impairment of endothelium-dependent brachial artery vaso-activity following a single high-fat meal. Journal of the American Medical Association. 278, 1682–1686.

Watson, R. R. & Leonard, T. K. (1986). Selenium and vitamins A, E, and C: nutrients with cancer prevention properties. Journal of the American Dietetic Association. 86, 505–510.

Allylic Sulfide

Food Source: Onions**, garlic*, strawberries, grapes, raspberries

Cooking Effects: Unaffected by cooking. Marinating onions may increase the concentration of quercetin.

Mechanism of Action:

- Detoxifies carcinogens
- Decreases initiation of cancer
- Increases activity of protective enzymes
- Lowers blood cholesterol
- Enhances immune function
- Decreases O_2 free radical activity

---

*Garlic is thought to be one of the most valuable foods on this planet. Garlic releases at least 100 sulfur-containing compounds and more than 400 garlic compounds with at least 30 linked to medicinal use. Most of garlic's medicinal constituents result from the breakdown of allicin when the garlic clove is cut. Allicin is highly unstable, half is degraded in 3 hours and all is degraded within 24 hours at room temperature. It degrades even faster when heated, but its degradation produces new compounds with a variety of medicinal uses. To obtain antibiotic effects, eat raw garlic, and to obtain blood-thinning or cholesterol-lowering properties, use raw, cooked, or a commercial variety. Every form of garlic has some cardiovascular benefit and anticancer properties.

Garlic:

lowers blood pressure
inhibits platelet aggregation
reduces risk of blood clots
reduces risk of cancer
stimulates activity of macrophages
stimulates activity of T-helper cells
prevents the liver from generating too much cholesterol by inhibiting HMG-Co A reductase–an enzyme associated with cholesterol production
is active against fungal infections such as athlete's foot
is beneficial for systemic candidiasis and yeast vaginitis
destroys viruses such as genital herpes and fever blisters
helps fight against the common cold and some influenza
improves circulation

**Onions contain more than 150 phytochemicals including many sulfur compounds, quercetin, an antioxidant, and prostaglandins that reduce blood pressure and reduce clots. Onions also increase the level of HDL, the good cholesterol.

For heart disease or cancer, take the equivalent of half of a whole clove/day. Garlic decreases platelet stickiness. It may increase bleeding during surgery and with ASA or coumadin use. Caution is advised.

Bibliography

Adler, A. J. & Holub, B. J. (1997). Effect of garlic and fish-oil supplementation on serum lipid and lipoprotein concentrations in hypercholesterolemic men. American Journal of Clinical Nutrition. 65, 445–450.

Anonymous. (1998). Garlic: can it keep your blood vessels young? Harvard Heart Letter. 8, (7), 6–7.

Bergner, P. (1996). The healing power of garlic. Rocklin, CA: Prima Publishing.

Etherton, P. M. (1997). Efficacy of multiple dietary therapies in reducing cardiovascular disease risk factors. American Journal of Clinical Nutrition. 65, (2), 560–561.

German, K., Kumar, U., & Blackford, H. N. (1995). Garlic and the risk of TURP bleeding. British Journal of Urology. 76, (4), 518.

Kasinath, R. T., Joseph, P. K., Hebron, K., Zhang, X. H., Connock, M. J., & Maslin, D. J. (1997). The effects of garlic oil upon serum indicators of liver function. Biochemical Society Transactions. 25, (3), 533S.

Lash, J. P., Cardoso, L. R., Mesler, P. M., Walczak, D. A., & Pollak, R. (1998). The effect of garlic on hypercholesterolemia in renal transplant patients. Transplantation Proceedings. 12, (4), 463–468.

Silagy, C. & Neil, A. (1994). Garlic as a lipid lowering agent meta-analysis. Journal of the Royal College of Physicians (London). 28, (1), 39–45.

Steiner, M., Khan, H., Holbert, D. & Lin, R. (1996). A double-blind crossover study in moderately hypercholesterolemic men that compared the effect of age garlic extract and placebo administration on blood lipids. American Journal of Clinical Nutrition. 64, 870.

Zhang, X. H., Maxwell, S. R., Thorpe, G. H., et al. (1997). The action of garlic upon plasma total antioxidant capacity. Biochemical Society Transactions. 25, (3), 523S.

INTERNET

Dharmananda, S. (1997) Garlic as the central herb therapy for AIDS www.centerforaids.org

Health World (Garlic The Great Protector) (The Chemistry of Garlic's Benefits) www.healthynet/library

Henahan, S. (1995) Garlic compound slows cancer growth— Access Excellence outcast.gene.com

The Garlic Information Centre (1996) An international information service on the medical benefits of garlic www.mistral.co.uk

Bioflavonoids

Bioflavonoids (flavonoids) are a group of more than 4,000 naturally occurring phenolic compounds (polyphenols) sharing a similar structure.

They are found widely in fruits and vegetables, beer, wine, tea, and coffee. Flavonoids are also a major constituent in medicinal plants used in herbal medicine around the world.

Additional facts and bodily uses of bioflavonoids:

- cannot be produced by the human body
- act synergistically with vitamin C to protect and preserve the structure of capillaries
- have antibacterial effect
- promote circulation
- stimulate bile production
- treat and prevent cataracts
- may be referred to as vitamin P
- limit cancer progression (animal studies only)
- prevent atherosclerosis
- may have hypolipidemic and antiatherosclerosis effects
- act as antioxidants

Flavonoids are divided into several categories:

1. anthocyanins: found in red-blue fruits
2. flavonols: green tea
3. flavonones: common to Chinese medicine and citrus fruits
4. isoflavonoids: found in legumes
5. catechins: bind to protein and are responsible for the astringency of food; found in pine bark and grape seeds.
6. flavones: celery, parsley

Food Source: Widely in fruits and vegetables, beer, wine, tea, coffee, and herbs

Cooking Effects: Unaffected by cooking.

Mechanism of Action:

- Antiallergy
- Conserving vitamin C
- O_2 free radical scavengers
- Inhibits platelet aggregation
- Antitumor activity

Bibliography

Armand, J. P., De Forni, M., Recondo, G., et al. (1998). Flavonoids: a new class of anticancer agents? Preclinical and clinical data of flavone acetic acid. Plant flavonoids in biology and medicine II. San Francisco, CA: Alan R.Liss, Inc. 235–241.

Jaeger, A., Walti, M., & Neftel, K. (1988). Side effects of flavonoids in medical practice. Plant flavonoids in biology and medicine II. Alan R. Liss, Inc. 379–394.

Kandaswami, C., Perkins, E., Soloniuk, D. S., et al. (1993). Ascorbic acid-enhanced antiproliferative effect of flavonoids on squamous cell carcinoma in vitro. Anti-Cancer Drugs. 4, 91–96.
Leibovity, B. E. (1994). Polyphenols & bioflavonoids: the medicines of tomorrow—Parts 1 & 2. Townsend Letters for Doctors. April–May, 12–20.

Bioflavanoids Anthocyanins

Food Source: Red-blue fruit
Cooking Effects: Unknown
Mechanism of Action:

- Protects GI system
- Interacts with estrogen receptor to block estrogen activity, thus decreasing incidence of breast cancer

Bibliography

Geboes, K., Spiessens, C., Nijs, G., et al. (1993). Anthranoids and the mucosal immune system of the colon. Pharmacology. 47, (Suppl 1), 9–57.
Phang, J. M., Poore, C. M., Lopaczynska, J., & Yeh, G. C. (1993). Flavonol-stimulated efflux of 7,12-dimethylbenz (a)anthracene in multidrug-resistant breast cancer cells. Cancer Research. 53, 5977–7981.
Sathyamoorthy, N., Wang, T. T. Y., & Phang, J. M. (1994). Stimulation of pS2 expression by diet-derived compounds. Cancer Research. 54, 957–961.

Bioflavonoids (Flavonols)

Food Source: Green tea*, citrus fruit, cucumbers, berries (cranberries), yams, apples, onions, kale, green beans, broccoli, endive, celery
Cooking Effects: Unaffected by cooking.
Mechanism of Action:

- Decreases activity of O_2 free radicals
- Inactivates mechanism of invasive human breast cancer cells
- Keeps cancer-causing hormones from latching onto cells in the first place

*Over the years, ingestion of tea has been demonstrated to decrease the risk of cancers (kidney, bladder, and upper and lower digestive system including the esophagus and colon). Tea contains polyphenols that act as antioxidants to capture free radicals. Black tea is produced from the fermentation and oxidization of green tea. Most authorities thought that the protective antioxidant properties of green tea were lost or destroyed in the process of producing black tea. Recent research indicates that black tea may be as beneficial. Remember though not to drink the tea too hot or with milk. Overly hot beverages are linked to an increase in esophageal cancer, and milk decreases the antioxidant effect. Adding sugar, lemon, or honey, at least at this time, appears to be OK.

- Stimulates enzyme systems that detoxify carcinogens
- Decreases risk of stroke by:
  - Inhibiting platelets from clumping together and forming clots
  - Blocking oxidation of LDL cholesterol (bad cholesterol) so it does not stick to vessel walls

Bibliography

Ali, M., Afzal, M., Gubler, C. J., et al. (1990). A potent thromboxane formation inhibitor in green tea leaves. Prostaglandins Leukotrienes and Essential Fatty Acids. 40, 281–283.

Balentine, D. A., Wiseman, S. A., & Bouwens, L. C. ()1997). The chemistry of tea flavonoids. Critical Reviews in Food Science & Nutrition. 37, (8), 693–704.

Halder, J. & Bhaduri, A. N. (1998). Protective role of black tea against oxidative damage of human red blood cells. Biochemical & Biophysical Research Communications. 244, (3), 903–907.

Hollman, P. C., Tijburg, L. B., & Yang, C. S. (1997). Bioavailability of flavonoids from tea. Critical Reviews in Food Science & Nutrition. 37, (8), 719–738.

Keli, S. O., Hertog, M. G. L., Feskens, E. J. M., et al. (1996). Dietary flavonoids, antioxidant vitamins and incidence of stroke. Archives of Internal Medicine. 154, 637–642.

Middleton, E. & Kandaswami, C. (1994). Potential health-promoting properties of citrus flavonoids. Food Technology. November, 115–119.

Miura, Y. H., Tomita, I., Watanabe, T., Hirayama, T., & Fukui, S. (1998). Active oxygens generation by flavonoids. Biological & Pharmaceutical Bulletin. 21, (2), 93–96.

Tijburg, L. B., Mattern, T., Folts, J. D., Weisgerber, U. M., & Katan, M. B. (1997). Tea flavonoids and cardiovascular disease: a review. Critical Reviews in Food Science & Nutrition. 37, (8), 771–785.

Bioflavanoids/Flavonones (Naringin)

Food Source: Chinese medicinals, citrus fruit
Cooking Effects: Unknown
Mechanism of Action:

- Antioxidant activity
- Decreases tumor initiation
- Decreases occurrence of chromosome aberrations
- Modifies allergic response by inhibiting release of histamine
- Decreases LDL (more than 10 servings a day)
- Antibacterial activity
- Enhances immune system function
- Protects teeth from decay
- Decreases hormones from resting on cell surface

Bibliography

Hollman, P. C. & Katan, M. B. (1998). Bioavailability and health effects of dietary flavonols in man. Archives of Toxicology. 20, 237–248.

Kuo, S. M. (1997). Dietary flavonoid and cancer prevention: evidence and potential mechanism. Critical Reviews in Oncogenesis. 8, (1), 47–69.

Matsukawa, Y., Yoshida, M., Sakai, T., et al. (1990). The effect of quercetin and other flavonoids on cell cycle progression growth of human gastric cancer cells. Planta Medica. 56, 677–678.

Bioflavonoids/Isoflavonoids (Daidzein)

Food Source: Legumes, soy*, tofu, beans, peas
Cooking Effects: Unaffected by cooking
Mechanism of Action:

- Inhibits angiogenesis and the proliferation of vascular endothelial cells or decreases the incidence of atherosclerosis
- Destroys cancer gene enzymes
- Inhibits cancer growth and division
- Inhibits estrogen receptor activity
- Blocks estrogen and testosterone in the development of cancer
- Decreases total cholesterol while increasing good "HDL" cholesterol
- Reduces menopausal symptoms such as hot flashes
- Acts as hormone regulators
- Acts as phytoestrogen
- Decreases rate of chronic disease
- Decreases osteoporosis
- Decreases platelet stickiness
- Increases abnormal cell death
- May improve migraines associated with hereditary hemorrhagic telangriectasia (HHT)

Excellent sources of soy:

Fresh soybeans	Tempeh
Miso	Canned/frozen soybeans
Soy flour	Soynuts
Soy protein powders	Soy milk
Textured vegetable protein	Tofu

Poor sources of soy (soy is too processed to be of much value):

Soy sauce	Soy cheese
Soy oil	Soy hot dogs
Canned soy drinks	Tofu desserts

*Soy is chock full of insoluble and soluble fiber, calcium, B vitamins, and phytoestrogens.

Bibliography

Adlercreutz, H. (1995). Phytoestrogens: epidemiology and a possible role in cancer protection. Environmental Health Perspective. 103, (Suppl 7), 103–112.

Barnes, S., Grubbs, C., Setchell, K. D. R., et al. (1990). Soybeans inhibit mammary tumors in models of breast cancer. In: Pariza, M, Ed. Mutagens and carcinogens in the diet. New York: Wiley-Liss. 239–253.

Cassidy, A., Bingham, S., & Setchell, K. (1994). Biological effects of a diet of soy protein rich in isoflavones on the menstrual cycle of premenopausal women. American Journal of Clinical Nutrition. 60, 333–340.

Ingram, D., Sanders, K., Kolybaba, M., & Lopex, D. (1997). Case-control study of phyto-estrogens and breast cancer. Lancet. 350, 990–994.

King, R. A. & Bursill, D. B. (1998). Plasma and urinary kinetics of the isoflavones daidzein and genistein after a single soy meal in humans. American Journal of Clinical Nutrition. 67, (5), 867–872.

Messina, M. & Barnes, S. (1991). The role of soy products in reducing risk of cancer. Journal of the National Cancer Institute. 83, (8), 541–546.

Bioflavonoids/Isoflavonoids (Silymarin)

Food Source: Artichokes
Cooking Effects: Unaffected by cooking.
Mechanism of Action:

- Antioxidant, may protect against skin cancer

Bibliography

Muriel, P., Garciniapina, T., Perez-Alvarez, V., et al. (1992). *Silymarin* protects against paracetamol-induced lipid peroxidation and liver damage. Journal of Applied Toxicology. 12, 439–442.

Yanagihara, K., Ito, A., Tonge, T., & Numoto, M. (1993). Antiproliferative effects isoflavones on human cancer cell lines established from the gastrointestinal tract. Cancer Research. 1, 53, (23), 581–521.

Bioflavonoids (Catchins)

Food Source: Pine bark, grape seeds, wine, green and black tea
Cooking Effects: Unaffected by cooking.
Mechanism of Action:

- Antioxidant effects against cancer
- Decreases cholesterol (eating grapes or drinking grape juice or wine—particularly purple juice or red wine)

Bibliography

Miyagi, Y., Miwa, K., & Inoue, H. (1997). Inhibition of human low-density lipoprotein oxidation by flavonoids in red wine and grape juice. American Journal of Cardiology. 80, (12), 1627–1631.

Capsaicin

Food Source: Hot peppers
Cooking Effects: Unaffected by cooking.
Mechanism of Action:

- Neutralizer of carcinogens
- Destroys bacteria in stomach associated with ulcer formation
- Decreases wound pain when applied topically
- Aids digestion
- Useful to decrease pain of arthritis
- Acts as a digestive stimulant

Bibliography

Dasgupta, P., Chandiramani, V., Parkinson, M. C., Bekett, A., & Fowler, C. J. (1998). Treating the human bladder with capsaicin: is it safe? European Urology. 33, (1), 28–31.
Lincoff, N. S., Rath, P. P., & Hirano, M. (1998). The treatment of periocular and facial pain with topical capsaicin. Journal of Neuro-Ophthalmology. 18, (1), 17–20.
May, A., Kaube, H., Buchel, C., et al. (1998). Experimental cranial pain elicited by capsaicin: a PET study. Pain. 74, (1), 61–66.
Yosipovitch, G. (1998). Adverse reactions of topical capsaicin. Journal of the American Academy of Dermatology. 38, (3), 503–504.

Carnosol or Carnosic Acid

Food Source: Rosemary
Cooking Effects: Unaffected by cooking.
Mechanism of Action:

- Blocks the effect of toxins from the environment
- Powerful antioxidant qualities
- Enhances cellular uptake of O_2
- Reduces tension
- Anti-inflammatory
- Increases flow of bile
- Aids fat digestion
- Mild analgesic, particularly good for headache
- Strengthens blood vessels

Bibliography

American Chemical Society. (1992). 204th Meeting, Washington, D.C. Abstract 107.
Flavor Chemistry of Fats & Oils. American Oil Chemical Society. p. 140. 1985.

Carotinoids

Carotinoids are a class of 600 compounds related to vitamin A. In some cases, they are precursors to vitamin A, and others act as antioxidants. The best known is beta carotene, but recent research has not shown much benefit from beta carotene and has shown increased benefit from some of the others. Not all carotenes are alike. Several varieties of carotenes are found: alpha, beta, lutein, and lycopene. See Table 4-8 for food sources high in carotinoids.

Food Source: Carrots, winter squash, sweet potatoes, apricots, spinach, kale, parsley, soy beans, cereal grains
Cooking Effects: Unaffected by cooking
Mechanism of Action:

- Antioxidant properties
- Stop or reverse osteoporosis
- Enhances immune function
- Decreases O_2 free radical activity
- Prevent formation of carcinogens

Carotenoid (Beta-carotene)

Food Source: Squash, pumpkin, watermelon, cucumber
Cooking Effects: Unaffected by cooking.
Mechanism of Action:

- Improves health of macula of eye
- Antioxidant properties

Bibliography

Seddon, J. M., Ajani, U. A., Sperduto, R. D., et al. (1994). Dietary carotenoids, vitamins A, C, and E, and advanced age-related macular degeneration. Journal of the American Medical Association. 272, 1413–1420.

Carotenoid (Lutein/Zeaxanthin)

Food Source: Kale, other dark green leafy vegetables
Cooking Effects: Unaffected by cooking.
Mechanism of Action:

- Antioxidant properties
- Decreases degeneration of macula

Carotenoid (Lycopene*)

Food Source: Tomatoes, watermelon
Cooking Effects: Tomatoes are probably best cooked. To assist absorption of lycopene in the intestine, oil should be combined with tomatoes
Mechanism of Action:

- Antioxidant, twice as good as beta carotene
- Decreases risk of prostate cancer
- Enhances immune function
- Decreases O_2 free radical activity
- Decreases macula degeneration, a leading cause of blindness
- Decreases cancer (stomach, colon, rectum)

Bibliography

Anonymous. (1996). Tomatoes fight cancer. PMA. 29, (3), 4.
Krinsky, N. I., Russett, M. D., Handelman, G. J., et al. (1990). Structural and geometrical isomers of carotenoids in human plasma. Journal of Nutrition. 120, 1654–1662.
Seddon, N. J., Ajani, U. A., Sperduto, R. D., et al. (1994). Dietary carotenoids, vitamins A, C, and E, and advanced age-related macular degeneration. Journal of the American Medical Association. 272, 1413–1420.

Curcumin

Food Source: Turmeric
Cooking Effects: Unknown
Mechanism of Action:

- Decreases inflammation, much like steroids
- Decreases inflammation in bowel, such as in ulcerative colitis, Crohn's disease
- Decreases inflammation in hepatitis and asthma
- Decreases symptoms of arthritis
- Causes malignant cells to shrink and die
- Interferes with blood clotting (interferes with thromboxanes)
- May protect liver during hepatitis

Bibliography

Agrez, M. V. & Bates, R. C. (1994). Colorectal cancer and the integral family of cell adhesion receptors: current status and future directions. European Journal of Cancer. 30A, (14), 2166–2170.

*Lycopene is the red pigment found in tomatoes. Recent research has suggested that 10 tomato meals/week can reduce man's risk of prostatic hypertrophy and cancer. Lycopene cannot be converted to vitamin A. Lycopene is not found in tomato juice.

Kuttan, R., Bhanumathy, P., Nirmala, K., et al. (1985). Potential anticancer activity of turmeric (Curcuma longa). Cancer Letters. 29, (2), 197–202.

Genistein

Food Source: Soy products*
Cooking Effects: Unaffected by cooking.
Mechanism of Action:

- Prevents a blood supply from being established to the tumor
- Inhibits platelet aggregation
- Induces cell death (particularly leukemia cells)
- Depresses action of tumor-promoting agents
- Assists with regulation of hormones
- Promotes the 2-hydroylation of estradiol, converting it to a weak estrogen with no carcinogenic capability

Bibliography

Fiedor, P., Kozerski, L., Dobrowolski, J. C., & Kawecki, R. (1998). Immunosuppressive effects of synthetic derivative of genistein on the survival of pancreatic islet allografts. Transplantation Proceedings. 30, (2), 537.

Geller, J., Sionit, L., Partido, C., et al. (1998). Genistein inhibits the growth of human-patient BPH and prostate cancer in histoculture. Prostate. 34, (2), 75–79.

Messina, M., & Barnes, S. (1991). The role of soy products in reducing risk of cancer. Journal of the National Cancer Institute. 83, (8), 541–546.

Peterson, G. & Barnes, S. (1993). Genistein and biochanin A inhibit the growth of human prostate cancer cells but not epidermal growth factor receptor tyrosine autophosphylatin. Prostate. 22, (4), 335–345.

Peterson, G. & Barnes, S. (1991). Genistein inhibition of the growth of human breast cancer cells: independence from estrogen receptors and the multi-drug resistance gene. Biochemical and Biophysical Research Communications. 179, (1), 661–667.

Sadowska-Krowicka, H., Mannick, E. E., Oliver, P. D., Sandoval, M., Zhang, X. J., Eloby-Childess, S., Clark, D. A., & Miller, M. J. (1998). Genistein and gut inflammation: role of nitric oxide. Proceedings of the Society for Experimental Biology and Medicine. 217, (3), 351–357.

Shao, Z. M., Alpaugh, M. L., Fontana, J. A., & Barsky, S. H. (1998). Genistein inhibits proliferation similarly in estrogen receptor-positive and negative human breast carcinoma cell lines characterized by P21WAF1/CIP1 induction, G2/M arrest, and apoptosis. Journal of Cellular Biochemistry. 69, (1), 44–54.

Glutathione

Food Source: Watermelon (also has a large amount of lycopene)
Cooking Effects: Unknown

---

*See also Flavenoids (Daidzein).

Mechanism of Action:

- O_2 free radical scavenger
- Enhances immune function
- Improves liver's ability to detoxify chemicals, drugs, and pollutants
- Enhances kidney and bladder function
- Helps defend body against effects of cigarette smoking, radiation, and chemotherapy
- Protects arteries from O_2 free radical damage

Bibliography

Davis, M., Wallig, M., & Jeffery, E. (1993). In vitro metabolism of cyanohydroxybutene: formation of a glutathione-Stransferase catalyzed product. Research Communications in Chemical Pathology and Pharmacology. 79, 343–353.

Prestera, T., Holtzclaw, W., Zhang, Y., & Talalay, P. (1993). Chemical and molecular regulation of enzymes that detoxify carcinogens. Proceedings of the National Academy of Sciences USA. 90, 2965–2969.

Sparnins, V. L., Venegas, P. L., & Wattenberg, L. W. (1982). Glutathione-S transferase activity: enhancement by compounds inhibiting chemical carcinogenesis and by dietary constituents. Journal of the National Cancer Institute. 68, 493–496.

Glycyrrhizin*

Food Source: Licorice root
Cooking Effects: Unknown
Mechanism of Action:

- Reinforces bodily cellular and antioxidant defenses
- Protects the digestive system from toxins
- Cleanses the colon
- Increases fluidity of mucous in lungs
- Has estrogen and progesterone activity
- Increases production of interferon
- Powerful anti-inflammatory
- Laxative
- Causes pseudoaldosteronism—may elevate blood pressure with long use
- Avoid during pregnancy because of its blood pressure effect
- Avoid with diabetes and heart disease

Indoles

Food Source: Cruciferous vegetables (broccoli, cauliflower, cabbage, Brussels sprouts, mustard greens)

*Glycyrrhizin is 50 times sweeter than sugar.

Cooking Effects: Unaffected by cooking.
Mechanism of Action:

- Promotes the 2-hydroylation of estradiol, converting it to a weak estrogen with no carcinogenic capability
- Protects against breast cancer, but be careful because large intake may increase risk of breast cancer
- Decreases risk of lung and colon cancer
- Prevents development of multidrug resistance in drug chemotherapy
- Increases the production of glutathione-S-transferase, which conjugates and clears carcinogens
- Enhances immune function and makes it easier for the body to excrete toxins
- May protect the body from environmental toxins

Bibliography

Elson, C. E. & Yu, S. G. (1994). The chemoprevention of cancer by mevalonate-derived constituents of fruits and vegetables. Journal of Nutrition. 124, 607–614.
Michnovicz, J. J., et al. (1990). Induction of estradiol metabolism by dietary indole-3—carbinal in humans. Journal of the National Cancer Institute. 82, 947–949.
Bogaards, J. J. P., Verhagen, H., Willems, M. I., Van Poppel, G., & Van Bladeren, P. J. (1994). Consumption of Brussels sprouts results in elevated alpha-class glutathione-S-transferase levels in human blood plasma. Carcinogenesis. 15, 1073–1075.

Isothiocyanatis

Food Source: Cruciferous vegetables (cabbage*, broccoli, watercress, turnips, radish)
Cooking Effects: Unaffected by cooking.
Mechanism of Action:

- Inhibits cancer process by detoxifying carcinogens
- May protect from carcinogens found in cigarettes
- May decrease incidence of stomach, breast, and lung cancer

Lignans

Food Source: Flaxseed**, walnuts
Cooking Effects: Unknown

*Cabbage also contains a lot of glutamine, an amino acid, that has been shown to heal ulcers.

**Do not take flaxseeds or flaxseed oil with niacin because a "flush" reaction can be triggered.

Mechanism of Action:

- Blocks hormones such as estrogen and testosterone that precipitate cancer
- Inhibits platelet aggregation
- Inhibits arachidonic acid cycle (part of clotting cycle)
- Reduces pain, inflammation, and swelling of arthritis (the oil: 1 tablespoon/day or 9 caps/day)
- Acts as bulk laxative
- Enhances healing of burns (applied topically)
- Decreases blood cholesterol (the fiber in the seed, not the seed); rich source of omega 3 oil
- Has antioxidant properties
- Removes carcinogens from the cell
- Source of vitamin A, B, D, and E

Flaxseeds are a rich source of omega 3 fatty acids. Usual dose is 25 to 30 grams of flaxseed daily or 3 tablespoons of whole or ground flaxseed. When grinding flaxseed, use a coffee grinder. The flaxseed powder quickly oxidizes so use within 30 minutes.

Bibliography

Clark, W. F., et al. (1995). Flaxseed: a potential treatment for lupus nephritis. Kidney International. 48, (2), 475–480.

Cunnane, S. C., et al. (1995). Nutritional attributes of traditional flaxseed in healthy young adults. American Journal of Clinical Nutrition. 61, (1), 62–68.

Jenab, M. & Thompson, L. U. (1996). The influence of flaxseed and lignans on colon carcinogenesis and beta-glucuronidase activity. Carcinogenesis. 17, (6), 1343–1348.

Phillip, W. (1995). Effects of flax seed ingestion on menstrual cycle. Journal of Clinical Endocrinology and Metabolism. 77, (5), 1215–1219.

Thompson, L. U. (1996). Flaxseed and its lignan and oil components reduce mammary tumor growth at a late stage of carcinogenesis. Carcinogenesis. 17, (6), 1373–1376.

Linolenic Acid

Food Source: Citrus fruits
Cooking Effects: Unknown
Mechanism of Action:

- Regulates production of prostaglandins within cells
- Inhibits histamine
- Anti-inflammatory effects
- Possibly inhibits clotting cascade

Monoterpenes*

Food Source: Citrus fruit, garlic, parsley, squash, basil, mint, eggplant, tomatoes, orange peel, citrus oils, caraway seed oil, grapefruit, lime, lemon.
Cooking Effects: Unknown
Mechanism of Action:

- Antioxidant properties
- Removes carcinogens from the cell

P-Coumaric/Chlorogenic Acid

Food Source: Tomatoes, green peppers, pineapple, strawberries, carrots
Cooking Effects: Unaffected by cooking
Mechanism of Action:

- Decreases formation of cancer-causing amines
- Decreases risk of prostate cancer in men (see Lycopene)
- Interferes with certain chemical unions that can create carcinogen
- Decreases prostaglandin synthesis
- Prevents formation of carcinogens
- Has antioxidant effect

Pectin

Food Source: All fruit (the cement of fruit cell walls)
Cooking Effects: Unaffected by cooking.
Mechanism of Action:

- Protective against prostate and lung cancer
- Slows absorption of food after meal, good for diabetics
- Removes toxins
- Helps lower cholesterol
- Reduces heart disease
- Reduces risk of gallbladder disease

---

*Two subtypes exist:
D-limonene found primarily in citrus fruit oils, coriander, cardamom, and mint
D-carvone found primarily in caraway seed oil

Polyacetylene

Food Source: Parsley*
Cooking Effects: Unknown
Mechanism of Action:

- Destroys potent cancer-causing substances
- Relieves gas and indigestion
- Freshens breath after onions and garlic
- Reduces blood pressure
- Acts as diuretic

Polyphenols

Food Source: Black tea†, green tea†‡, artichokes, grapes**
Cooking Effects: Unaffected by cooking.
Mechanism of Action:

- Decreases inflammatory reactions with exposure to chemical tumor promoters
- Protects cholesterol from oxidative damage, thereby protecting artery walls
- Protects skin from solar radiation
- Antioxidant
- O_2 free radical scavengers
- Inhibits formation of carcinogens in upper GI tract

Bibliography

Ho, C., Huang, M., Eds. (1995). Food phytochemicals for cancer prevention, II: teas, spices, and herbs. (ACS Symposium Series 547). Trends in Food Science Technology. 6, 216–217.

---

*Rich in vitamins A, C, iron, calcium, and K^+ . Contains essential oils of limonene, cumarins, and flavonoids. Do not use large amount of parsley seed if pregnant or with kidney disease because of its effect on blood pressure and kidneys.

†One polyphenol-epigallo cathechin 3 gallage (EGCG) inhibits an enzyme urokinase. Because urokinase plays an important role in the growth and spread of malignant tumors, it is understandable that tumors decrease in size and may completely remiss. It seems that EGCG selectively destroys cancer cells but spares healthy ones.

†‡When drinking tea, do not drink it too hot because extremely hot liquids are linked to cancer of the esophagus. Do not drink tea with milk because some of the antioxidant effect is lost. Black tea may also decrease the risk of certain cancers. At the University of Minnesota, a study conducted over 8 years found women who drank two cups of tea daily were 60% less likely to develop cancer of the kidney and bladder and had a 32% lower risk of GI cancer; and those who drank four cups or more a day were even less prone to cancer development.

**Grapes made into wine seem to slow the oxidation of LDL and inhibit the blood from clotting. This fact may give cardiac patients protection from worsening heart disease.

Anonymous. (1992). Physiological and pharmacological effects of Camellia sinensis (tea): First Symposium. New York City, March 4–5, 1991. Preventive Medicine. 21, (3), 379–391.
Wany, Z. Y., Huang, M. T., Ferraro, T., et al. (1992). Inhibitory effect of green tea in the drinking water on tumorigenesis by ultraviolet light and 12-O-tetradecanoylphorbol-13-acetate in the skin of SKH-1 mice. Cancer Research. 52, (5), 1162–1170.

Polyphenols (Ellagic Acid)

Food Source: Walnuts, strawberries, cranberries, blackberries, apples, raspberries
Cooking Effects: Unknown
Mechanism of Action:

- O_2 free radical scavengers that inhibits cells from becoming malignant
- Antiaging effects
- Antioxidant
- Inhibits enzymes that cancer cells need to grow
- Protease inhibitor, suppresses enzyme production in cancer cells, therefore slows tumor growth
- Phytoesterol content, lowers cholesterol, lowers Ca^{++}, and inhibits cell reproduction in GI tract

Proanthocyanidins (procyanidins)

Food Source: Red grapes, blueberries, blackberries, cherries, raspberries, grape seed extract, pycnogenol (see separate heading)
Cooking Effects: Unknown
Mechanism of Action:

- Decreases circulatory disorders
- Decreases varicose veins
- Decreases atherosclerotic heart disease (ASHD)
- May be an antioxidant

Saponins*

Food Source: Kidney beans, chick peas, soy beans, lentils
Cooking Effects: Unaffected by cooking
Mechanism of Action:

*Increasing fiber to 28 grams/day decreases incidence of breast cancer (Journal of Cancer [1994] 56); decreases incidence of heart disease and lowers blood sugar levels (20 grams/day) in the diabetic patient. Most of the fiber in these studies has come from fruits and vegetables, not from cereal and grains. Use the label to help guide you to cereal and grain products. High fiber means 5 grams of fiber per serving.

- Prevent cancer cells from multiplying in GI tract, thereby decreasing cancer colon risk
- May decrease diverticuli formation
- Decreases estradiol levels by increasing fecal excretion

Bibliography

Aruna, K. & Sivaramakrishnan, V. M. (1990). Plant products as protective agents against cancer. Indian Journal of Experimental Biology. 28, 1008–1011.

Block, G., Patterson, B., & Subar, A. (1992). Fruit, vegetables, and cancer prevention: a review of the epidemiological evidence. Nutrition in Cancer. 18, 1–29.

Parson, T. J., Van Dusseldorp, M., et al. (1997). Reduced bone mass in Dutch adolescents fed a macrobiotic diet in early life. Journal of Bone and Mineral Research. 12, (9), 1486–1494.

Sulforaphane

Food Source: Broccoli*, cauliflower, Brussel sprouts, turnips, kale
Cooking Effects: Not affected by cooking.
Mechanism of Action:

- Boosts synthesis of anticancer enzymes
- Destroys carcinogens
- Enhances removal of toxic substances from cells

3-N-Butylphthalide

Food Source: Celery
Cooking Effects: Unaffected by cooking.
Mechanism of Action:

- Regulates hormones that trigger increased blood pressure in some people

Bibliography

Anonymous. (1998). USDA finally tackles "organic" definition and proposes national standards. Environmental Nutrition. 21, (2), 3.

Anonymous. (1997). Glucosamine for osteoarthritis. Medical Letter on Drugs and Therapeutics. 39, (1010), 91.

Anonymous. (1995). Position of the American Dietetic Association. Journal of the American Dietetic Association. 95, (4), 493–6.

Anonymous. (1998). Plastic & microwaves. Environmental Nutrition. 21, (8), 7.

Anonymous. (1998). Sucralose—A new artificial sweetener. The Medical Letter. 40, (1030), 67–68.

Anonymous. (1996). Dehydroepiandrosterone (DHEA). The Medical Letter. 38, (985), 91.

---

*To obtain the greatest benefit from broccoli, eat approximately 2 lb a week of the plant or 2 oz of broccoli sprouts. According to a 1997 study at the Mayo Clinic in Minnesota, broccoli sprouts contain 50 times the sulforaphane than broccoli fruit.

Bland, J. (1996). Phytonutrition, phytotherapy, and phytopharmacology. Alternative Therapies. 2, (6), 73–75.

Forman, A. (1998). Food as medicine: will nutraceuticals take over? Environmental Nutrition. 21, (2), 1, 6.

Ingram, D., Sanders, K., et al. (1997). Case-control study of phyto-estrogens and breast cancer. Lancet. 350, 990–994.

Jensen, B. & Anderson, M. (1990). Empty harvest. New York: Avery Publishing.

Lieberman, S. & Bruning, N. (1997). The real vitamin & mineral nook. New York: Avery Publishing.

Nicholson, A. (1996). Diet and the prevention and treatment of breast cancer. Alternative Therapies. 2, (6), 32–38.

Nygard, O., et al. (1997). Plasma homocysteine levels and mortality in patients with coronary artery disease. New England Journal of Medicine. 337, 230–236.

Palwak, L. & Freedman, M. (1998). Precious metals. Emeryville, CA: Biomed Publication.

Parson, T. J., et al. (1997). Reduced bone mass in Dutch adolescents fed a macrobiotic diet in early life. Journal of Bone & Mineral Research. 12, (9), 1486–1494.

Reichelt, A., Forster, K. K., et al. (1994). Efficacy and safety of intramuscular glucosamine sulfate in a placebo-controlled, double-blind study. Arzneimittelorschung. 44, (1), 75.

Reiter, R. & Robinson, J. (1995). Your body's natural wonder drug melatonin. New York: Bantam Books.

Simone, C. (1992). Cancer nutrition. New York: Avery Publishing.

Somer, E. (1995). Food and mood: the complete guide to eating well and feeling your best. New York: Henry Holt. 184–185.

Wang, H., Cao, G., Prior, R. L. (1996). Total antioxidant capacity of fruits. Journal of Agricultural & Food Chemistry. 44, (3), 701–705.

Walsh, J. (1998). How your hormones are affected by what you eat. Environmental Nutrition. 21, (2), 1, 4.

Walters, R. (1992). Options, the alternative cancer therapy book. New York: Avery Publishing.

Ward, E. (1998). Can a multi offer one-stop shopping for vitamins and minerals? Environmental Nutrition. 21, (8), 4–5.

Webb, D. (1997). Coenzyme Q10 miracle nutrient or merely promising? Environmental Nutrition. 20, (11), 1, 4.

Worthington, V. (1998). Effect of agricultural methods on nutritional quality: a comparison of organic with conventional crops. Alternative Therapies. 4, (1), 58–64.

Further Reading

Anderson, R., et al. (1998). Chromium content of selected breakfast cereals. Journal of Food Com and Analysis. 1, 303–308.

Anonymous. (1997). An analysis of colloidal mineral claims: parts 1 & 2. Health Counselor. IMPAKT Communications, Inc.

Appel, L. J., et al. (1997). A clinical trial of the effects of dietary patterns on blood pressure. New England Journal of Medicine. 336, 1117–2411.

Balch, J. & Balch, P. (1997). Prescription for nutritional healing. New York: Avery Publishing.

Bragg, P. & Bragg, P. (1997). The miracle of fasting. CA: Health Sciences.

El-Bayoumy, K., et al. (1995). Chemoprevention of cancer by organoselenium compounds. Journal of Cell Biochemistry. 22 (Suppl), 92–100.

Harris, S. S. & Dawson-Hughes, B. (1994). Caffeine and bone loss in healthy postmenopausal women. American Journal of Clinical Nutrition. 60, 573–578.

Ingram, D., et al. (1997). Case-control study of phyto-oestrogens and breast cancer. Lancet. 350, 990–994.

Karakucuk, S., et al. (1995). Selenium concentrations in serum, lens and aqueous humour of patients with senile cataract. Acta Ophthalmologica Scandinavica. 73, 329–332.

Kuczmarski, R. J. (1994). Increasing prevalence of overweight among U.S. adults. Journal of the American Medical Association. 207, 205.

Laitinen, K., et al. (1993). Is alcohol an osteoporosis-inducing agent for young and middle-aged women? Metabolism: Clinical and Experimental. 42, 875–881.
Nygard, O., et al. (1997). Plasma homocysteine levels and mortality in patients with coronary artery disease. New England Journal of Medicine. 337, 230–236.
Shelton, H. (1991). Fasting can save your life. FL: American Natural Hygiene.
Tranquilli, A. L, et al. (1994). Calcium, phosphorus and magnesium intakes correlate with bone mineral content in postmenopausal women. Gynecology and Endocrinology. 8, 55–58.
Trent, L. K. & Thieding-Cancel, D. (1995). Effects of chromium picolinate on body composition.
Journal of Sports Medicine and Physical Fitness. 35, 273–280.
Van Straten, M. (1997). Healing foods. Great Britain: Ivy Press.
Walker, N. (1978). Fresh vegetable and fruit juices. AZ: Norwalk Press.
Wilson, B. E., & Gondy, A. (1995). Effects of chromium supplementation of fasting insulin levels and lipid parameters in health, non-obese young subjects. Diabetes Research Clinical Practice. 28, 179–184.

INTERNET

The Vegetarian Society
www.veg.org/veg

The Vegetarian Resource Group
www.vrg.org

Ask The Dietician
www.dietician.com

American Cancer Society
www.cancer.org

National Cancer Institute
www.nci.nih.9ou

Organic Foods
http://www.ecomall.com/
http://allorganic.com/

Ornish
http://www.ccnet.com/~newmed/ornish.htm
http://www.altavista.digital.com/cgi-

Pritikin
http://www.pritikin.com/contents.html
http://www.pritikin.com/pantry.html

CHAPTER 5

MIND AND BODY CONTROL

AROMATHERAPY

What Is Aromatherapy?

When people hear the term "aromatherapy," they think about fragrance and perfumes, an alluring world of imagination, magic, religion, and fantasy; but aromatherapy consists simply of using essential oils obtained from plants for healing. Aromatherapy uses essential oils obtained directly from the roots, flowers, bark, leaves, and the rind of fruits from a variety of plants. Modern aromatherapy is an expansion of the ancient practice of using and studying the effects of certain aromas on the body and mind. Over the last several decades, aromatherapists have compiled formulas and extracts to use in specific ways for selected conditions and ailments. Aromatherapy has been popularized in recent years so that the average person has access to essential oils for home use.

WHAT IS AN ESSENTIAL OIL?

An essential oil:

- Plays a key role in the biochemistry of the plant
- Is a hormone-like substance located between cells that acts as a regulator and messenger (estrogen—sage, parsley, hops)
- Plays a role in plant protection, fertilization, and response to stress. Assists the plant to adapt to its environment
- May contain as many as 200 to 3,000 constituents
- Controls multiplication and renewal of cells, has cytophilactic and healing effects (lavender, geranium, Italian Everlastin)

- May have anticarcinogenic properties
- Is a part of the plant's sexual system releasing fragrances that mimic insect pheromones to facilitate pollination
- Also has the power to repel insects that could be harmful (citronella and geranium repel mosquitoes; lavender spike repels fleas and mites)
- Acts as selective weed killers and does not allow other plants to grow near by
- Is a part of the plant's immune system—plays a part in protection against the sun (frankincense bushes are surrounded by a thin cloud of essential oils that filters the sun's rays and freshens the air)
- Is stored in specific areas and the plant retrieves them in a dilute form as needed
- Contains carbonic chains of 10 carbons or more. These chains are lypophilic, which means they are readily absorbed by vegetable oils, waxes, or fats. This characteristic allows for the extraction process called enfleurage.
- Is hydrophobic, which means they do not mix with water. Essential oils float to the surface in water. Essential oils are soluble in alcohol.
- Are found primarily in outer leaves, in the skin of citrus fruits, and in the bark of certain trees; therefore, essential oils have an affinity toward our outside—the skin.
- Produced by solar activity in plants, many of which grow in dry, hot areas. (Some say essential oils are produced by the plant's cosmic self.)

WHERE DO ESSENTIAL OILS WORK?

Essential oils work:

- On the body with an allopathic action caused by their chemical composition—stimulant (peppermint, lemon), calming (lavender, marjoram, ylang-ylang), analgesic (clove, birch), antispasmodic (cramps, PMS), and cough (tarragan, lavender)
- At the information level (it has a pleasant odor)
- On the skin as antiseptics (tea tree oil), astringent (geranium, lemon grass), protectant (sandalwood, myrrh), cellular stimulant (rose, lavender, geranium), and as a soother (chamomile, rose, ylang-ylang)
- In the mind on an emotional level (relaxing)
- At the spiritual level in rituals. All major religions use incenses and scented oils in their rituals and ceremonies
- At the energy level and are used with great efficiency in energy work such as acupressure, shiatsu, and chakra work—crown (rose), third eye (mugwort, sandalwood), throat (geranium), heart (rose, melissa),

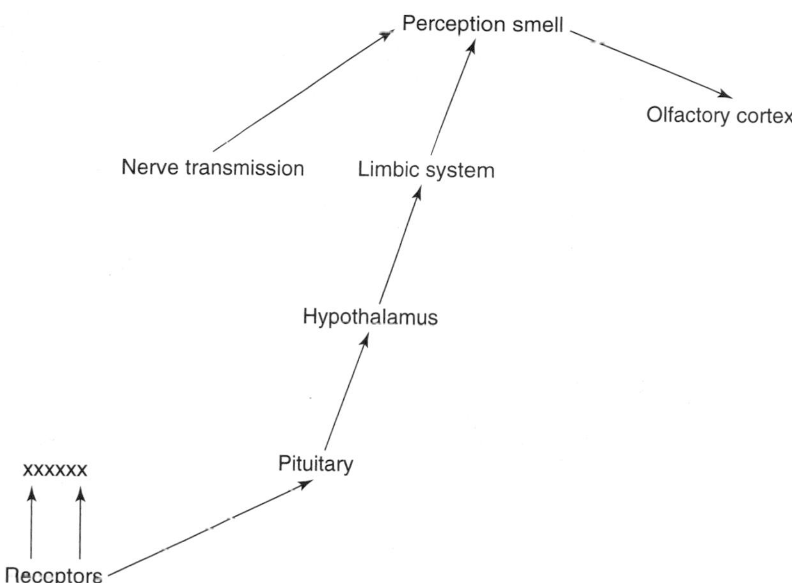

FIGURE 5-1
Nervous receptors in the nose send messages through the nerves to the olfactory cortex and to the limbic system where past information on scents is stored. From the limbic system, messages also travel to the hypothalamus and pituitary.

solar plexus (rosemary, ginger), navel (jasmine, ylang-ylang), and root (angelica, ginger, spruce).

- By inhalation. The cells of the nose are replaced every 30 to 40 days and the sense of smell is 10,000 times more acute than other senses. The essential oil is inhaled, travels to the lungs, enters the blood stream, and because of its small size, easily penetrate body tissues (Fig. 5-1). Essential oils may circulate for 30 minutes to 24 hours. At the same time, the essential oil binds to the olfactory epithelium at the top of the nose, which creates a neurochemical response. This response travels to the olfactory bulb in the base of the brain and to the limbic system. The limbic system (primitive brain) interprets emotion, moods, desires, motivation, memory, intuition, and well being. The essential oil may also travel to the thalamus, which releases endorphins, and to the pituitary, which releases serotonin. Research has indicated the smell is closely related to memory and persons with anosmia (lack of smell) often suffer from depression.

HOW ARE ESSENTIAL OILS PREPARED, AND WHAT IS THEIR STRUCTURE?

- Essential oils are prepared by several techniques
- Oil infusion (the "red oil" of St. John's wort)
- Enfleurage (fresh flowers are used and the end product, although not an essential oil, is particularly suited for preparing perfumes). Enfleurage describes a process in which fresh flowers are soaked in animal fat, with fresh flowers added every few days. The concentrated *pommade* is then added to alcohol, which absorbs the fragrance when the alcohol is distilled off. The resulting product is known as an "absolute through enfleurage."
- Cold expression (citrus oil)
- Distillation (lavender, hyssop)
- Extraction by solvents followed by dilution in alcohol, double filtration, and double concentration (roses, neroli [orange blossoms], jasmine, honeysuckle, carnation). Structure of oils includes volatility, either low or high. For example, place several drops of vegetable oil on a cloth. The oil will remain and stain the cloth. Place several drops of essential oil on a cloth. It will eventually evaporate completely, leaving no stain. (Except when the oil is more viscous or has dark color.) The volatile quality is also what allows us to smell essential oils.
- Volatile oils (high speed of absorption) have an energizing effect on the body
- Low volatility oils promote calmness

WHAT ARE THE MAJOR METHODS OF USING ESSENTIAL OILS?

- Through the skin (massage, bath, friction)
- Through inhalation
- Skin care and cosmetic use (facial, compresses, masks, lotions, creams)
- Hair care
- Ingestion: Essential oils should not be taken internally unless under the direct supervision of a professional.

WHAT DO ESSENTIAL OILS CONTAIN?

The chemistry of essential oils is complex. The essential oils vary during the day and throughout the year, depending on the part of the plant being processed (root, bark, leaves, buds, flowers, seeds) and the variety of plant, soil, and climate. Essential oils contain vitamins, hormones, antibiotics, or antiseptics. The oils are mainly constituted of terpenes, sesquiterpenes, esters, alcohols, phenols, aldehydes, ketones, and organic acids.

WHAT IS THE YIELD OF THE MOST COMMON ESSENTIAL OILS?

The yield of essential oils varies from one plant to another. To make 1 kg of essential oil, it takes approximately:

20 kg clove buds

30 kg eucalyptus leaves

150 kg lavender

300 kg peppermint

500 kg red thyme

600 kg French rosemary

800 kg clary sage

1,000 kg chamomile

3,000 kg rose

10,000 kg melissa

The difference in yields leads to variations in price from one essential oil to another. Euculyptus oil will be rather inexpensive, whereas rose oil is going to be costly (Lavabre, M. *Aromatherapy Workbook*. Healing Arts Press. 1997.)

The History of Aromatherapy

Since earliest man, aromatics have been used in rituals and religious ceremonies. The rituals were most often healing ceremonies in which the plant was burned, releasing its antiseptic effect into the air to bring about physical healing. The origin of aromatherapy dates back to ancient Egypt and India with the very precious frankincense and myrrh.

The Egyptians are considered the inventors of western medicine, pharmacy, and cosmetology. Paralleled with medicine and pharmacy, the Egyptians developed refined techniques for skin care. Cleopatra was legendary for her use of cosmetics. The Egyptians also practiced the art of massage with scented oils, unguents, creams, and aromatic wines. They also used perfumes, resins, and fragrant preparations for embalming. The antiseptic and preserving power of their essential oils was so powerful that human tissues remain preserved thousands of years later—the mummies.

India is the only place in the world where the traditions of aromatherapy have not been lost. The "Vedas," the most sacred books of India and the oldest known books, mention more than 700 different products for liturgical and therapeutic purposes, among them cinnamon, coriander, ginger, myrrh, and sandalwood.

The birthplace of modern aromatherapy was France in the 1920s. A French perfumer, René Maurice Gattefosse, burned his hand in an explosion and plunged his hand into a vat of lavender oil. The pain disappeared instantly and he recovered so quickly, he decided to investigate further the healing effects of essential oils. Gattefosse coined the term "aromatherapy."

Aromatherapy is the most commonly used complementary therapy in the United Kingdom. England, France, Switzerland, and New Zealand have professional licensing standards, and physicians can prescribe oral doses of essential oils.

In the United States, there seems to be two movements: the "genuine approach," and the "mass-market approach." The genuine approach is education driven and based on the study of essential oils as chemical substances. The genuine approach integrates body, mind, and spirit and is geared more for maintaining health rather than curing disease. The mass-market approach looks for a new trend, which often focuses on fragrances (not necessarily natural essential oils) for their mood-enhancing properties. The mass-market approach is often driven by entrepreneurs as a new way of producing large profits.

What Research, Reviews, or Comments Exist?

After attempting to analyze the research relating to aromatherapy, it appears there has been little clinical research undertaken. Most of the trials were methodologically poor or inadequately reported. Aromatherapy appears theoretically to be a promising treatment, and hopefully there will be some good quality empirical evidence to justify current practice in the near future.

PRO

Several clinical studies suggest that aromatherapy may have emotional and physical benefits. Balacs (1992) reports that there are hundreds of receptor cells that have been discovered in the nose that relay smells to the brain. Balacs also suggests that lavender has been demonstrated to increase alpha brain wave activity, which is associated with relaxation and meditative states. Rose and Behm (1994), in a controlled study, found that inhaling the vapor from black pepper extract significantly reduced cigarette smokers' craving for tobacco and seemed to improve their mood. Wilkinson (1995) concluded that by adding Roman Chamomile to massage oil for 51 patients with cancer, anxiety was reduced and there was an improvement in self-reported quality of life. These changes were greater in the study group than in the control group in which unscented oil was used. Welsh (1997) found similar results.

Stevenson (1994) found that cardiac surgery patients (unspecified number) had greater and more long-lasting psychological benefits when their feet were massaged with neroli oil (derived from orange flowers) than when unscented oil was used. Tate (1997), using a three-condition experimental design, determined that postoperative patients inhaling peppermint oil had less nausea and required less pain medication than the control group.

CON

Weiss and James (1997) have reported allergic contact dermatitis from essential oils. Tong, et al (1992) studied tea tree oil in a randomized, double-blind trial in 104 patients to determine the efficiency in treating tinea pedis. Tea tree oil appeared to be no more effective than placebo in achieving a cure. Lindsay, et al (1997) looked at the effects of massage and aromatherapy on patients with severe learning disabilities. The researchers concluded that the technique did not improve concentration scores, and may even have made the scores worse.

Lis-Balchen, et al (1997) concluded that the action of single essential oils and combination essential oils is different, and the difference cannot be predicted from animal studies; therefore, human studies must be done. Lis-Balchen concludes that there is a possible danger in the indiscriminate usage of mixes on some susceptible patients, e.g., asthmatics and patients who are pregnant or in labor.

What Is Aromatherapy Used to Treat or Improve?

Aromatherapy is a routine part of medical treatment in Europe. English nurses routinely use oils to stimulate the skin, heal wounds, and encourage sleep. Aromatherapy can be used to treat:

- Bacterial/viral infections
- Herpes simplex and zoster
- Arthritis
- Skin conditions
- Muscular disorders

- Insomnia
- Anxiety, depression
- Complications of cancer treatment (Nelson, 1997)
- Anorexia (lime, geranium, lemon grass)
- Hair loss (cedar wood, rosemary)
- Anxiety and fear (melissa, bergamot)
- Aches and pains (rosemary and lavender)

Specific application for selected oils can be found in the discussion of each oil (to follow).

What Happens During Aromatherapy?

- The practitioner takes a complete health history identifying sleep and exercise habits, dietary patterns, allergies, and any problems. Aromatherapy uses essential oils to affect the body through inhalation, external application, or ingestion.
- Through a diffuser: The diffuser projects drops of essential oils into a nebulizer, which uses air as a propellant. The nebulizer acts as an expansion chamber, where the drops of oil are broken into a thin mist. These ionized droplets remain suspended for several hours. This system is particularly effective because it diffuses the oils without altering or heating them. Essential oils can be used to achieve beneficial results in respiratory conditions, or to simply change the air with the mood-lifting or calming qualities of the fragrance.
- Through a spray: Sprayers are easy to use and portable. Sprayers create fairly large droplets, which are present for a short period of time. The area covered depends on the type of sprayer.
- External application: Oils are readily absorbed through the skin. Convenient applications are baths, massages, hot and cold compresses, or a simple topical application of diluted oils. Essential oils in a hot bath can stimulate the skin, induce relaxation, and energize the body. Using certain essential oils, such as rosemary (always use diluted rosemary and use no more than five drops) in the bath, can stimulate the elimination of toxins through the skin. In massage, the oils can be worked into the skin and, depending on the oil and the massage technique, can calm or stimulate an individual. When used in compresses, essential oils soothe minor aches and pains and reduce swelling.

Caution: Approximately 5% of the population will exhibit a dermatitis reaction to oils when applied to the skin. Occasionally, irritation can also occur from overuse of certain oils. This is nontoxic and will disappear when use of the oil is discontinued. A 1% to 3% concentration of essential oil in a base carrier oil is recommended in massage.

- Floral waters: These can be sprayed into the air or sprayed on skin that is too sensitive to touch.
- Internal application: For certain conditions (such as organ dysfunction or disorder), it can be advantageous to take oils internally, but not recommended because essential oils can be toxic to the liver. It is essential to receive proper medical guidance for internal use of oils. Such professional guidance is difficult to obtain in the United States.

Caution: Certain essential oils, such as those derived from thuja, wormwood, mugwort, tansy, hyssop, and sage, can cause a toxic reaction if taken internally. However, their toxicity is much lower when applied externally. Other essential oils with a high phenol (disinfectant) content, such as oregano and savory, should not be taken internally for any prolonged period of time (exceeding 10 to 21 days). Doing so may have negative implications on certain aspects of liver metabolism. Clove and cinnamon should also be used with caution because they are known allergens.

Natural Versus Synthetic Essential Oils

Aromatherapists believe that molecules produced through the processes of life are more active in a living context than their synthetic counterparts are, although the synthetic counterparts cannot be chemically differentiated from their natural cousins. A natural extract is often found to be more efficient than its main active ingredient. Therefore, until more research is performed, it is suggested by aromatherapists that natural essential oils are the best to use. (Lavabre, M. *Aromatherapy Workbook*. Healing Arts Press. 1997.)

The information regarding aromatherapy presented next is obtained from books written on aromatherapy. Most of this information, particularly the medical uses, are not research based, but anecdotal, passed on from generation to generation of aromatherapists.

Application of Selected Essential Oils

BERGAMOT

Name: Citrus bergamia
Family: Rutaceae
Produced in: Italy, Ivory Coast, Guinea

Process: Cold pressure—rind of fruit
Essential Oil: Yellow to emerald green
Fragrance: Sweet, citrus, floral, refreshing
Comments: Each tree is extremely prolific, can produce more than 100 fruits, and is deeply rooted
Current medicinal uses:

- Antiseptic: skin
- Antispasmodic: GI cramps, colic, stomatitis
- Skin care as a tonic

CHAMOMILE

Name: Roman Chamomile (Anthemis Nobilis)
German Chamomile (Chamomile Matricaria)
Blue Chamomile (ormenis multicolis or tannacetum anum)
Family: Compositae
Produced in: France, Monaco, Spain, Egypt
Process: Distillation of flowers
Essential Oil: Roman and German—yellow
Blue—blue because of Azulene
Fragrance: Refreshing, aromatic
Comments: Azulene has the greatest anti-inflammatory effect (decreases redness, irritation, allergic reaction, and pain). German Chamomile, the mother herb, is also used in female disorders (painful menses, irregular periods, menopause). Chamomile likes light; it grows in open fields, in light, sandy soil.
Current medicinal uses:

- Anti-inflammatory (especially matricaria)
- Antidepressant
- Antiemetic
- Antiseptic
- Hair care—adds luster and silkiness
- Stress reducer—a drop rubbed on the solar plexus can bring rapid relief of mental and physical stress

EUCALYPTUS

Name: Eucalyptus globulus
Family: Myrtaceae
Produced in: Australia, Spain, Portugal
Process: Distillation of leaves
Essential Oil: Yellow to red
Fragrance: Fresh, balsamic, camphor like

Comments: One of the tallest trees in world, fast growing with deep root system, likes fresh water

Current medicinal uses:

- General antiseptic (especially pulmonary and urinary) (Minski, 1996)
- Expectorant, decongestant
- Antiviral
- Bug repellent

GERANIUM

Name: Pelargonium graveolens
Family: Geraniaceae
Produced in: Egypt, Monaco
Process: Distillation
Essential Oil: Green-yellow
Fragrance: Strong, sweet, rose-like; best when diluted
Comments: Geranium can develop a variety of chemotypes and can be made to imitate a variety of other fragrances. This ability seems to indicate a strong adaptability, indicative of immunostimulant properties.

Current medicinal uses:

- Affects adrenal cortex by calming catecholamine release
- Affects central nervous system (CNS), balances mind and body
- Astringent for skin care
- Antiseptic antivirals with healing properties
- Hair care—tones scalp, decreases oiliness
- Insect repellent

JASMINE

Name: Jasminum grandflorium
Family: Oleaceae
Produced in: France, Northern Africa, India
Process: Solvent extraction of flowers
Essential Oil: Brown/red
Fragrance: Deep, sweet, warming, exotic
Comments: Blends well with rose, nerolic, citrus, geranium, and others; referred to by Hindus and Muslims as “oil of romance”; considered a “noble oil” of perfumery

Current medicinal uses:

- Aphrodisiac. Relieves inhibition, liberates imagination, develops playfulness, stimulates sexual chakra (energy centers) (see Ayurvedic section for more information)
- Relieves anxiety, depression

LAVENDER

Name: Lavandula angustifolia
Family: Labiatae
Produced in: France, Spain, and others, the finest quality grows approximately 3000 feet in the Alps
Process: Distillation of flowers
Essential Oil: Clear-yellow-green
Fragrance: Clean, appeasing
Comments: Dates back to the early Romans who used it in their baths. Has a high ester content. Lavender oil has been found to penetrate the skin during massage and be present in the body within 5 minutes of finishing the massage. The maximum concentration was measured in 20 minutes and most of the lavender was eliminated in 90 minutes. (Jager, et al, 1992)
Current medicinal uses:

- Tones and soothes the CNS (relieves anxiety and depression); calming, helps to relax and induce sleep (because of high ester content). A drop in a cup of water at the bedside helps to induce sleep. Also spraying the bed sheets with lavender oil has a calming, soothing effect on the CNS.
- In skin care as an antiseptic, good for dermatitis, acne, eczema; enhances wound healing, stimulates growth of new cells
- In respiratory diseases, to increase mucous elimination
- In hair care, tones and balances the scalp
- In migraine headache relief, add a few drops of lavender to a cold compress, apply to forehead and migraine pain may be lessened

MINT

Name: Peppermint (mentha piperita), Spearmint (mentha viridis)
Family: Labiatae
Produced in: All over the world, United States is the biggest producer
Process: Distillation of the plant
Essential oil: Clear to green
Fragrance: Refreshing, aromatic, soothing, warming
Comments: 20 different species of mint; likes abundant light and deep, humid soil
Current medicinal uses:

- Stimulates CNS, awakens the mind. A drop placed externally at base of brain just under hairline enhances learning, comprehension, and creativity
- Decongestant and expectorant for colds, coughs, flu

- Relaxes GI system, relieves cramps, improves digestion, relieves dyspepsia, improves appetite, relieves nausea

NEROLI (ORANGE BLOSSOMS)

Name: Citrus Vulgaris
Family: Rutaceae
Produced in: France, Spain, North Africa, United States
Process: Distillation of orange blossoms
Essential Oil: Clear to orange
Fragrance: Sweet, delicious, slightly euphoric
Comments: A native tree to China, dating back to the 1500s. Widely used as a perfume and in pastry making. Stimulates the heart chakra (see Ayurvedic section for more information)
Current medicinal uses:

- Antidepressant, for hysteria, anxiety, depression, palpitations, grief
- Antispasmodic, for GI cramps, colic
- Sedative, to enhances sleep

ROSE

Name: Rosaceae, Rose centifolia
Family: Rosaceae
Produced in: Bulgaria, Turkey
Process: Distilled (rosebuds are picked during a few morning hours only, right after the dew, and processed immediately)
Essential oil: Yellow to yellowish green
Fragrance: Sweet, refreshing
Comments: Expensive. Pure rose oil is used only in high-grade perfumes. Rose oil is most often adulterated with synthetics. Stimulates heart chakra (energy centers) (see Ayurvedic medicine section for more information)
Current medicinal uses:

- In skin care, as an astringent, for prevention of wrinkles, eczema, inflammation, and redness
- Female reproductive system
- As an antidepressant for anxiety and grief

ROSEMARY

Name: Rosamarimus officinalis
Family: Labiatae
Produced in: All over the Mediterranean Sea

Process: Distillation of the herb
Essential oil: Almost colorless
Fragrance: Aromatic, invigorating, fiery
Comments: Loves rocky, sunny slopes, grows from sea level to 2,000 feet, dates back thousands of years. Chemotypes depend where the rosemary grows (Barker, 1997). During the middle ages, the monks made a rejuvenating liquor from rosemary.
Current medicinal uses:

- Restores blood in anemia and increased menses
- Stimulates metabolism, increases digestion, acts on liver
- Antiseptic
- Acts as diuretic
- Acts on skin to heal wounds, burns, remove scabies and pediculoses, decreases painful joints of arthritis

SANDALWOOD

Name: Santalum album
Family: Santalaceae
Produced in: India (Sacred Tree), Indonesia, China
Process: Distillation of inner wood
Essential oil: Thick yellow
Fragrance: Wood, sweet, spicy, oriental
Comments: Often used as a fixative with other oils. Old recorded use in religion and cosmetics. Used as incense.
Current medicinal uses:

- Antidepressant
- Antiseptic for urinary system
- As an aphrodisiac because of its phergmore odor

TEA TREE OIL

Name: Malaleuca Alternifolia
Family: Myrtaceae
Produced in: Australia
Process: Distillation of leaves
Essential oil: Yellowish
Fragrance: Strong camphor-like, pungent
Comments: Caution: Approximately 1% to 5% of the population will exhibit a dermatitis reaction to this oil when applied to the skin, but comparatively low when ingested (in moderate doses). Occasionally, irritation can also occur from overuse of a certain oil. This is not hazardous and will disappear when use of the oil is discontinued.

Current medicinal use:
- Immunostimulant activities when used to treat acne, psoriasis, herpes
- Insect repellent for lice and mosquitoes.
- Antifungal for ringworm, athletes foot, thrush

YLANG-YLANG

Name: Unona odorantissimum
Family: Anonaceae
Produced in: Java, Madagascar, Philippines
Process: Distillation of flowers
Essential oil: Yellowish and syrupy
Fragrance: Sweet, voluptuous, exotic
Comments: Tree grows to 60 feet and produces beautiful yellow flowers
Current medicinal uses:
- In skin care, it soothing, reduces oiliness, softens, balances all skin types
- As an antiseptic for all skin diseases
- In hair care, stimulates growth
- For CNS as sedative, reduces depression, relieves insomnia
- For cardiovascular system, relieves tachycardia and reduces blood pressure, probably by reducing anxiety

MANY OTHER ESSENTIAL OILS ARE ALSO USED

Frankincense (Boswellia Carteri) is used for breast inflammation, uterine disorders, pregnancy and birth preparation, and as a respiratory expectorant.

Myrrh (Commiphora Myrrha) is used as an expectorant, astringent, anti-inflammatory, tonic, and sedative.

Everlasting (Helichrysum italicum) is used by skin care professionals in dilutions of 2% or lower for its tissue-regenerating qualities on scars. Applied topically, it is a powerful anti-inflammatory agent, and can prevent hemorrhaging and swelling after sports injuries or bruising. Because of its ketone content, this oil should only be used topically and in concentrations not exceeding 2%.

Mandarin (Citrus reticulata) has calming properties and universally pleasing fragrance that make it a top choice to release anxiety. It is typically dispersed in a room with a diffuser.

Niaouli (Melaleuca quinquenervia viridiflora) calms respiratory allergies, is a vitalizing, balancing agent for overactive and oily skin, and helps with hemorrhoids (in the nonacute stage).

Palmarosa (Cymbopogon martinii) is a staple in many different homemade aromatherapy compositions. Palmarosa's pleasant fragrance and excellent antiseptic and antiviral activity have uses in skin care and in the treatment of herpes.

Spikenard (Nardostachys jatamansi) is from the root of a plant from the Himalayan mountains. It has an open life cycle and a theoretically endless life span. One belief is that the spikenard oil embodies the life energy of the plant. For that reason it is often used at the core of aromatherapy blends that are aimed as much toward benefitting the psyche as they are the skin.

Risks, If Any, That Are Involved With the Therapy

Aromatherapy is a safe practice as long as the correct dose is used for the correct condition, but all oils can have adverse effects. Persons with asthma, lung disease, or pregnant women should not inhale oils. Careful use of oils on the skin is important to determine skin sensitivity. If oils get into the eyes, flush immediately with normal saline. See cautions throughout this section.

Essential oils that should be completely avoided:

Bitter almond
Yellow camphor
Horseradish
Mustard
Mugwort
Pennyroyal (may cause abortion if pregnant)
Sassafras
Tansy
Sage

All of these oils are likely to cause toxic skin reactions, or if absorbed, can cause severe systemic symptoms such as liver toxicity. Research into aromatherapy is in its infancy. No research yet exists on potential interaction with drugs and foods and other oils.

The Training Required of the Practitioner

Aromatherapy can be self-taught. The practitioner could be educated by taking seminars offered by various organizations and schools around the country (see listing at end of section.) The Natural Association of Holistic Aromatherapists is working to put training and licensing standards in place. The organization believes that to practice aromatherapy, one must be familiar with chemistry, botany, and physiology.

Bibliography

Balacs, T. (1992). Research reports. International Journal of Aromatherapy. 4, (1), 28–29.

Barkers, A. (1997). The herb of remembrance: exploring the chemotypes of rosemary. Aromatherapy Quarterly. (51), 9–11.

Burton Goldberg Group. (1995). Alternative medicine: the definitive guide. Fife, WA: Future Medicine Publishing.

Cerrato, P. (1998). Aromatherapy: is it for real? RN. 98, (6), 51.

Jager, W., et al. (1992). Percutaneous absorption of Lavender oil from a massage oil. The International Journal of Aromatherapy. 43, 49–54.

Lavabre, M. (1997). Aromatherapy workbook. Healing Arts Press.

Lindsay, W. R., Pitcaithly, D., Geelen, N., Buntin, L., Broxholme, S., & Ashby, M. A (1997). comparison of the effects of four therapy procedures on concentration and responsiveness in people with profound learning disabilities. Journal of Intellectual Disability Research. 41, (Pt.), 201–207.

Lis-Balchin, M., Deans, S., & Hart, S. (1997). A study of the changes in the bioactivity of essential oils used singly and as mixtures in aromatherapy. Journal of Alternative & Complementary Medicine. 3, (3), 249–256.

Minski, R. L. (1996). The benefits of eucalyptus oil. Australian Nursing Journal. 4, (2), 5.

Nelson, N. J. (1997). Scents or nonsense: aromatherapy's benefits still subject to debate. Journal of the National Cancer Institute. 89, (18), 1334–1336.

Packham, C. L. (1997). Essential oils and 'aromatherapy': their role in healing. Journal of the Royal Society of Health. 117, (6), 400.

Rose, J. E. & Behm, F. M. (1994). Inhalation of vapor from black pepper extract reduces smoking withdrawal symptoms. Drug and Alcohol Depending 34, 225.

Stevenson, C. (1994). The psychophysiological effects of aromatherapy massage following cardiac surgery. Complementary Therapies in Medicine. 2, (1), 27.

Tate, S. (1997). Peppermint oil: a treatment for postoperative nausea. Journal of Advanced Nursing. 26, (3), 543–549.

Tong, M. M., Altman, P. M., & Barnetson, R. S. (1992). Tea tree oil in the treatment of tinea pedis. Australas Journal Dermatology 33, (3), 145–149.

Weiss, R. R. & James, W. D. (1997). Allergic contact dermatitis from aromatherapy. American Journal of Contact Dermatitis. 8, (4), 250.

Welsh, C. (1997). Touch with oils: a pertinent part of holistic hospice care. American Journal of Hospice & Palliative Care. 14, (1), 42–44.

Wilkinson, S. (1995). Aromatherapy and massage in palliative care. International Journal of Palliative Nursing. 1, (1), 24.

Further Reading

Rose, J. The aromatherapy book: applications and inhalations. Berkely, CA: North Atlantic Books, 1992.

Price, S. Aromatherapy for common ailments. New York: Simon & Schuster, 1991.

Tisserand, R. Aromatherapy, to heal and tend the body. Santa Fe, NM: Lotus Light Press, 1988.

Lavabre, M. Aromatherapy workbook. Rochester, VT: Healing Arts Press, 1990.

Tisserand, R. B. The art of aromatherapy. Rochester, VT: Destiny Books, 1987.

Fisher-Rizzi, S. The complete aromatherapy handbook: essential oils for radiant health. NY: Sterling Press, 1991.

Valnet, Jean. The practice of aromatherapy. Rochester, VT: Inner Traditions, 1990.

The International Journal of Aromatherapy. PO Box 746, Hove, East Sussex, BN3 3XA, UK.

Scholes, M. Answers to commonly asked questions on aromatherapy. Aromapress. 1992. Available exclusively through the Michael Scholes School of Aromatic Studies. Los Angeles, CA. (800) 677-2368.

RESOURCES

Michael Scholes School for Aromatic Studies
117 North Robertson Blvd.
Los Angeles, CA 90048
310 276-1191, 800 677-2368, Fax 310 276-1156
E-mail: mnscholes@aol.com

The Pacific Institute of Aromatherapy
P.O. Box 6842
San Rafael, CA 94903
(415) 479-9121
Lotus Light
P.O. Box 1008
Wilmot, WI 53170
(414) 889-8501

National Association of Holistic Aromatherapy
P.O. Box 17622
Boulder, CO 80308
Jeanne Rose Aromatherapy
219 Carl Street
San Francisco, CA 94117
(415) 564-6337

The New England Center for Aromatherapy
60 Myrtle Street, Suite 1
Boston, MA 02114
(617) 720-4585

Smell and Taste Treatment and Research Foundation
Water Tower Place
845 North Michigan Avenue, Suite 990W
Chicago, IL 60611
(312) 938-1047

SUPPLIES

Aroma Vera (Manufacturer)
5901 Rodeo Road
Los Angeles, CA 90016-4312
(800) 669-9514, (310) 280-0407, Fax: (310) 280-0395

Frontier Cooperative Herbs (Manufacturer)
1 Frontier Rd.
Norway, IA 52318
(319) 227-7996

Original Swiss Aromatics (Manufacturer)
P.O. Box 606
San Rafael, CA 94915
(415) 479-9120

SELECTED AROMATHERAPY TREATMENT CENTERS

A Place To Relax
1410 Guerneville Road, Suite 11
Santa Rosa, CA 95410
(707) 573-3910

Preston Wyn Salon
14567 Big Basin Way
Saratoga, CA 95070
(408) 741-5525

Hair Studio 2000
955 West Lancaster Road
Orlando, FL 32809
(407) 857-0223

Carapan
96 5th Avenue, #9L
New York, NY 10011
(212) 633-6220

The Summit Aesthetic Spa
Park Lane Mall
5657 Spring Garden Road
Halifax, Nova Scotia, Canada B3J 3R4
(902) 423-3888

INTERNET

Office of Alternative Medicine
http://altmed.od.nih.gov/
E-mail list
send "subscribe aromatherapy-1 your name" to listserv@netcom.com

BIOFEEDBACK

What Is Biofeedback?

Biofeedback training is a method of learning how to consciously regulate normally unconscious bodily functions (such as breathing, heart rate, and blood pressure) to improve overall health. It refers to any process that measures and reports back immediate information about the biologic system of the person being monitored so he or she can learn to consciously influence that system, and thus gain control over activities that are not usually thought to be controllable. At first, equipment with audio or visual response is used to train the individual to control bodily functions and then eventually the control is performed without the equipment. With continued practice, the skills continue to improve. Biofeedback has been supported by much research and is used today by traditional and complementary practitioners.

Biofeedback:

- Trains the individual to relax and pay attention to body responses
- Can be measured by skin temperature (thermal), muscle tension (electrodermal), heart rate (EKG), brain wave activity (electroencephalographic), or respiratory rate
- Uses various techniques (meditation, relaxation, visualization) to effect the desired response

What Is the History of Biofeedback?

Biofeedback is a relatively new technique, first presented by Dr. H. Mowrer in 1938. Dr. Mowrer used an alarm system to stop bed wetting in children. In 1960, at the Menninger Foundation in Topeka, KS, Dr. E. Green identified that yogis could control breathing and alter their state of consciousness using EEG feedback. News of this research along with subjects being able to achieve a "drugless high" piqued public interest. The altered state of consciousness could now be measured.

What Research, Reviews, and Comments Exist?

Much research has been performed (at least 3,000 research articles and more than 100 books) on biofeedback demonstrating its effectiveness. Biofeedback is an approved treatment for headache control, chronic pain syndromes, attention deficit disorders, hot flashes, incontinence, and Raynaud's disease. Selected research is presented.

PRO

Moser, et al (1997) demonstrated that in a single session, patients with advanced heart failure were able to increase finger temperature and cardiac output and decrease systemic vascular resistance and respiratory rate, without any effect of systemic levels of catecholamines or O_2 consumption. Moreland, et al (1998) performed a meta-analysis on published studies from 1976 to 1995, and found that all studies indicate that EMG biofeedback is superior to conventional therapy alone for improving ankle dorsiflexion muscle strength. Linden, et al (1996) used biofeedback to improve the IQ and intellectual functioning and decrease the inattention behaviors in a group of children with attention deficit disorders and learning disabilities. Glia, et al (1998) used biofeedback to significantly improve fecal incontinence. Positive results were still present at follow-up 21 months later. Payne (1998) used biofeedback to improve urinary incontinence in women and Mathewson-Chapman (1997) used biofeedback to improve urinary incontinence in men after prostatectomy. Both studies have demonstrated a statistically significant result over the control group.

CON

Vander Plas, et al (1996) found that biofeedback training did not result in a higher success rate in treating 200 children with constipation.

What Is Biofeedback Used to Treat or Improve?

There are at least 150 uses for biofeedback:

- Sleep disorders, insomnia
- Hyperactivity in children
- Behavioral disorders
- Postural problems
- Pain control (back ache, headache)
- Temporal mandibular joint syndrome
- Heart disorders, hypertension
- Reduction and control of stress and anxiety
- GI disorders (ulcers, irritable bowel syndrome)
- Urinary and fecal incontinence

What Happens During Biofeedback?

- A device is used to measure some autonomic body response (skin temperature, heart rate, brain wave activity, or muscle tension).

- The practitioner interprets the signals and guides the patient through mental and physical exercises to achieve the desired response.
- The patient learns to recognize the pattern during the practice sessions.
- A stressor is added and the patient learns to recognize the stress response.
- The patient is then instructed to use various techniques such as meditation, relaxation, and visualization to return the measurement to normal.
- Patient practices the techniques to achieve the desired response.
- Seven to twelve 30-minute training sessions are generally recommended.

Are There Any Risks Involved With Biofeedback?

Few risks exist. Local irritation to the electrodes may be experienced by some patients. Patients with low blood pressure should be monitored throughout the procedure because the relaxation response may lower blood pressure.

Biofeedback is contraindicated in patients with dementia, severe depression, or severe attention or memory deficits.

Biofeedback is used cautiously with persons with psychoses, seizures, hyperactive conditions, and diabetes. Relaxation exercises in persons with diabetes can beneficially reduce blood sugar, but hypoglycemic reactions may occur.

What Training Is Required of the Practitioner?

The practitioners of biofeedback must have a complete understanding of physiology and psychology. Most practitioners are psychologists, but other health professionals, including nurses, may use biofeedback. Practitioners are certified by the Biofeedback Certification Institute of America.

Bibliography

Glia, A., Gylin, M., Akerlund, J. E., Lindfors, U., & Lindberg, G. (1998). Biofeedback training in patients with fecal incontinence. Diseases of the Colon and Rectum. 41, (3), 359–364.

Linden, M., Habib, T., & Radojevic, V. (1996). A controlled study of the effects of EEG biofeedback on cognition and behavior of children with attention deficit disorder and learning disabilities. Biofeedback & Self Regulation. 21, (1), 35–49.

Mathewson-Chapman, M. (1997). Pelvic muscle exercise/biofeedback for urinary incontinence after prostatectomy: an education program. Journal of Cancer Education. 12, (4), 218–223.

Moreland, J. D., Thomson, M. A., Fuoco, A. R. (1998). Electromyographic biofeedback to improve lower extremity function after stroke: a meta-analysis. Archives of Physical Medicine & Rehabilitation. 79, (2), 134–140.

Moser, D. K., Dracup, K., Woo, M., & Stevenson, L. (1997). Voluntary control of vascular tone by using skin-temperature biofeedback-relaxation in patients with advanced heart failure. Alternative Therapies. 3, (1), 51–59.

Payne, C. K. (1998). Biofeedback for community-dwelling individuals with urinary incontinence. Urology. 51, (Suppl 2A), 35–39.

Vander Plas, R. N., Benninger, M. A., Buller, H. A., et al. (1996). Biofeedback training in treatment of childhood constipation: a randomized controlled study. Lancet. 348, 776–778.

RESOURCES

Micro Straight, Inc.
2709 Cherry Street
Kansas City, MO 64108
(816) 474-0144, (800) 238-2225

Tools for Exploration
4460 Redwood Highway, Suite 2
San Rafael, CA 94903

Center for Applied Psychophysiology Menninger Clinic
P.O. Box 829
Topeka, KS 66601-0829
(913) 273-7500, ext. 5375

Association for Applied Psychophysiology and Biofeedback
10200 West 44th Avenue, Suite 304
Wheat Ridge, CO 80033
(303) 422-8436

Biofeedback Certification Institutes of America
10200 West 44th Avenue, Suite 304
Wheat Ridge, CO 80033
(303) 420-2902

INTERNET

Association of Applied Psychophysiology and Biofeedback
http://aapb.org

"If you can laugh at it, you can live with it."

—AUTHOR UNKNOWN

DANCE THERAPY

What Is Dance Therapy?

Dance movement therapies emphasize the holism of human beings. The combination of movement and breathing engages the body and mind. The continuous interchanges of weight-bearing and non–weight-bearing legs enhances balances and effects motor control and coordination in the brain. Dance may range in physical intensity from low, moderate, and high so it may also be a method of improving cardiovascular fitness. Dance therapy:

- Offers exercise and many physical benefits
- Is primarily used for psychotherapeutic purposes in groups
- Groups are a safe setting to express internal fears, anger, rage, joy, and sorrow
- Is used to recreate feeling states

What Is the History of Dance Therapy?

Dance is one of the oldest art forms used to heal the sick and celebrate major events in many cultures. Dance therapy was first accepted as a medical therapy in the United States in 1942. Dance teacher, M. Chace worked with disturbed psychiatric patients in Washington, D.C., and T. Schoop worked with noncommunicative patients in California. Both had excellent results with their patients. The American Dance Therapy Association was formed in 1956 to promote research, create and monitor dance therapists, and develop guidelines for dance educators.

What Research, Reviews, and Comments Exists?

PRO

Hanna (1995) and Serlin, et al (1997) identified that dance therapy was a healing process that allowed persons to gain a sense of control in their life. Kudlacek, et al (1997) demonstrated that a 12- month dance program could increase spinal and peripheral bone mass. Lewis and Scannel (1995) and Adams, et al (1991) identified that dance therapy had a positive impact on improving body image. Participants were more satisfied with their appearance, fitness, and body parts after participating in a dance program. Heber (1993) demonstrated that dance therapy improved the emotional, psychological, and physical well-being of psychiatric patients.

CON

No evidence of con research was found when a Medline search was performed.

What Is Dance Therapy Used to Treat or Improve?

- As psychotherapy to draw out clients and improve their ability to communicate
- To retrain body parts in rehabilitation programs for patients with stroke or brain injury
- For chronic disease such as Alzheimer's to retain muscle tone
- For autistic, emotionally disturbed, or learning-disabled children to enhance communication
- For patients with cancer to express their loss
- To reduce and control stress
- To improve flexibility, strengthen muscles, and improve cardiovascular and respiratory function, particularly in the elderly
- To promote socialization and sense of connectedness with one's own body and the group
- To diminish shyness, and improve self-esteem and body image

What Happens During Dance Therapy?

- Movements may be spontaneous or choreographed sequences
- The therapist interacts with each participant and guides movement and discusses feelings
- Adequate space and enjoyable music are selected
- Faster music is chosen to stimulate the group and slower music provides a calming effect

Are There Any Risks Involved With Dance Therapy?

Dance therapy is safe for most people. A complete physical should be performed on everyone before beginning dance therapy, particularly if aerobic activity is included. Dizziness may be a complaint of some persons when rapid up and down movements are used. Vigorous exercise may also result in sore muscles and muscle strains.

What Training Is Required of the Practitioner?

American Dance Association offers graduate degrees in dance therapy. Teachers must be qualified in psychiatry or social work to handle any issues or problems that arise during the sesions.

Bibliography

Adams, D. D., Radell, S. A., Johnson, T. C., & Cole, S. P. (1991). Physical fitness, body image, and locus of control in college women dancers and nondancers. Perception and Motor Skills. 72, (1), 91–95.

Hanna, J. L. (1995). The power of dance: health and healing. Journal of Alternative & Complementary Medicine. 1, (4), 323–331.

Heber, L. (1993). Dance movement: a therapeutic program for psychiatric clients. Perspectives in Psychiatric Care. 29, (2), 22–29.

Kudlacek, S., Pietschmann, F., Bernecker, P., Resch, H., & Willvonseder, R. (1997). The impact of a senior dancing program on spinal and peripheral bone bass. American Journal of Physical Medicine and Rehabilitation. 76, (6), 477–481.

Lewis, R. N. & Scannell, E. D. (1995). Relationship of body image and creative dance movement. Perception and Motor Skills. 81, (1), 155–160.

Serlin, I., Frances, B., Vestevich, K., Bailey, T., & Lavaysse, L. (1997). The effect of dance/movement therapy on women with breast cancer. Alternative Therapies Symposium Abstracts. 3, (2), 103.

RESOURCES

American Dance Therapy Association
2000 Century Plaza, Suite 108
Columbia, MD 21044
(301) 997-4040

If you want others to be happy, practice compassion.
If you want to be happy, practice compassion.

—DALAI LAMA

GUIDED IMAGERY

What Is Guided Imagery?

Imagery is a mind-body technique based on the principle that the mind and body are interconnected and can be encouraged to work together to treat disease and heal. Imagery, guided imagery, self-hypnosis, and visualization are all synonymous terms. Imagery:

- Is a flow of thoughts that one can see, hear, feel, or taste in one's imagination
- Directly affects physiology
- Provides insight into health through association and synthesis of mental processes
- Represents an experience, fantasy, and is highly personal
- Always reflects internal reality and may reflect external reality
- Is a natural way the nervous system stores, accesses, and processes information
- Maintains a constant dialogue between mind and body, which is a source of the body's power in the healing process
- Can affect heart and respiratory rate, GI function, sexual arousal, and levels of hormones and neurotransmitters
- Has an intimate relationship with emotions
- Can assist with accessing emotions and consciously altering their effect
- Is part of almost all relaxation and stress-reduction techniques
- Is a method of treating people, not symptoms or diseases

What Is the History of Guided Imagery?

Imagery has been used since at least the Middle Ages, when Tibetan monks tried to visualize the Buddha healing disease. In recent times, bidirectional therapy (the mind affects the body, the body affects the mind) was first proposed in the late 1800s by William James, the father of American psychology. During the last 30 years, there has been a powerful scientific movement to explore the mind's ability to influence the body.

What Research, Reviews, and Comments Exist?

PRO

In 1993, Rossman demonstrated with positron emission tomography (PET) that the same areas of the brain are activated whether people imagine or experience an event. Benson (1993) found that relaxation makes the mind more receptive to new information. McKinney, et al (1997) found that persons who taught guided imagery had a significant self-reported decrease in depression, fatigue, and total mood disturbances after 6 weeks of daily practice. Spiegel and Moore (1997), in a 10-year trial, found that women who were taught and practiced daily imagery had a longer survival from cancer. Richardson, et al (1997) also found that guided imagery reduced stress and improved quality of life and coping ability in women with breast cancer. Syrjala, et al (1995) identified that use of relaxation and guided imagery reduced cancer treatment pain significantly. Tusek, et al (1997) found that guided imagery, taught preoperatively, significantly reduced postoperative anxiety, pain, and narcotic requirements after colorectal surgery.

CON

Field, et al (1997) found the guided imagery was no more beneficial or successful in reducing job stress than social support or muscle relaxation techniques.

What Is Guided Imagery Used to Treat or Improve?

Imagery is a complementary treatment for just about all conditions, including injuries or illness. Specifically, imagery can be used to:

- Reduce acute and chronic pain
- Treat (maybe cure) cancer
- Relieve headaches and all types of discomforts
- Relieve premenstrual syndrome
- Assist with smoking and drug withdrawal
- Relieve and eliminate allergies
- Relieve benign arrhythmias
- Lower high blood pressure
- Relieve anxiety
- Accelerate healing of sprains, strains, and fractures
- Relieve acute symptoms of colds and flus
- Enhance immune system function
- Enhance self-esteem
- Bring about a behavior change

What Happens During Guided Imagery?

Directions are given by a coach, teacher, or audio tape:

- Expect to sit quietly, breathe deeply, and with each breath imagine you are taking in calmness and peacefulness.
- As you breathe, relax each part of your body from your feet up to your head (deep relaxation is necessary for imagery because it reduces muscle tension and promotes images).

- Now imagine yourself in a favorite place. Visualize how restful, peaceful, and quiet it is. Notice what you feel, hear, and smell.
- Now you may image a decrease in disease, decrease in symptoms, and so on.
- When you are ready, allow the image to fade, stretch, and open your eyes.
- Sessions may last 10 to 15 minutes to 1 hour.
- Music or scents may be used during the experience.
- Guided imagery involves imaging through any sense and usually uses all six senses—visual, aural, tactile, olfactory, proprioceptive, and kinesthetic.

Are There Any Risks Involved With Guided Imagery?

Guided imagery is mostly considered to be safe, but some dialogue audio tapes may bring up powerful negative thoughts that may be confusing or frightening.

- Imagery is contraindicated in psychotic patients because of the negative thoughts that may be provoked.
- Imagery is used cautiously with person with underlying lung disease because respiratory distress may occur.

What Training Is Required of the Practitioner?

Guided imagery may be self-taught through books or tapes or be taught by a trained professional. There is a 150-hour certification program available for teachers.

Bibliography

Benson, H. (1993). The relaxation response. In: Goleman, D. & Gurin, J. Eds. Mind/body medicine. 233–258. Yonkers, NY: Consumers Union.

Field, T., Quintero, O., Henleff, T., et al. (1997). Job stress reduction therapies. Alternative Therapy in Health & Medicine. 3, (4), 54–56.

McKinney, C. H., Tims, F. C., Kumar, A. M., & Kumar, M. (1997). The effect of selected classical music and spontaneous imagery on plama beta-endorphin. Journal of Behavioral Medicine. 20, (1), 85–99.

McKinney, C. H., Antoni, M. H., Kumar, M., Tims, F. C., & McCabe, P. M. (1997). Effects of guided imagery and music (GIM) therapy on mood and cortisol in healthy adults. Health Psychology. 16, (4), 390–400.

Rees, B. L. (1995). Effect of relaxation with guided imagery on anxiety, depression, and self-esteem in primiparas. Journal Holistic Nursing. 13, 255–267.

Richardson, M. A., Post-White, J., Grimm, E. A., Moye, L. A., Singletary, S. E., & Justice, B. (1997). Coping, life attitudes, and immune responses to imagery and group support after breast cancer treatment. Alternative Therapies in Health & Medicine. 3, (5) 62–70.

Rossman, M. (1993). Imagery: learning to use the mind's eye. In: Goleman D., & Gurin, J. Eds. Mind/body medicine. 291–300. Yonkers, NY: Consumers Union.

Spiegel, D. & Moore, R. (1997). Imagery and hypnosis in the treatment of cancer patients. Oncology. 11, (8), 1179–1189; discussion 1189-95, 1997.

Syrjala, K. L., Donaldson, G. W., Davis, M. W., Kippes, M. E., & Carr, J. E. (1995). Relaxation and imagery and cognitive-behavioral training reduce pain during cancer treatment: a controlled clinical trial. Pain. 63, 189–198.

Tusek, D. L., Church, J. M., Stong, S. A., et al. (1997). Guided imagery: a significant advance in the care of patients undergoing elective colorectal surgery. Diseases of the Colon and Rectum. 40, (2), 172–178.

Further Reading

Bresler, D. Free yourself from pain. Topanga, CA: The Bresler Center, 1992.

Fexler, W. Total visualization. New Jersey: Prentice Hall, 1992.

Jaffe, D. Healing from within. New York: (Fireside) Simon and Schuster, 1988.

RESOURCES

The Academy for Guided Imagery
P O. Box 2070
Mill Valley, CA 94942
(800) 726-2070

American Holistic Medical Association and American Holistic Nurses Association
4101 Lake Boone Trail, Suite 201
Raleigh, NC 27607
(919) 787-5146, (800) 878-3373

Simonton Cancer Center
P.O. Box 890
Pacific Palisades, CA 90272
(310) 459-4434

Center for Applied Psychophysiology
Minninger Clinic
P.O. Box 829
Topeka, KS 66601-08829
(913) 273-7500 Ext. 5375

INTERNET

Mind-Body Healing
http://www.wholeness.com/

http://www.queendom.com/main.html
http://ayurvedahc.com/aycertif.htm

Office of Alternative Medicine
http://altmed.od.nig.gov/

The next major advance in the health of the American people will be determined by what the individual is willing to do for himself.

—John Knowles, Former President of the Rockefeller Foundation

HYPNOTHERAPY

What Is Hypnotherapy?

Hypnotherapy uses the power of suggestion and trance-like states to access the deepest levels of the mind to effect positive changes in a person's behavior and to treat a wide range of conditions. Under hypnosis, patients can experience relaxation and changes in vital signs. Hypnosis can lead to positive changes in behavior. Hypnotherapy is a state of attentive and focused concentration that leaves people relatively unaware of their surroundings.

There are three major components of hypnosis:

- Absorption involves the complete attention that the individual pays to the words or images presented by the therapist
- Dissociation involves the person leaving his or her ordinary consciousness and surroundings
- Responsiveness involves the person becoming responsive to the therapist

All hypnosis is ultimately self-hypnosis. The therapist is a facilitator; there can be no hypnosis unless the client is a willing participant in the process. The person always enters a hypnotic state in a natural way. During hypnosis, the person has a heightened receptivity to suggestion.

People who benefit most believe that hypnosis is not surrender of control, but only an advanced form of relaxation.

There are two states of hypnosis:

- Superficial state, in which a person accepts suggestions, but may not carry them out.
- Somnambulistic state, a deeper state of relaxation in which a person accepts the suggestions and carries them out after the session.

What Is the History of Hypnotherapy?

Hypnotherapy has been part of healing dating back to ancient Greece and Persia. Hypnotherapy was a central part of healing in the Greek temples. The power of suggestion and trance-like states assisted people in the search for health. Modern application dates to the 18th Century to Dr. F. Mesmer with his use of hypnotherapy to treat headaches, joint pain, hysterical blindness, and other physiologic and psychologic disorders. Mesmer's principles became the foundation for Sigmund Freud who also used hypnotherapy in his early practice.

The British Medical Association recognized hypnotherapy as a valid medical treatment in 1955, and the American Medical Association did the same in 1958. The American Society of Clinical Hypnotists began in 1957 and has grown to thousands of members who use hypnotherapy alone or in conjunction with other therapies. The organization, based on research performed by its members, suggests that 94% of patients benefit from hypnotherapy, even if its only benefit is relaxation.

What Research, Reviews, and Comments Exist?

PRO

Ashton, et al (1997) found that self-hypnosis relaxation techniques created a more restful, complication-free postoperative period in patients having coronary artery bypass surgery. Olness, et al (1997) found that children taught self-hypnosis had a significant reduction in the number and severity of migraine headache episodes. LaVorgner-Smith (1997) found that teaching women with osteoporosis self-hypnosis techniques improved quality of life and improved well-being.

Johnson, et al (1996) found that hypnotherapy was able to improve the immune response on biochemical assay; therefore, hypnotherapy may be able to enhance resistance to disease. Horton-Hausknecht (1995) reviewed 115 studies, all of which cited strong evidence for a bidirectional interaction between the CNS and the immune system, leading to the belief that hypnosis was capable of enhancing immune system function.

CON

No evidence of con research was found when a Medline search was performed.

What Is Hypnotherapy Used to Treat or Improve?

Hypnotherapy can be used to treat psychological and physical conditions. It can:

- Decrease phobias and anxiety states
- Decrease all types of headaches in severity and number
- Gain control over depression
- Improve self-esteem
- Control pain, acute and chronic (arthritic, surgical, menstrual)
- Enhance the healing process
- Gain control over some fear or anxiety (fear of flying)
- Assist with habit control (cigarette smoking, eating)
- In surgical procedures (increase relaxation, control pain, reduce bleeding)
- Shorten labor and decrease pain of delivery

What Happens During Hypnotherapy?

There are numerous ways that can be used to induce hypnosis. All require:

- Rapport between the therapist and the client
- Comfortable, quiet environment
- Willingness on the part of the client to be hypnotized
- Acceptance on the part of the client that the therapist's words and suggestions are descriptions of reality
- Acceptance of the suggestions without criticism or analysis

In addition:

- A complete history is obtained.
- The therapist addresses any concerns that the client may have and perhaps illustrates how suggestions work in everyday life.
- A session lasts 60 to 90 minutes and usually 2 to 12 sessions are required.
- The therapist is a facilitator. The therapist leads the client to a state of deep relaxation. During this state, the therapist makes suggestions that will take effect after the patient awakens.

Are There Any Risks Involved With Hypnotherapy?

Hypnotherapy is a safe practice in the hands of a qualified practitioner. It should not be used in organic psychiatric conditions, antisocial personality disorders, and patients with psychoses. It should never be performed by amateurs.

If the client becomes frightened, anxious, or aggressive, the therapist will direct them to a more pleasant, safe memory and terminate the session.

Some clients may experience lightheadedness and dizziness after the session. The client should lie quietly for several minutes after the session until these sensations end. The therapist stays with the client through the entire session.

What Training Is Required of the Practitioner?

Professional psychologists, nurses, or physicians take additional training and become certified by the American Society of Clinical Hypnosis

Bibliography

Ashton, C., Whitworth, G. C., Seldomridge, J. A., et al. (1997). Self-hypnosis reduces anxiety following coronary artery bypass surgery: a prospective, randomized trial. Journal of Cardiovascular Surgery. 38, (1), 69–75.

Horton-Hausknecht, J. R. (1995). The effect of clinical hypnosis and relaxation techniques on the functioning of the immune system: new directions for psychoneuroimmunology research and practice. Forschende Komplementarmed. 2, 196–202.

Johnson, V. C., Walker, L. G., Heys, S., Whiting, P. H., & Eremin, O. (1996). Can relaxation training and hypnotherapy modify the immune response to stress, and is hypnotizability relevant? Contemporary Hypnosis. 13, (2), 100–108.

LaVorgna-Smith, M. (1997). Hypnotherapy/meditation and mind/body healing: a phenomenological study of women with osteoporosis. (Paper presented, San Diego, CA. 1997). Alternative Therapies Conference 3, (2), 97.

Olness, K., Hall, H., Schmidt, W., & Theoharides, T. (1997). Mast cell activation in child migraine patients before and after training in self regulation. (Paper presented at San Diego, CA 1997). Alternative Therapies Conference. 3, (2), 100.

RESOURCES

The American Institute of Hypnotherapy
1805 East Garry Avenue, Suite 100
Santa Ana, CA 92705
(714) 261-6400

The American Society of Clinical Hypnosis
2200 East Devon Avenue, Suite 291
Des Paines, IL 60018
(708) 297-3317

International Medical and Dental Hypnotherapy Association
4110 Edgeland, Suite 800
Royal Oak, MI 48073
(313) 549-5594, (800) 257-5467

The National Guild of Hypnotists
P.O. Box 308
Merrimack, NH 03054

INTERNET

Office of Alternative Medicine
http://altmed.od.nig.gov/

MEDITATION

What Is Meditation?

Meditation is defined in several ways: a systematic and continued focusing of the attention on a single target perception—a sound or mantra—or continually holding a specific attention set; or a technique that allows a person to investigate the process of his or her consciousness and experiences to discover the more basic underlying qualities of existence; or simply any activity that keeps the attention pleasantly anchored in the present moment. Meditation is a way we learn to access the relaxation response.

There are two basic approaches to meditation: concentrative and mindfulness meditation. Concentrative meditation involves focusing on an image, sound (mantra), or one's own breathing. Transcendental Meditation (TM), popular in the 1960s, is a form of concentrative meditation, as well as the relaxation response of Dr. Herbert Benson of Harvard Medical School. When other thoughts enter the mind, the person is taught to notice them and gently return to his or her mantra. Concentrating on the mantra usually prevents any distracting thoughts. Mindful meditation focuses on awareness of feelings, images, thoughts, sounds, and smells that pass through the mind without concentrating on them. The goal of mindful meditation is a calmer, clearer, nonreactive state of mind.

Many meditations are actually forms of imagery and visualization that can be guided to heal old traumas, confront death, finish "old business," learn to forgive, and enhance self-esteem. The longer one meditates, the further is the expansion of self-understanding. Meditation is:

- A technique that actively keeps the attention pleasantly anchored in the present.

- When the mind is not preoccupied with memories of the past or preoccupied with plans for the future.
- Research has demonstrated that reactions are faster, creativity is greater, and comprehension is broader after meditation.

What Is the History of Meditation?

Meditation arose out of the practice of yoga (see Yoga for more information) and Eastern religions hundreds of years ago. Meditation can be done sitting quietly as in yoga, or moving.

Moving meditation includes Tai Chi of China, Aikido of Japan, or the walking meditation of the Zen Buddhist. Christian prayer, saying the rosary or the "Our Father," is also a form of meditation.

Dr. Hans Seley, the Canadian stress researcher, suggested that an individual who is aware of his own reaction to stress, is more in control of his stress. Meditation provides the person with that internal sense of control over stress.

Dr. Herbert Benson developed his "relaxation response" and did much research in the 1960s in patients with cardiac problems to determine its benefits. Today, well-known physicians, Dean Ornish, Larry Dossey, Deepok Chapra, Bernie Siegel, and Norman Shealy, advocate meditation for total well-being and improvement in the physiologic, psychologic, and spiritual domains.

What Research, Reviews, and Comments Exist?

PRO

Dr. Herbert Benson, in his book, *The Relaxation Response* (1975), studied the relaxation response and identified that it significantly lowered blood pressure in hypertensive individuals. A recent study completed at W. Oakland's Health Center in California, observed 100 people, 55 and older, with hypertension. After being taught TM and practicing TM daily for 3 months, all had a significant decrease in blood pressure. Some were able to discontinue their medications and thus the side effects of medication and possible other drug interactions were eliminated. Schneider, et al (1998) found that persons practicing TM for years (average 16.5 years) had a lowered serum lipid peroxide level. High lipid peroxide levels may contribute to atherosclerosis and other chronic diseases. Cole (1997) used meditation in palliative care to decrease the anxiety of impending death with great success. Walton, et al (1995) demonstrated that the more meditation was practiced on a daily basis, the lower the stress level and the lower the blood pressure. Harte, et al (1995) found that meditation increases plasma corticotrophin-releasing hormone, which itself is significantly associated with circulating B-endorphins and a calming effect. This effect was previously thought only to be activated by exercise. Much research was performed in the 1980s (Frenn, et al 1986; Guzzetta, 1989; Melville, 1987; Moreno, 1987) to examine the use of meditation in patients with coronary conditions in the CCU. All studies demonstrated positive results finding that meditation lowered apical heart rates, increased peripheral temperatures, and overall, patients experienced fewer complications.

Studies on meditation over the years have shown such sufficient promise that the NIH allocated $3 million in 1998 to further study meditation's effect on hypertension.

CON

No evidence of con research was found when a Medline search was performed.

What Is Meditation Used to Treat or Improve?

- Used to clear the mind and enhance mental functioning
- May enhance immune function and assist with treating chronic disease
- May be part of a life plan to reverse heart disease (Dr. Dean Ornish)
- Reduces signs and symptoms of asthma
- Relieves acute and chronic pain
- Reduces anxiety with acute conditions such as surgery, myocardial infarction, or diagnostic tests
- Desensitizes for phobias
- Reduces incidences and symptoms of headache
- Reduces insomnia
- Promotes menstrual comfort
- Reduces signs and symptoms of posttraumatic stress syndrome.
- Reduces blood pressure and possibly the need for antihypertensive medications

What Happens During Meditation?

Meditation can be taught by anyone experienced with the technique, or self taught. Many audio tapes are available to take one into a meditative state. During meditation:

- Sit in a relaxed position, in a private, quiet environment
- Close the eyes
- Focus on breathing slowly and deeply
- Relax muscles sequentially from feet to head
- Clear the mind of all thoughts by concentrating on breathing or repeating a word
- If the mind wanders, gently bring it back to your breathing or word
- Spend 15 to 20 minutes one to two times a day in meditation

Persons should be taught to maintain a passive attitude and permit relaxation to occur at its own pace. Anyone can meditate, but success at meditation takes practice.

Are There Any Risks Involved With Meditation?

- Meditation is relatively safe, but it should not be used alone to treat acute or chronic conditions.
- Persons are encouraged to rest for several minutes after meditation to decrease risks of orthostatic hypotension when rising.
- Meditation should not be used with patients with schizophrenia or patients with attention deficit disorder because these conditions may worsen.

What Training Is Required of the Practitioner?

- Can be self-taught or taught by a qualified instructor.

Bibliography

Benson, H. (1975). The relaxation response. New York: Avon Books.

Cole, R. (1997). Meditation in palliative care—a practical tool for self-management. Palliative Medicine. 11, (5), 411–413.

Frenn, M., et al. (1986). Reducing the stress of cardiac catheterization by teaching relaxation. Dimensions of Critical Care Nursing. 5, (2), 108–116.

Guzzetta, C. E. (1989). Effects of relaxation and music therapy on patients in a coronary care unit with presumptive acute myocardial infarction. Heart Lung. 18, (6), 609–616.

Harte, J. L., Eifert, G. H., & Smith, R. (1995). The effects of running and meditation on beta-endorphin, corticotropin-releasing hormone and cortisol in plasma, and on mood. Biology and Psychology. 40, 251–265.

Melville, S. B. (1987). Relaxation techniques in acute myocardial infarction: the theoretic rationale. Focus on Critical Care. 14, (1), 9–11.

Moreno, C. K. Concepts of stress management in cardiac rehabilitation. Focus on Critical Care. 14, (5), 13–19.

Schneider, R. H., Nidich, S. I., Salerno, J. W., et al. (1998). Lower lipid peroxide levels in practitioners of the Transcendental Meditation program. Psychosomatic Medicine. 60, (1), 38–41.

Walton, K. G., Pugh, N. D., Gelderloos, P., & Macrae, P. (1995). Stress reduction and preventing hypertension: preliminary support for a psychoneuroendocrine mechanism. Journal of Alternative and Complementary Medicine. 1, (3), 263–283.

Further Reading

Benson, H. The relaxation response. New York: Outlet Books, Inc., 1993.

Benson, H. & Procter, W. Beyond the relaxation response. NY: Putnam/Berkley, Inc., 1984.

Hendricks, G. Conscious breathing. New York: Bantam Books, 1995.

Kabat-Zinn, J. Full catastrophe living. New York: Delacorte Press, 1990.

Mills, J. Mind, body, and soul balance. California: Mills Publishing, 1993.

Roth, R. Transcendental meditation. New York: Donald I. Fine, Inc., 1988.

Wallace, R. K. The neurophysiology of enlightenment. Fairfield, IA: Maharishi International University Neuroscene Press, 1986.

RESOURCES

Stress Reduction Clinic
University of Massachusetts Medical Center
55 Lake Avenue, North
(508) 856-2656

INTERNET

Office of Alternative Medicine
http://altmed.od.nig.gov/

Meditation
http://www.syda.org/glossary.html
http://www.sivananda.org/meditati.htm
http://www.diamondway-buddhism.org/meditations/me-e-gy.htm
http://www.geocities.com/RodeoDrive/1415indexc.html

We must take responsibility for our happiness and stop blaming and directing control outside of ourselves. Grab hold of all that you are. Discover new and different aspects of yourself and life—Through a happy, positive set of glasses—They are there, waiting for you to put them on.

—HELENE NAWROCKI

QIGONG

What Is Qigong?

Qigong (pronounced chee-gong) is a combination of two words, "Qi" or "chi," meaning energy and "gong" meaning work or exercise (for more information, see Oriental Medicine section). Therefore, Qigong is exercising with your vital energy. Qigong is also referred to as "Breathing Exercise," "Longevity Method," and "Internal Training." There are thousands of varieties of Qigong, but usually it is classified into several schools:

- Daoist Qigong consists of soft, internal relaxation and steady, gentle training movements with postures moving from soft to hard.
- Buddhist Qigong consists of strong, active, dynamic, and external movements with postures moving from hard to soft.
- Dao and Buddhist Qigong aim to achieve an equal balance of yin and yang and empty the mind.
- Confucian Qigong is rare. Its methods are basic and simplistic.
- Medical Qigong is concerned with theory not practice, concerned with acupuncture points and channels.
- Martial Art Qigong has internal training and uses either or both Daoist and Buddhist techniques.

There are two ways to practice Qigong—active or passive (discussed later). The practice of Qigong is most important to one part of the body—the *Dantien*. ("Dan" means crystal or essence of energy, "tien" means field or area for the essence of energy). It is the area of the body that stores our Chi to balance the body. The Dantien can be related to the sun in our solar system, the father in a family, or the capital of a country. The practice of Qigong, then, allows the body to cultivate and build Chi and store the Chi in the Dantien. By cultivating and building Chi, the body builds resistance to disease and helps cure disease, and the Chinese say that once Chi cures disease, the disease will never return because the body has developed immunity.

Qigong:

- Uses breathing techniques, specific movements, and meditation to stimulate the flow of Chi (Qi) (energy)
- Cultivates inner strength, calms the mind, and restores or maintains body in natural state of health
- Creates energy flow directed along the acupuncture meridian pathways to maintain health

What Is the History of Qigong?

Qigong is one of the most ancient health exercises that has been passed down from generation to generation for more than 3,000 years. Qigong was developed as a way of enhancing energy flow throughout the body. In approximately 250 BC, a famous Chinese doctor, Hwa Tou, created "Five Animal Play." He watched how wild animals lived and moved and maintained their bodies' natural balance; and he further saw how man had lost his natural ability. Five Animal Play was designed to help people relearn this skill to cure illness and strengthen the body. Hwa Tou explained that when you raised your arms above your head, as if they were the horns of a deer, it stimulated the Chi circulation of the liver; when you stretched your arms out like a bird spreading its wings, it was good for the heart and relieving tension; rubbing and slapping yourself and moving like a monkey was good for the spleen; stretching your arms out in front of you while exhaling, like a tiger, was good for releasing the tension in the lungs; and bending forward like the bear was good for the back and the kidneys. Hwa Tou used the names of animals because it made the exercises easier to remember and by using wild animals, instead of domestic ones, he made the exercises sound exhilarating. All these movements help the Chi flow along the channels, strengthening the body and promoting vitality. They also balance the circulation and stimulate the internal organs.

The famous 17th Century BC philosopher Lao Zi advised people to relax their hearts (meaning their chests) and to firm their stomachs, by which he meant that they should concentrate their minds on the center (Dantien). And so these techniques continued to be used, with great effect, for hundreds of years.

In the 20th Century, while Western medicine was relying heavily on new drugs, improved surgical techniques, and so on, this ancient and proven method of healing was still highly valued in the East. The first Qigong therapy clinic was established at China in 1955. That Qigong was taken seriously even in official quarters is evidenced by the fact that in 1959 the Ministry for Public Health held the First National Meeting for the Exchange of Qigong Experiences. It was attended by approximately 64 groups from 17 provinces, municipalities, and autonomous regions from within a country as large as the United States. Today, Qigong is practiced by more than 200 million Chinese daily.

What Research, Reviews, and Comments Exist?

PRO

Agishi (1998) successfully used Qigong exercises to bring warmness and improve blood flow to persons with arterosclerotic obstruction in the lower extremities. Singh, et al (1998) found Qigong exercises and meditation to be effective adjunctive therapies for patients with fibromyalgia. Reuther and Aldridge (1998) use Qigong exercises to improve airway capability to decrease illness severity in patients with asthma.

CON

No evidence of con research was found when a Medline search was performed.

What Is Qigong Used to Treat or Improve?

- Pain relief from chronic pain, cancer pain, low back pain
- May prevent, treat, and even cure cancer
- Improves strength, health, and energy level
- Improves posture, attitude, and coordination
- Enhances self-healing, reduces stress, and enhances calmness
- Reduces depression
- Enhances sleep and insomnia
- Enhances weight loss and body toning
- Improves chronic complaints, such as asthma, arthritis, headaches
- Reduces hypertension
- Helps maximize physical meditation performance
- Meditation form improves problem solving, sleep, and heightens receptivity

Much research in China has demonstrated the Qigong masters can transmit their Chi to heal others. The treated individual will quickly lose the Chi and return to the diseased state, so it is important for individuals to be learning and practicing Qigong to develop and build their own Chi. Qigong practice has also been found to develop the potential of children.

The Chinese National Research team is researching the relationship with human development. It is suggested that the practice of Qigong may be the link between the ancient legends of Chinese Gods and their use of magic and reality.

What Happens During Qigong?

Qigong is practiced in a relaxed way for 20 minutes/day, longer if wished. Any time of day is fine, but the keen practitioner of Qigong recommends approximately zi time (11:00 PM to 1:00 AM) and Mao time (5:00 AM to 7:00 AM). These times relate to liver and lungs; the liver is connected to the blood and its circulation, and the lungs are connected to the breathing and Chi. Because there are many exercises, the individual can pick and choose the ones that are needed by the body. Each exercise is usually repeated in multiples of six (12, 18, 24) times.

ACTIVE AND PASSIVE QIGONG

Active Qigong (Dong Gong) involves movements that relate to acupuncture points and channels and strengthens the internal organs.

Passive Qigong (Jing Gong) consists of meditation in any body position, which helps to cultivate and store Chi in the Dantien. It works on the internal body and cleans the mind.

BREATHE TRAINING

Breathing is performed in time with movements. Inhaling brings positive Chi in and exhaling releases negative Chi. Breathing exercises include:

- Natural breathing in which you breathe naturally
- Normal breathing in which you breathe in (expand the abdomen) and breathe out (contract abdomen). (The Dandien is in the abdomen, so this breathing stimulates the Dandien.)
- Reverse breathing is the opposite of normal breathing. With reverse breathing, you inhale (contract abdomen) and exhale (expand abdomen).

DIRECTION TO FACE

The four points of the compass relate to different internal organs: east is liver, west is lungs, north is kidneys, and south is heart.

If there is a health problem in any of these areas, face the appropriate direction. If there is a problem in the stomach, it is the center, so the individual can face any direction. Health problems are also connected to yin (weak energy) and yang (too much energy). So if a person has a bad temper because of bad circulation, it means the liver is too yang. Face west (note the opposite direction for liver conditions) to decrease excessive liver energy or Chi. (See Oriental Medicine section for a more complete discussion of yin, yang, and organ systems.)

DAOIST QIGONG EXERCISES

Balancing Exercises

Daoist Qigong includes balancing gong exercises that mainly imitate the movements and daily life of animals, such as:

- Roc extends its wings (Fig. 5-2)
- Monkey Walk (Fig. 5-3)

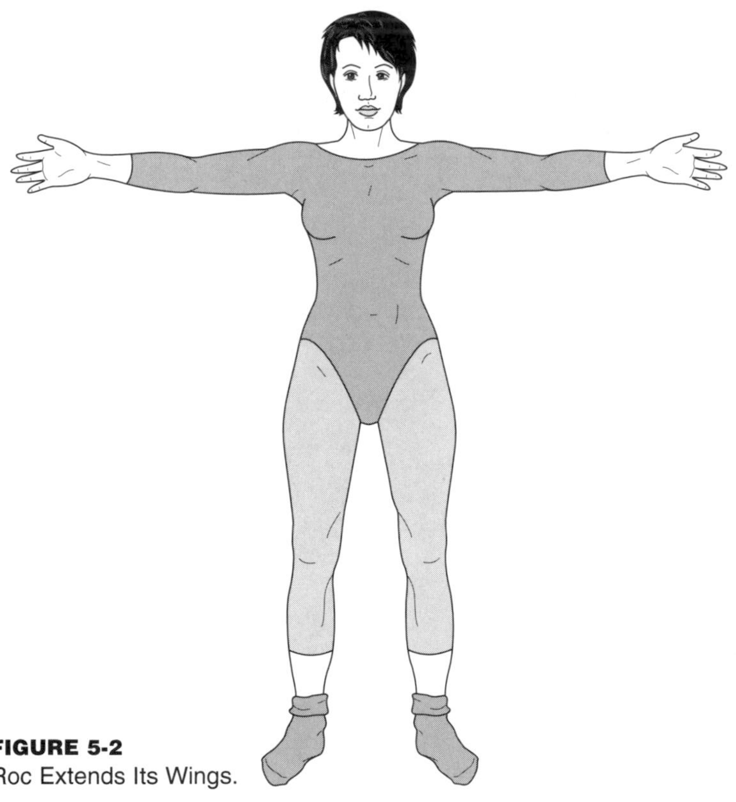

FIGURE 5-2
Roc Extends Its Wings.

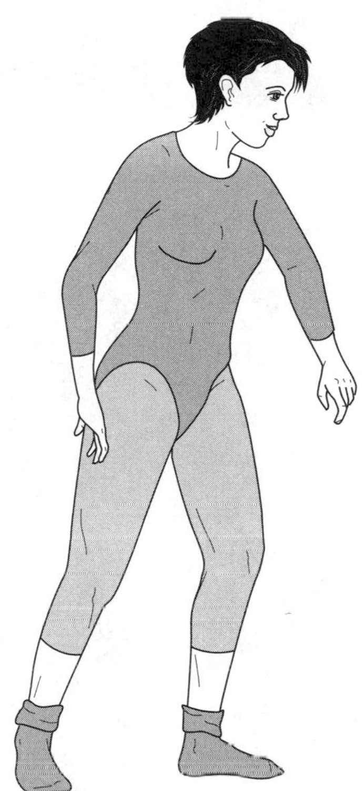

FIGURE 5-3
Monkey Walk.

Starting Exercises

Starting exercises stimulate the Dantien:

- Holding the Dantien
- Dantien: up and down
- Opening and closing the Dantien

Continuing Exercises

- Turning the head and twisting the tail
- Beautiful woman turns her waist
- Peeping monkey (Fig. 5-4)
- Big bear stretches
- Supporting the sky
- Cloud steps

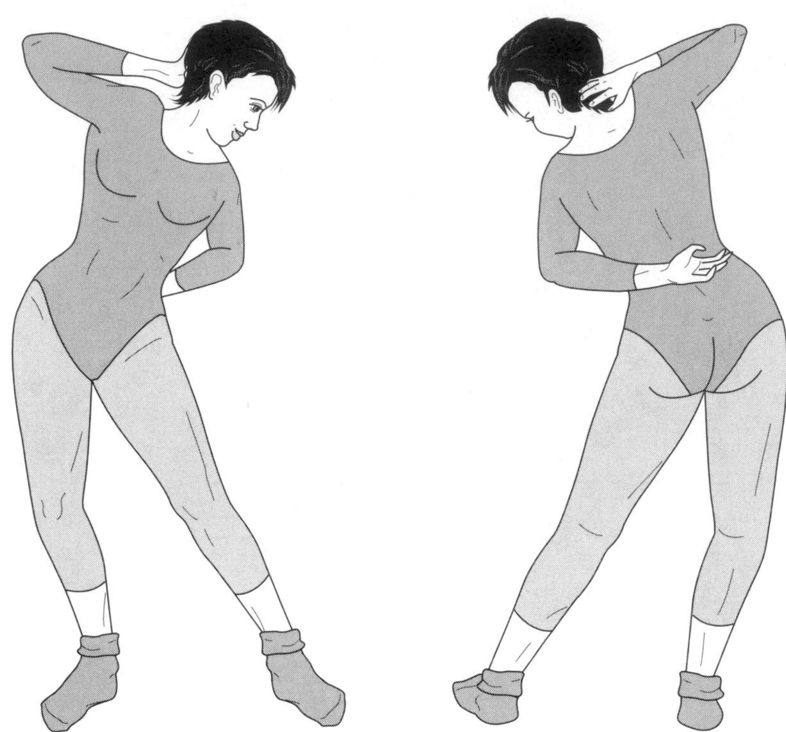

FIGURE 5-4
Peeping Monkey. 1. Stand naturally and relax your whole body. 2. Lean to the left, bend your right leg, and relax your left leg. 3. Raise your right arm and with your fingers, touch the Yarmen point on the back of the neck. At the same time, bring the left hand to the back, so the left Hegu point touches the Mingmen point on your back. 4. Repeat for the other side.

Closing Exercise

At the end of each practice, the Sho Gong exercise is performed. It brings all the Chi back to the Dantien and stores it there.

SPONTANEOUS MOVEMENT

Spontaneous movement *qigong* is common in China. Instead of following a prescribed set of instructions, each individual is guided to move about or not move at all by an internal sense of the body's needs, a sense of the *Chi*. Some people seem to be doing nothing or almost nothing, others may be sitting and moving their arms about in coordination with the breath, and others may be dancing about in a deeply energized state.

QIGONG MEDITATION

This practice can be done standing, sitting, or lying down. In the severely ill, it can mobilize important healing resources. If the person is healthy, it can help maintain health and coordinate body, mind, and spirit.

In this practice, natural forces accelerate through breathing, relaxation, intention, and visualization. On inhalation, visualize a concentration of chi in the abdominal area. On exhalation, visualize these resources circulating out from the center to all the parts of the body: extremities, organs, tissues, and glands. Continue, through thought and visualization, to circulate healing energy with deep breathing and deep relaxation.

Are There Any Risks Involved With Qigong?

- Qigong may be used by anyone, even those with a chronic disease.
- During pregnancy, some of the moves may need to be eliminated or practiced at the level of comfort.

What Training Is Required of the Practitioner?

Qigong may be self-taught. Teachers are trained at centers that teach Chinese philosophy.

Bibliography

Agishi, T (1998). Effects of the external qigong on symptoms of arteriosclerotic obstruction in the lower extremities evaluated by modern medical technology. Artificial Organs. 22, (8), 707–710.

Reuther, I. & Aldridge, D. (1998). Qigong Yangsheng as a complementary therapy in the management of asthma: a single-case appraisal. Journal of Alternative and Complementary Medicine. 4, (2), 173–183.

Singh, B. B., Berman, B. M., Hadhazy, V. A., & Creamer, P. (1998). A pilot study of cognitive behavioral therapy in fibromyalgia. Alternative Therapies in Health and Medicine. 4, (2), 67–70.

Further Reading

Chia, M. Chi self-massage: the Taoist way of rejuvenation. Huntington, NY: Healing Tao Books, 1986.

Chang, S. T. The complete system of self-healing: internal exercises. San Francisco, CA: Tao Publishing, 1986.

Jahnke, R. The most profound medicine. Santa Barbara, CA: Health Action Books, 1990.

Tse, M. Qigong for health & vitality. NY: St. Martin's Griffin, 1995.

Qigong Magazine. Pacific Rim Publishers, Inc. PO Box 31578, San Francisco, CA. 94131. (800) 924-2433.

QI: The Journal of Traditional Eastern Health and Fitness. PO Box 22143, Chantilly, VA 22022. (800) 787-2600.

RESOURCES

American Foundation of Traditional Chinese Medicine
505 Beach Street
San Francisco, CA 94133
(415) 776-0502

The Healing Tao Center
P.O. Box 1194
Huntington, NY 11743
(516) 367-2701

Health Action
243 Pebble Beach
Santa Barbara, CA 93117
(805) 682-3230

Qigong Institute/East-West Academy of the Healing Arts
450 Sutter Street, Suite 916/2104
San Francisco, CA 94108
(415) 788-2227

INTERNET

Office of Alternative Medicine
http://altmed.od.nig.gov/

When we laugh, muscles are activated. When we stop laughing, these muscles relax....Many people with arthritis, rheumatism and other painful conditions benefit greatly from a healthy dose of laughter.

—WILLIAM FRY, MD

TAI CHI

What Is Tai Chi?

Tai Chi is a Chinese martial art and meditation that combines a choreographed series of slow movements with mental concentration and some coordinated breathing. Most of the forms of Tai Chi have been passed down from generation to generation, and have assumed the name of a particular family. Each may be slightly different, but all follow the same basic principles. Two distinct types of Tai Chi are practiced today in the United States. Tai Chi Chuan, originated in China has a short form, which uses 37 movements (takes 10 to 15 minutes), and a long form, which uses108 movements (takes 20 to 25 minutes). Tai Chi Chih (joy through movement) was recently developed by Justine Stone in the United States with 20 simple movements (takes 30 minutes). Tai Chi Chih can be performed by anyone, regardless of age, and even done by people in a wheelchair.

Tai Chi emphasizes self-awareness and circulates and balances the body's internal energy. Chi is defined as the vital force (see Oriental Medicine). Breathing assists the movement of Chi around the body. Tai Chi is a powerful centering activity, and may be a prelude for meditation or prayer or vigorous physical or mental activity. Tai Chi is similar to other body and mind therapies such as biofeedback, in which the individual learns control over some bodily functions and quiets the mind.

Characteristics of Tai Chi:

- It is moving meditation. Each movement has symbolic meaning and all have descriptive names such as:
  - Tai Chi Chuan: grasp the bird's tail, embracing tiger, parry punch, green dragon dropping water
  - Tai Chi Chih: base drum, around the platter, pulling taffy, push-pull
- It is moderate movement and exercise that produces several biologic changes within the body including improved maintenance of joint mobility, cardiovascular fitness, and release of B-endorphins producing a sense of well-being.
- Emphasizes strength and flexibility rather than muscle mass.
- Performed without strain.
- Movements are carried out in pairs, negative (yin) and positive (yang), to maintain and promote energy balance in the body.
- Movements involve flexing knees, weight transfer, and raising and lowering the arms.
- Sometimes breathing is coordinated with the movement.
- Gentle movements massage the internal organs and enhance their functioning.
- Enhances energy flow (Chi) throughout the body.
- With each posture, the weight alternates between the left and right side causing the leg muscles to contract and expand, improving blood flow.
- Increases joint flexibility, making Tai Chi an excellent practice for persons with arthritis.
- Helps to align the body with gravity. It helps straighten the spine and alleviates tension, so it is particularly good for persons with back problems

- Balances the mind, helps empty the mind while practicing Tai Chi and therefore allows person to see the "big picture" in his or her life
- On a spiritual level, it can be a wonderful meditation in movement.
- Promotes serenity and inner peacefulness and focus.

What Is the History of Tai Chi?

Tai Chi originated in China thousands of years ago and is based on the Taoist principle of yin and yang (see Oriental Medicine) and Buddhism. According to the Taoist view, good health requires a balance of opposing forces within the body. Tai Chi is also related to the martial arts. Tai Chi was introduced into the west in the 19th Century, but it was not until the 1970s that Tai Chi became well-known in the United States.

What Research, Reviews, and Comments Exist?

PRO

Bhatti, et al. (1998) found that 6 weeks of Tai Chi reduces pain intensity of persons with chronic low-back pain better than conventional care. In addition, a statistically significant improvement in mood was also found. Wolf, Coogler, & Xu (1997) are exploring the effects of Tai Chi Chuan in the elderly. From the original 108 forms, they have selected 10 as being the easiest to perform and best to evaluate. Jacobson, et al (1997) studied films of persons practicing the 108 forms of Tai Chi. They found that Tai Chi presents a low-stress method to enhance stability, improve kinesthetic sense, and strengthen knee extension. Lan, et al (1996) found that Tai Chi has benefits for health-related fitness, and it may be prescribed as a suitable conditioning exercise for the elderly. Lumsdem, et al (1998) found that Tai Chi was beneficial to enhance mobility of patients with osteoarthritis. Tai Chi did not activate joint pain, and patients reported they had less discomfort.

CON

Wolf, et al (1997) found that Tai Chi did not enhance postural stability and therefore did not affect level of falling in a trial with elderly clients. A slight benefit may be that Tai Chi exercises promoted confidence by facilitating a reduction in sway-based measures.

What Is Tai Chi Used to Treat or Improve?

- Enhances health and wellness
- Enhances respiratory function
- Enhances balance, coordination, and gracefulness
- Provides socialization because Tai Chi is usually performed in a group
- May alleviate pain
- Reduces stress
- Improves energy and endurance
- Helps to maximize physical, spiritual, and emotional potential
- Helps control blood pressure
- Enhances body toning of muscles, improves circulation
- Enhances serenity and provides beautiful meditation
- Provides a sense of body control
- Silent activity allows one the opportunity to open up and grow to enhance self-awareness
- Cultivates strength through softness

What Happens During a Visit?

Tai Chi is often done with a partner to help understand another person's energy.

- Each movement flows from the previous one, which results in one continuous series of movements (Figs. 5-5–5-8).
- Movements are effortless and smooth.
- Gradual mental detachment usually occurs.
- Energy is contained by the body and gently released in a systematic way.

Are There Any Risks Involved With Tai Chi?

There are no specific dangers. Movements are slow and gentle and can be performed by someone with a chronic disease or in a wheelchair. There are no quick, jerky movements or pounding of the floor as with aerobic dance or jogging.

- It is important to warm up before Tai Chi to prevent stretching injuries.
- Single stance procedures may result in falls
- Wear appropriate non-skid footwear.

What Training Is Required of the Practitioner?

Tai Chi can be self-taught, but qualified teachers are available.

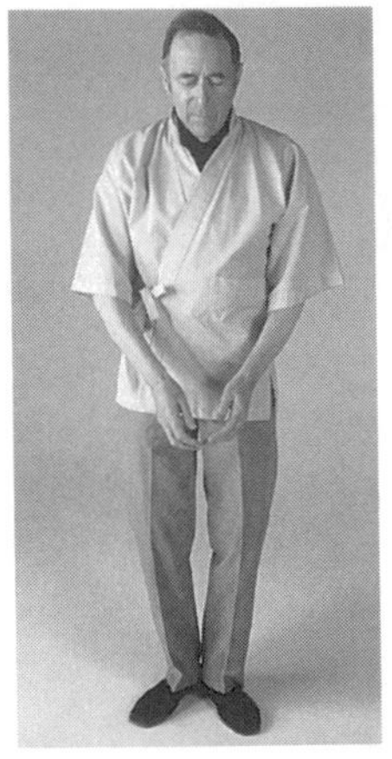
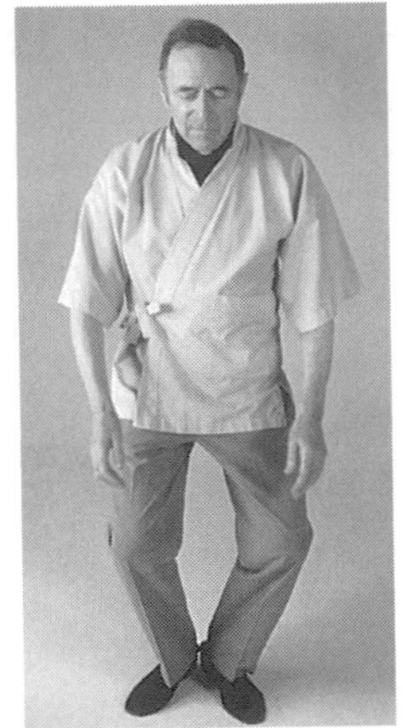
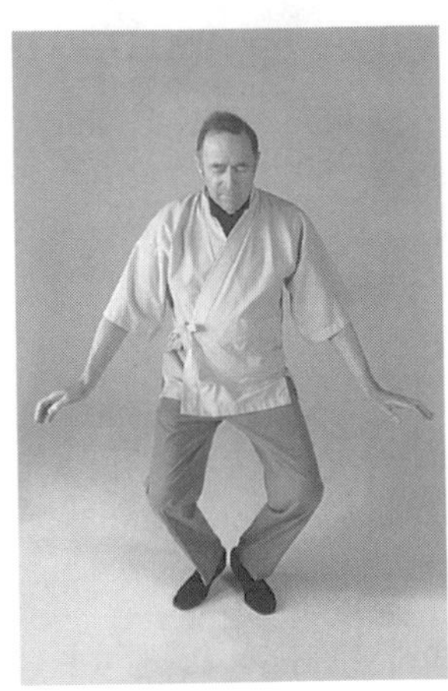

FIGURE 5-5
Bird Flapping Its Wings. (With permission of Stone, J. [1996]. Tai chi chih! Joy through movement. Fort Yates, ND: Good Karma Publishing.)

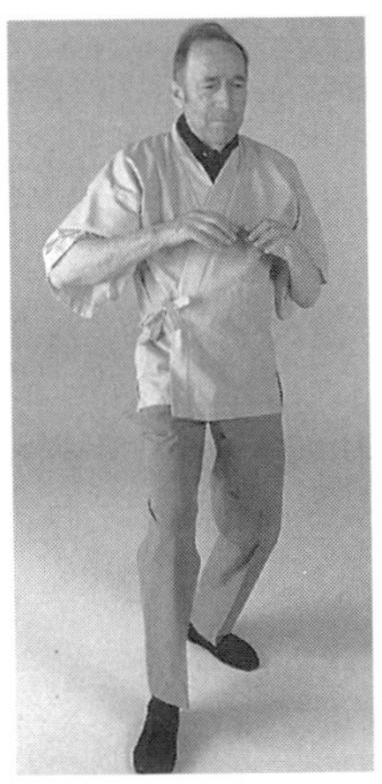
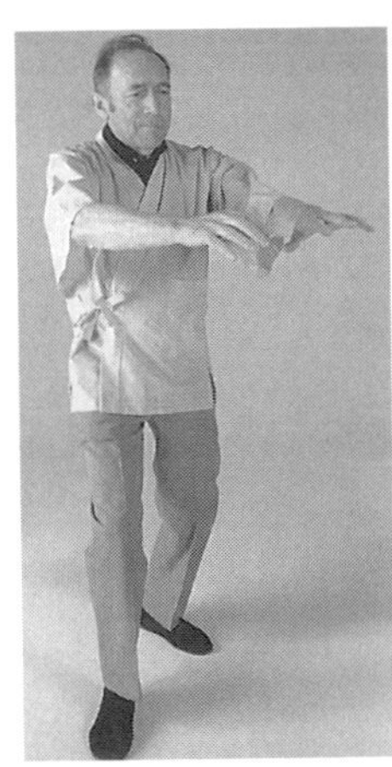
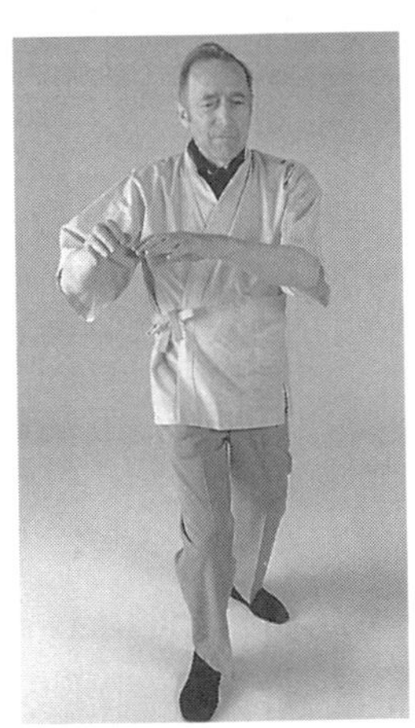

FIGURE 5-6
Around the Platter (right). (With permission of Stone, J. [1996]. Tai chi chih! Joy through movement. Fort Yates, ND: Good Karma Publishing.)

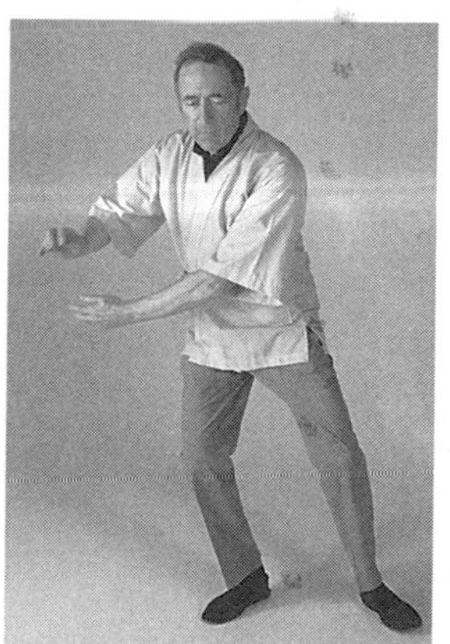
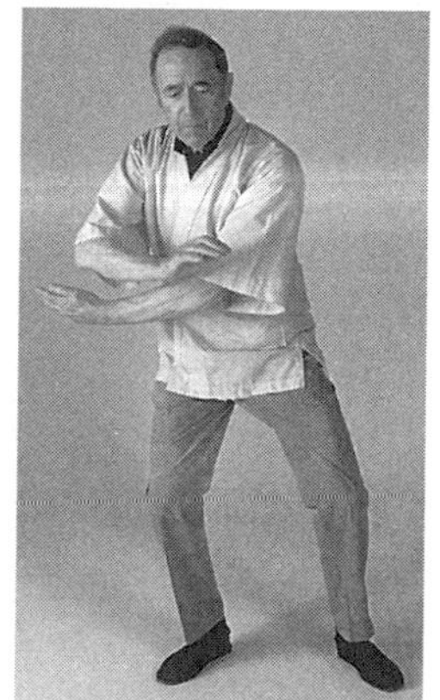
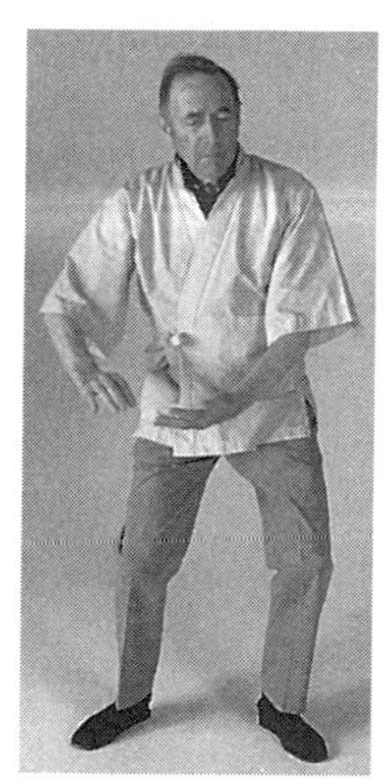

FIGURE 5-7
Pulling Taffy. (With permission of Stone, J. [1996]. Tai chi chih! Joy through movement. Fort Yates, ND: Good Karma Publishing.)

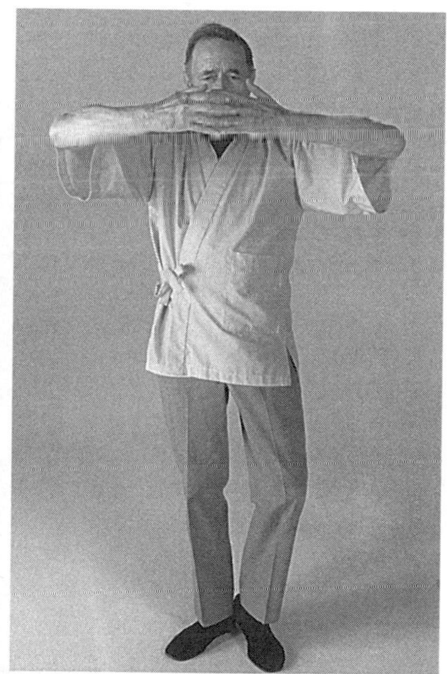

FIGURE 5-8
Cosmic Consciousness Pose. (With permission of Stone, J. [1996]. Tai chi chih! Joy through movement. Fort Yates, ND: Good Karma Publishing.)

Bibliography

Bhatti, T. I., Gillin, J. C., Atkinson, J. H., et al. (1998). Tai chi chih as a treatment for chronic low back pain. Alternative Therapies. 4, (2), 90.

Jacobson, B. H., Chen, H. C., Cashel, C., & Guerrero, L. (1997). The effect of Tai Chi Chuan training on balance, kinesthetic sense, and strength. Perceptual & Motor Skills. 84, (1), 27–33.

Lan, C., Lai, J. S., Wong, M. K., & Yu, M. L. (1996). Cardiorespiratory function, flexibility, and body composition among geriatric Tai Chi Chuan practitioners. Archives of Physical Medicine & Rehabilitation. 77, (6), 612–616.

Lumsden, D. B., Baccala, A., & Martire, J. (1998). Tai Chi for osteoarthritis: an introduction for primary care physicians. Geriatrics. 53, (2), 84, 87–88.

Stone, J. (1996). Tai Chi Chih: joy thru movement. Good Karma Publishing Inc..

Wolf, S. L., Coogler, C., & Xu, T. (1997). Exploring the basis for Tai Chi Chuan as a therapeutic exercise approach. Archives of Physical Medicine & Rehabilitation. 78, (8), 886–892.

Wolf, S. L., Barnhart, H. X., Ellison, G. L., & Coogler, C. E. (1997). The effect of Tai Chi Quan and computerized balance training on postural stability in older subjects. Physical Therapy. 77, (4), 371–381.

Further Reading

Darling, Kemdersely, McFarlane, S: The Complete Book of Tai Chi. 1997.

Kirstein A: Tai-Chi Chuan. Archives of Physical Medicine & Rehabilitation. 79(4):471. April, 1998.

Lam P: New horizons-developing tai chi for health care. Australian Family Physician. 27(1-2):100-1, Jan-Feb. 1998.

Levitt R, Shuff P: Balance and harmony: the essence of tai chi. Nursing Spectrum. 7(18):14, Sept.8, 1997.

Liao, W: Tai Chi Classics.Shambhala Publishing, 1990.

Mooton, C: Tai Chi for Beginners. Perigel Books: New Uork, 1996.

YOGA

What Is Yoga?

Yoga has many meanings, but essentially has come to mean a union, a uniting or a method of discipline. Yoga comes out of an oral tradition in which the teaching was transmitted directly from teacher to student. Yoga teaches basic principles of mind and body unity. If the mind is chronically restless, and agitated, the health of the body is compromised, and if the body is in poor health, mental strength and clarity are adversely affected. The practice of yoga can restore physical and mental health.

Man is seen as an energetic being within a larger energy system of the universe. The *prana* or vital life force (Chi to the Asians) is considered to be an extension of the same cosmic energy that sustains and directs the universe. The *chakras* (seven wheels) in the yoga tradition, are considered energy centers that transform the universal energy into usable human forms of energy. The purpose of yoga, particularly hatha yoga, is to balance the prana and allow it to ascend through all the chakras until it emerges from the Crown Chakra and one achieves self-realization (see Ayurvedic Medicine for additional information).

Yoga is organized into eight limbs and six branches. All are systematically arranged to outline lifestyle, hygiene, detoxification regimens, physical, and psychological practices.

THE LIMBS OF YOGA

The eight limbs are the eight basic guidelines regarding how to live a meaningful and purposeful life. They are prescriptions for moral and ethical conduct, self-discipline, one's health, and to assist us to acknowledge the spiritual aspects of our nature.

The first four limbs concentrate on refining personality, gaining mastery over the body, and developing an energetic awareness of one's self; all of which prepares one for the second half of the journey, which deals with the senses, the mind, and attaining a higher state of consciousness.

- Yama: ethical standards, sense of integrity. "Do unto others as you would have them do unto you."
- Niyama: self-discipline and spiritual observances, attending religious services or daily meditation.
- Asana: postures of yoga that, when used, develop the habit of discipline and the ability to concentrate.
- Pranayama: breath control recognizes the connection between breath, the mind and the emotions. Pranayama means "life force extension."
- Pratyahara: withdrawal or sensory transcendence in which we make a conscious effort to draw awareness away from the external world and external stimuli; allows us to step back and observe ourselves.
- Dharana: concentration. Precedes meditation in which we focuses attention on an object, a place inside ourselves, an image, or a silent repetition of a sound. Extended periods of concentration lead to meditation.
- Dhyana: uninterrupted flow of concentration. The mind is quiet and in its stillness produces few or no thoughts.
- Samadhi: state of ecstasy. The person comes to realize a profound connection to the divine, an interconnectedness with all living things. This step is the completion of the yogic path.

THE BRANCHES OF YOGA

From ancient times, yoga is referred to as a tree, a living entity with roots, a trunk, branches, blossoms, and fruit. Each branch has its distinct function and represents a particular approach to life. Involvement may be in one branch or several.

- Hatha yoga (yoga of activity), the "force of determined effort." A powerful method of self-transformation. It is the most practiced form in the United States because it fits in with the American physical fitness industry.
- Raja yoga (meditation yoga). Members of religious orders and spiritual communities dedicate themselves to this branch of yoga.
- Karma yoga (path of service yoga). Karma is the path of self-transcending action. We practice Karma yoga each time we perform our work and live our lives in a selfless fashion.
- Bhakti yoga (path of devotion). Cultivation and acceptance of everyone we come in contact with is the goal of Bhakti yoga, the yoga of the heart.
- Jnana yoga (path of the mind, of wisdom for the sage or scholar). Requires the development of the intellect with serious study.
- Tantra yoga (pathway of ritual that includes consecrated sexuality). This pathway is often associated with celibacy. It is the most esoteric of all the yoga branches.

What Is the History of Yoga?

The uses of postures and breathing exercises for spiritual and physical well-being dates to 3000 BC in India. The first written records were in 1500 BC with references in other texts in 400 BC.

The first detailed description comes from the classic *Yoga Sutras* written approximately 300 BC by Patanjali. Patanjali outlines the eight limbs of yoga. In the 10th Century, breathing and postures became associated with Ayurvedic medicine.

Yoga philosophy came to the United States in 1893. In the beginning, the yoga was philosophical in nature with little attention paid to hatha yoga. In the 1920s, hatha yoga was introduced in the physical fitness movement in the United States. In the 1960s, Maharishi Mahesh Yogi's Transcendental Meditation became the order of the day to fill the growing need for the spiritual awakening of America.

What Research, Reviews, and Comments Exist?

PRO

Yoga breathing has been studied and found to increase spatial memory scores in the trained groups by 84% (Naveen, et al, 1997), but it did not increase verbal scores as was previously thought. Yoga was also found to have a positive effect (86%) on decreasing optical illusions in a group of people who practiced yoga for 1 month. (Telles, et al, 1997). Yoga has demonstrated a significant effect in lowering heart rate in the elderly. This effect was more significant than when aerobic exercise was performed for the same time period (Bowman, et al, 1997).

Yoga techniques taught in an asthma and allergy clinic resulted in patients experiencing a greater degree of relaxation, a more positive attitude, better tolerance to exercise, and a reduced usage of beta adrenergic inhalers (Vedanthan, et al, 1998). Pulmonary and autonomic function was shown to improve significantly in patients with asthma (Khanam, et al, 1996). Patients did not show improvements in their volumes or expiratory flow rate, but showed improvement in pulmonary ventilation by way of relaxation of voluntary inspiratory and expiratory muscles. Yoga breathing and relaxation techniques have been shown to lessen labor pain (Fields, 1995; Miller, 1996).

Yoga has been used in rehabilitation in many areas. Yoga has been shown to reduce anxiety in visually impaired children; significantly improve sleep, appetite, and general well-being in prisoners in jail; decrease substance abuse; and improve general sense of well-being in persons who are HIV-positive (Telles & Naveen, 1997).

CON

Shaffer, LaSalvia, and Peter (1997) found that yoga is not more effective than conventional psychotherapy methadone treatment. However, 80 patients experienced a benefit. The authors suggest that further research is necessary to determine the characteristics that identify patients who might benefit from the use of yoga.

What Is Yoga Used to Treat or Improve?

- Back pain
- Arthritis
- Migraines and headaches
- Menstrual problems
- Sexual dysfunction
- Hypertension (reduces blood pressure, but not the need for medication)
- Heart disease (Bowman, et al, 1997)
- GI problems (ulcers)
- Respiratory diseases (asthma, bronchitis) (Vedanthan, et al, 1998; Khanan, et al, 1996)

- Obesity
- Diabetes (reduces insulin requirements)
- Cancer
- Addictions (tobacco, alcohol) (Telles & Naveen, 1997)
- Reduces anxiety
- Enhances sense of well-being in elderly
- Reduces serum cholesterol
- Enhances spatial memory (Naveen, et al, 1997)
- Reduces labor pain (Fields, 1995)
- Improves sense of well-being in patients with multiple sclerosis (MS) (Saperia, et al, 1997)

What Happens During a Visit?

There are three primary types of yoga practices in the United States: yoga postures (asana), breath control (pranayama), and meditation.

YOGA POSTURES

There are many yoga postures that can be learned: standing, seated, prone, supine, and inversions. Each asana is composed of the movement to reach the pose and a phase in which the pose is held. Thus each asana alternates between activity and rest. The asana helps regulate the circulatory, endocrine, and nervous systems. Some postures are used for warm-up, toning, or to stimulate various organ systems. Several are described as to the posture and its benefits.

Corpse (Shavasana)

Pose: relaxation

Posture: Lie on your back with our arms spread out approximately 12 to 18 inches from your side, palms open and up, and your feet spread about as wide as your shoulders. Place a folded blanket or towel behind your head and neck. Close your eyes and relax, breathing slowly and deeply, allowing the abdomen to expand with each inhalation and to fall with each exhalation (Fig. 5-9).

Benefits:

- An excellent relaxation technique that aids circulation and improves the functioning of the nervous system
- Helps relax the skeletal muscles, enabling one to go further into the postures while reducing the likelihood of injuries
- Reduces fatigue

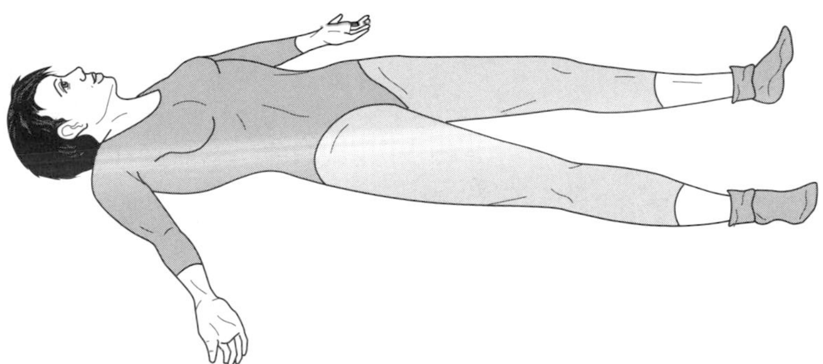

FIGURE 5-9
Corpse (Shavasana).

Child's Pose (Balasana)

Pose: prone

Position: Sit in a kneeling position, with top of feet on floor and buttocks resting on feet. Relax the arms and rest the hands on the floor. Exhaling slowly, bend forward from the hips until the stomach and chest rest on the thighs. Keep the body completely relaxed. The body is kept compact. Do not hold this posture longer than 5 minutes because it decreases circulation to the legs (Fig. 5-10).

Benefits:

- Enhances circulation to the lower back
- Stimulates the organs of the pelvic area
- Relieves lower back tension

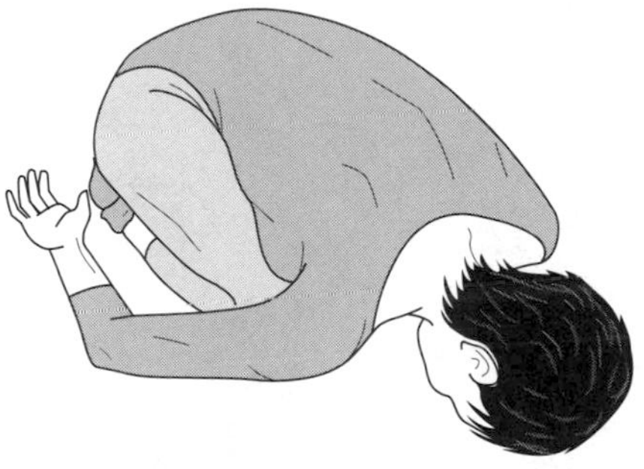

FIGURE 5-10
Child's Pose (Balasana).

Posterior Stretch (Paschimottanasana)

Pose: seated

Posture: Sit with your head, neck, and trunk straight and your legs together extended in front of your body. Inhaling, raise your arms overhead, stretch up, and expand the chest.

Exhaling, with your back straight and head between the arms, bend forward as far as possible, placing the hands comfortably on the legs. The back of your knees should remain on the floor. Relax, breathe evenly, and hold for 5 to 10 seconds.

To further the stretch, remain in position, inhale, and stretch forward from the base of the spine to the crown of the head. Exhaling, bring the head further down toward the legs. Relax and breathe evenly (Fig. 5-11).

Benefits:

- Stimulates the peristaltic movement of materials through the digestive tract and prevents constipation
- Stimulates the entire abdominal area: kidney, liver, stomach, spleen, and pancreas
- Relieves indigestion and poor appetite
- May be therapeutic in the treatment of diabetes
- Stretches the hamstring muscles of the thighs and the muscles and ligaments of the back
- Gently massages the intervertebral discs, develops flexibility of the spinal column

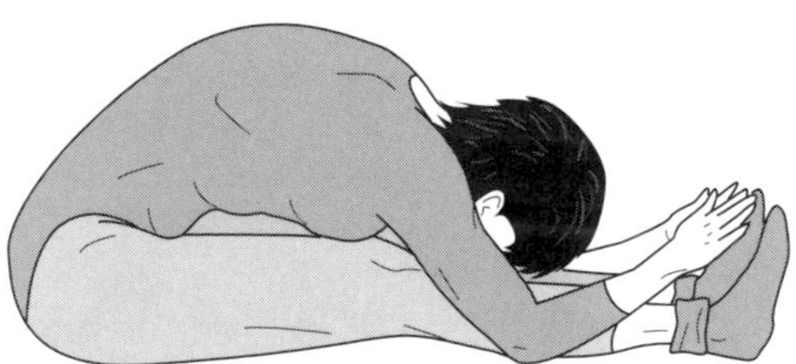

FIGURE 5-11
Posterior Stretch (Paschimotanasana).

Cobra (Bhujangasana)

Pose: prone

Position: Lie on your stomach with your forehead resting on the floor, legs and feet together, your body fully extended and relaxed. Bend the elbows, keeping them close to the body, and place your hands, palm down, beside your chest, aligning the fingertips with the nipples.

Inhaling, slowly begin to raise your head, allowing first the nose and then the chin to touch the floor as the head is stretched forward and upward. Without using the strength of the arms or hands, slowly raise the shoulders and chest; look up and bend back as far as possible. Breathe evenly; hold for 5 seconds.

Exhaling, slowly lower the body until the forehead rests on the floor. Relax.

In this posture the navel remains on the floor. Do not use the arms and hands to push your body off the floor, use the muscles of the back only. Keep the feet and legs together and relaxed (Fig. 5-12).

Benefits:

- Strengthens the muscles of the shoulders, neck, and back
- Develops flexibility of the cervical vertebrae
- Improves posture
- Corrects deviations of the spine
- Improves circulation to the intervertebral discs
- Expands the chest and develops elasticity of the lungs
- May help low back pain, constipation, stomach pains, gas pains, and backaches

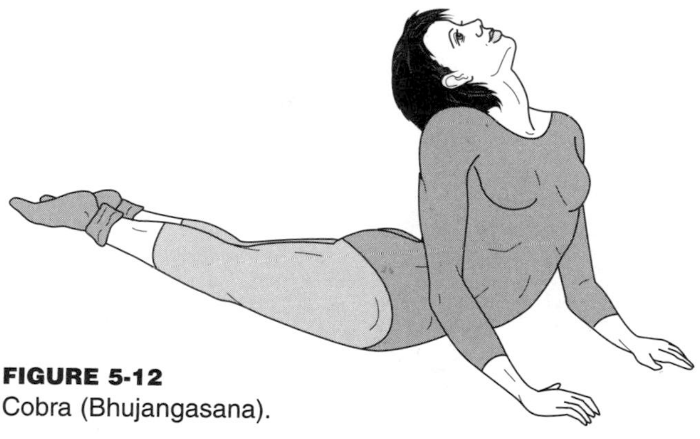

FIGURE 5-12
Cobra (Bhujangasana).

Locust (Shalabhasana)

Pose: prone

Position: Lie on your stomach with your legs together and your arms extended along the sides of your body; place the chin on the floor. Make fists with the hands, placing the thumbs and the forefingers on the floor. Keeping the arms straight, place the fists under the tops of the thighs.

Inhaling, raise both legs as high as possible. Breathe evenly; hold for 5 seconds.

Exhaling, slowly lower the legs and relax (Fig. 5-13).

Benefits:

- Strengthens the muscles of the lower back
- Reduces lower back pain tendencies

Half Spinal Twist (Ardha Matsyendrasana)

Pose: seated

Position: Sit with your head, neck, and torso straight with your legs together and extended in front of your body.

Bend the left leg and place the left foot on the floor at the outside of the right knee. Twist the body toward the left and place the left hand approximately 4 to 6 inches behind the left hip, fingers pointing away from the body. Bring the right arm over the outside of the left leg and grasp the

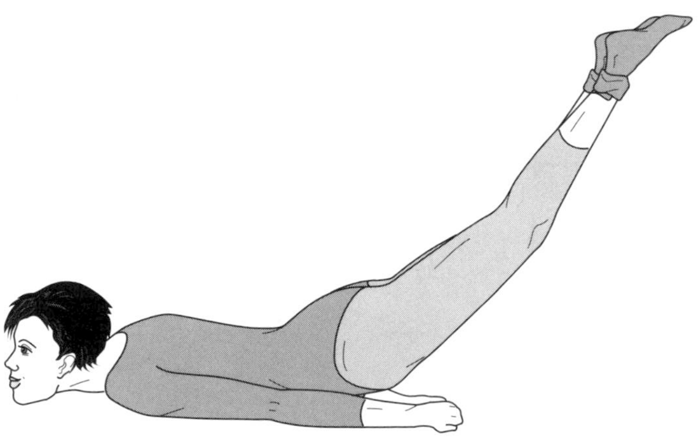

FIGURE 5-13
Locust (Shalabhasana).

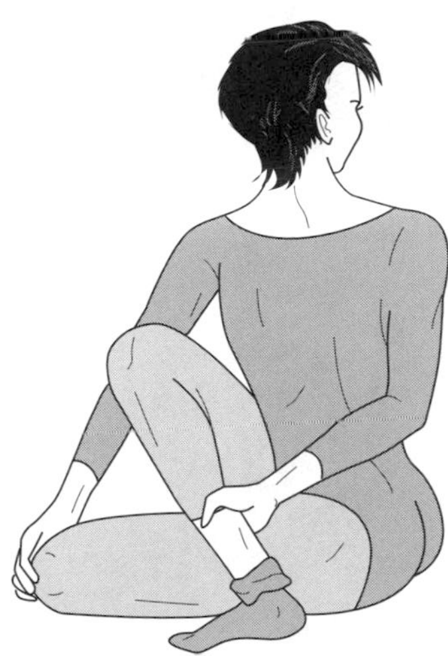

FIGURE 5-14
Half Spinal Twist (Ardha Matsyendrasana).

left foot with the right hand. When bringing your arm over your leg, you may bend slightly forward if necessary; however, do not arch your back and then twist your body.

Keeping the back straight, turn to the left, twisting from the lower spine, and look over the left shoulder. Do not use the arms to force your body further into the twist, use them only for balance.

Breathe evenly; hold for 5 seconds. Repeat on the opposite side (Fig. 5-14).

Benefits:

- Provides twist to the spinal column, stretching and lengthening the muscles and ligaments and keeping the spine elastic and healthy
- Alternately compresses each half of the abdominal region, squeezing the internal organs and promoting better circulation through them
- Combats constipation, reduces fat, and improves digestion

Shoulder Stand (Sarvangasana)

Pose: standing

Position: Lie on your back with your legs together, flat on the floor. Bend the elbows and place the hands as close to the shoulders as possible, with fingers pointing toward the small of the back and the elbows firmly on the floor. Raise both legs until they are perpendicular to the floor, lifting the

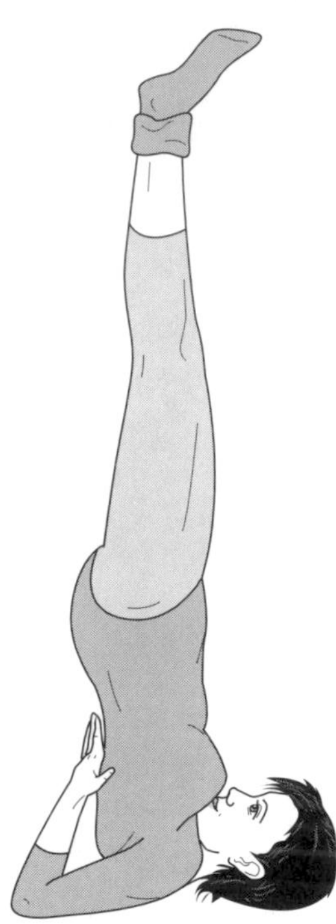

FIGURE 5-15
Shoulder Stand (Sarvangasana).

hips toward the ceiling. Press the breastbone against the chin, gently at first and more firmly with experience. Keep the legs straight, relaxed, and perpendicular to the floor.

Breathe evenly; hold for 20 to 30 seconds. Slowly increase your capacity until you can hold this posture comfortably for 1 minute (Fig. 5-15).

Benefits:

- As implied in the literal translation of sarvangasana, "all member posture" or "entire body posture," this exercise benefits all parts of the body: the shoulders, arms, legs, head, neck, back, and internal organs
- Strengthens arms, chest, and shoulders
- Strengthens the back and abdominal muscles
- Places gentle traction on the cervical vertebrae, keeping this important area healthy and flexible
- Venous drainage of the legs occurs quickly and completely, especially benefitting those persons with varicose veins

- Diaphragmatic breathing is easily observed and learned
- Causes higher blood pressure and simple mechanical pressure in the neck; said to rejuvenate the thyroid and parathyroid glands, making them function optimally
- Reduces the occurrence of acute and chronic throat ailments
- Increases the blood supply to all the important structures of the neck
- Fights indigestion, constipation, degeneration of the endocrine glands, and problems occurring in the liver, the gallbladder, the kidney, the pancreas, the spleen, and the digestive system

Half Fish (Matsyasana)

Pose: prone

Position: Sit with your head, neck, and trunk straight, legs together and extended in front of your body. Lean back and place the elbows and forearms on the floor in line with the body and legs. Arch the back, expanding the chest, and stretch the neck backward, placing the crown of the head on the floor. Increase the stretch by further arching your back and pulling your head as far as you can toward the back. Be sure to keep the mouth closed to maintain the stretch in the neck.

Breathe evenly; hold for 15 to 20 seconds. Gently lower the body to a prone position. Relax. Once again, conclude with corpse posture to ensure complete relaxation and prevent fatigue (Fig. 5-16).

Benefits:

- Provides a stretch to the cervical vertebrae complementary to that of the shoulder stand. It amplifies the effects of the shoulder stand and eliminates the slight stiffness in the neck and back that results from doing the shoulder stand alone
- Expands the chest, promoting deep inhalation, giving good ventilation to the top of the lungs and increasing lung capacity

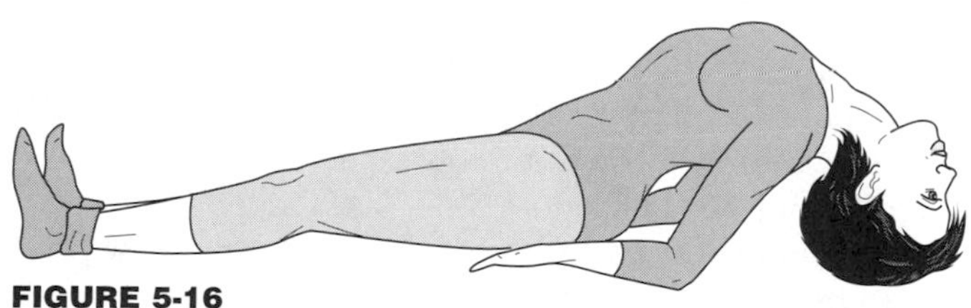

FIGURE 5-16
Half Fish (Matsyansana).

TABLE 5-1 BRAIN ACTIVITY

Left	Right
Male	Female
Logical thinking	Intuition
Investigation	Compassion
Inquiry	Love
Aggression	Art, Poetry, Music
Competitiveness	Humor
Judgement	Religion
Right Breathe	Left Breathe
Cycle is →	
Dominants →	

Breathing Techniques

Breathing takes on an additional importance in the yoga philosophy because prana is drawn in with each breath and circulates within the body. Controlling the breath, or learning to breathe correctly, is called pranayama, which literally means "regulating the life force." In the traditional interpretation, the sun controls the breath through the right nostril and the moon controls the breath through the left nostril. Proper breathing is essential for the mental concentration necessary for meditation.

Just as the right side of our body is controlled by the left side of our brain, breathing better through the left nostril activates the right brain and vice versa. See Table 5-1 for activities of the left and right brain. The secret of prana is the secret of handling male and female energy. When alternate nostril breathing is conducted, the male and female energies are balanced, the neutral energy is awakened, and one experiences pure awareness.

Several examples of pranayamas include:

Alternate nostril pranayama

- Sit comfortably
- Close the right nostril with your right thumb, and inhale through the left nostril. Inhale into the belly, not into the chest.
- Hold your breath for just a moment
- Exhale through your right nostril while closing the left with the ring and little finger of your right hand
- Repeat

Cooling Breath (Shitali Pranayama)

Purpose:

- Lowers the oral temperature, makes the saliva cool, helps to quench thirst, and improves digestion, absorption, and assimilation.
- Effective for high blood pressure, burning throat or tongue, and a burning sensation in the eyes
- Cools the entire body

Technique:

- Curl tongue into a tube
- Inhale slowly through the curled tongue, swallow, and then exhale normally through the nose, keeping the mouth closed
- Incoming air cools your saliva, your tongue, and the oral mucous membranes

Breath of Fire (Bhastrika Pranayama)

Purpose:

- Increases the vital capacity of the lungs, relieves allergies and asthma, and helps make the lungs strong and healthy
- Heats the body

Technique:

- Inhale passively through the nose, but exhale actively and with a little force
- Start slowly and increase the speed
- Do one round of 30 strokes or exhalations, then rest for 1 minute
- You can do up to five such rounds in the morning and five in the evening

Humming Breath (Bhramari Pranayama)

Purpose:

- Improves the melodiousness of the voice
- Humming vibrates the nervous system and is a form of sound therapy for the brain
- Good for the thyroid, thymus, and parathyroid glands

Technique:

- On inhalation, constrict the epiglottis so as to create a humming sound

- On exhalation, the sound is long and low
- On inhalation, the sound is more high-pitched
- Do 10 cycles

Breath of Victory (Ujjayi Pranayama)

Purpose:

- Brings great joy
- Calms the mind, relaxes the intercostal muscles, really brings a sense of victory
- Helps to reestablish constitutional balance
- Promotes longevity

Technique:

- Sit in Lotus posture, with you hand resting on your knees, palms up. Keep your head, neck, and chest in a straight line
- Lower your head into a slight chin lock by moving your head in and down, toward your chest
- Without actually swallowing, start the action of swallowing, to raise the trachea upward
- At the same time, while constricting your epiglottis, as in silently "saying" the letter "e", slowly and deeply inhale into the belly. Inhaled air will create a soft, gentle whispering sound of rushing air as it brushes the throat, trachea, heart, and diaphragm.
- After inhaling, swallow and hold your breath at the belly for a moment, then slowly exhale the air by again constricting the epiglottis
- Do 12 cycles at a time

Are There Any Risks Involved With Yoga?

There are no specific dangers, although some postures should be avoided in certain patients, e.g., if you have a back injury, certain postures are avoided until strength and flexibility have been built. If exercise has not been done for a long time, yoga should be started slowly and a movement should never be forced.

Contraindications:

Sciatica. *Do not do* forward bends or intense stretching.

Menstruation. *Do not do* inverted poses.

Hypertension. *Do not do* breath retentions or inverted poses.

Glaucoma. Ear congestion. *Do not do* breath retentions or inverted poses.

Pregnancy. *Do not do* breath retentions, inverted poses, or breath suspensions.

What Training Is Required of the Practitioner?

Yoga can be self-taught through books, tapes, and so on. Yoga can also be taught by yoga teachers. There is no national certification.

Bibliography

Bowman, A. J., Clayton, R. H., Murray, A., Reed, J. W., Subhan, M. M., & Ford, G. A. (1997). Effects of aerobic exercise training s without lateralized effects. Psychological Reports. 81, 2), 555–561.

Fields, N. (1995). Teaching the gentle way to labor. Nursing Times. 91, (6), 44-45.

Khanam, A. A. Sachdeva, U., Guleria, R., & Deepak, K. K. (1996). Study of pulmonary and autonomic functions of asthma patients after yoga training. Indian Journal of Physiology & Pharmacology. 40, (4), 318-324.

Miller, C. (1996). Making a difference: yoga in pregnancy. Birth Gazette. 13, (1), 34-35.

Naveen, K.V., Nagarantha, R., Nagendra, H. R., & Telles, S. (1997). Yoga breathing through a particular nostril increases spatial memory scores without lateralized effects. Psychological Reports. 81, (2), 555-561.

Saperia, D., Jessum, R., Cooper, P., & Martelli, K. (1997). Influence of the practice of Hatha Yoga on functional recovery and perceived health status in individuals with multiple sclerosis. Alternative Therapies. 3, (2), 102.

Shaffer, H., LaSalvia, T., & Stein, J. (1997). Comparing Hatha Yoga with dynamic group psychotherapy for enhancing methadone maintenance treatment. Alternative Therapies in Health and Medicine. 3, (4), 57–66.

Telles, S., Nagarathna, R., Vani, P. R., & Nagendra, H. R. (1997). A combination of focusing and defocusing through yoga reduces optical illusion more than focusing alone. Indian Journal of Physiology & Pharmacology. 41, (2), 179–182.

Telles, S., Naveen, K. V. (1997). Yoga for rehabilitation: an overview. Indian Journal of Medical Sciences. 51, (4), 123–127.

Vedanthan, P. K., Kesavalu, L. N., Murthy, K. C., et al. (1998). Clinical study of yoga techniques in university students with asthma: a controlled study. Allergy & Asthma Proceedings. 19, (1), 3–9.

Further Reading

Devereux, G. The elements of yoga. Massachusetts: Element, 1994.

Iyengar, B. Light on pranayama. New York: Crossroad Publishing, 1992.

Morris, K. (1998). Meditating on yogic science. Lancet. 351, (9108), 1038.

Samskrti & Veda. Hatha Yoga: manual I. 2nd Ed. Honesdale, PA: The Himalayan International Institute, 1985.

Schatz, M. P. Back care basics: a doctor's gentle yoga program for back and neck pain relief. Berkeley, CA: Rodmell Press, 1992.

Taylor, E. (1995). Yoga and meditation. Alternative therapies in health and medicine. 1, (4), 77–78.

Vishnudevananda, S. The complete illustrated book of yoga. New York: Harmony Books, 1980.

Yoga Journal. 2054 University Ave. Berkeley, CA 94794. (510) 841-9200.

RESOURCES

Himalayan Institute of Yoga, Science, and Philosophy
RRI Box 400
Honesdale, PA 18431
(800) 822-4547

The International Association of Yoga Therapists
109 Hillside Avenue
Mill Valley, CA 94941
(415) 383-4587

Sivananda Yoga
5178 South Lawrence Boulevard
Montreal, Quebec, Canada H2T 1R8
(514) 279-3545

INTERNET

Office of Alternative Medicine
http://altmed.od.nig.gov/

Meditation and Yoga
http://www.syda.org/glossary.html
http://www.sivananda.org/meditati.htm
http://www.diamondway-buddhism.org/meditations/me-e-gy.htm
www.geocities.com/RodeoDrive/1415indexc.html

Maharishi University
www.mum.edu/

Beginning with the early dawn each day, I will radiate joy to everyone I meet. I will be mental sunshine for all who cross my path. I will burn candles of smiles in the bosoms of the joyless. Before the unfading light of my cheer, darkness will take flight.

—PARAMAHANSA YOGANANDAJ

CHAPTER 6

ALTERNATIVE SYSTEMS OF MEDICAL PRACTICE

ACUPUNCTURE

What Is Acupuncture?

Acupuncture, a 3,000-year-old Chinese medical treatment, has gained great popularity in the United States. Acupuncture is one of the most popular complementary modalities, with approximately 10 to 13 million visits to acupuncturists annually. Acupuncture balances the flow of vital life energy throughout the body. It is a complete system of medical care that provides effective treatment for numerous conditions, from the common cold and flu to addiction and chronic fatigue syndrome. Acupuncture is based on the belief that health is determined by a balance of energy flow or Chi (Qi). The Asians believe that health is the reflection of harmony with heaven and represents a state of balance in the complementary and opposing forces of the universe. Disease occurs as an imbalance in these forces, producing excesses or deficiencies of basic life energy in particular organs. If the energy force is not corrected, physical changes in the body occur.

Because Chinese medicine sees all illness as a process of energetic disharmony, which acupuncture helps to reestablish, there are no disorders for which this form of treatment is inappropriate. Special needles are inserted into acupoints (just under the skin), to help correct and rebalance the flow of energy and consequently relieve pain and restore health. The needles draw energy away from organs with excess and redirect it to organs with deficiency.

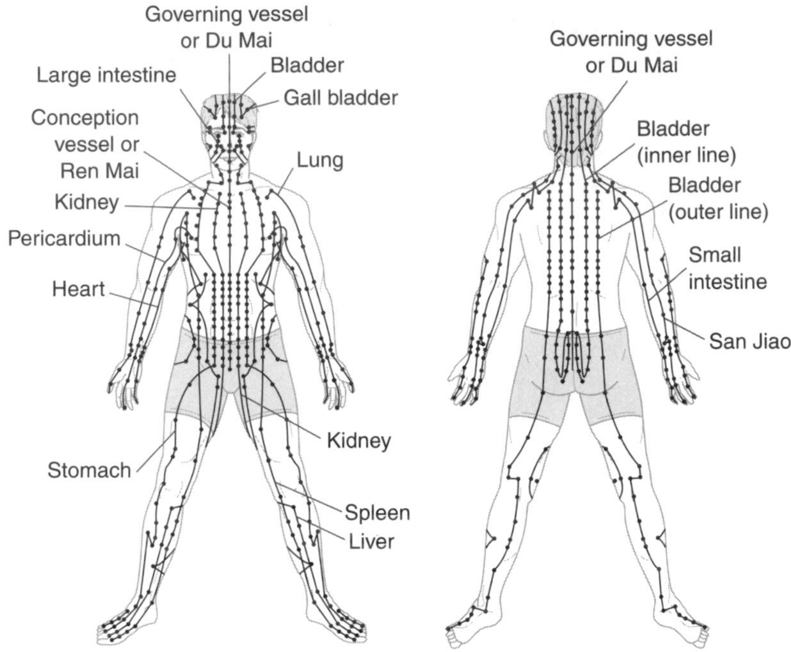

FIGURE 6-1

The Meridians. Meridians are invisible channels along which Chi or energy flows around the body. There are 14 main meridians.

Acupuncture is believed to work through various mechanisms: improved microcirculation by vasodilating arteries and veins; relaxation of muscle groups; release of endorphins, enkephalins, serotonin, adrenocorticotropic hormone (ACTH), and other humoral factors; activation of B and T lymphocytes; and improvement in the complete blood cell (CBC) count. The CBC count begins to change in 4 hours and becomes significant by 24 hours after a treatment. CBC count changes are only obvious when preacupuncture and postacupuncture studies are drawn.

Acupoints influence the 12 organs that are connected by lines called meridians (See Oriental Medicine for further explanation) (Fig. 6-1). Each organ has a superficial meridian with many numbered points. The meridians end and begin at the fingers and toes, where the polarity of chi is said to change. Needling is frequently done below the elbows and knees because energy circulation is most easily influenced near the origins and terminations of the meridians.

Identification of the point is based on strict anatomic criteria and requires precision and practice. Even a slight error in placement results in an ineffective treatment. A proper diagnosis within the principles of oriental medicine is essential to obtain the best results from acupuncture.

The History of Acupuncture

Acupuncture is an ancient technique that traditionally is believed to have begun 3,000 years ago in China. Before the end of the Stone Age, people in China used stone needles, animal bones, or bamboo to treat illness and had identified the specific points through which symptoms could be influenced. Two thousand years ago a Chinese story relates a tale about wounded warriors sometimes recovering from chronic diseases after being shot with arrows in combat. These healings provided clues to acupuncture and its potential for healing. Sometime between 400 and 200 BC, *The Yellow Emperor's Canon of Internal Medicine* was compiled and became the first book on acupuncture. Another major book, the *Classic of Acupuncture and Moxibustion*, was written in the 3rd Century AD. By the Tang Dynasty in the late 600s AD, China had universities and medical schools. Chinese doctors had to pass a three-part medical board to practice medicine.

Over time, the initial practice of inserting needles into points where pain was experienced (ashi points) was systematically developed. Energy flows were mapped as the meridians of the body. Specific points were identified and their actions recorded. The theory of acupuncture continues to develop and be refined. More than 2,000 acupuncture points have been discovered and confirmed.

Interest in the United States began in the early 1970s, when front page publicity in the *New York Times* told a story of a reporter who required an emergency appendectomy while in China. The reporter was given acupuncture to relieve a bowel obstruction, and his postoperative pain was relieved and the technique was successful. This publicity created an instant curiosity and demand for acupuncture.

Acupuncture has recently (March, 1998) received support from the U.S. Food and Drug Administration (FDA) and was upgraded from "experimental" to "tool" (same category as scalpels and syringes) from the National Institutes of Health (NIH) in 1998.

What Research Exists?

PRO

Research has been ongoing since the 1960s to prove the existence of meridians. Isotopes injected into the acupuncture meridians traveled

30 cm in 4 to 6 minutes. Isotope injected into random parts of the body did not travel in the same manner, indicating that meridians comprise a system of separate pathways within the body (Gerber, 1988; De Vernejoul, et al, 1985). In the 1970s, under a grant from the NIH, Becker, et al (1985 & 1990) found that electricity flowed along the Chinese meridians. Recently, DeSmul (1996) demonstrated the restoration of immunologic parameters and balance between coagulation and fibrinolysis by using small microwave frequencies at acupuncture points along meridians. Deng, et al (1996) found that mast cell activity was increased in and near the acupuncture point after being stimulated, suggesting that mast cells play an important role in the functions of the meridians. Pomeranz (1996), who has studied acupuncture for many years, has proven that acupuncture stimulates peripheral nerves that send messages to the brain to release endorphins, which then block the pain pathway. The NIH consensus statement on acupuncture developed by a panel of experts convened by NIH in 1998, stated that acupuncture is effective for the treatment of postoperative pain, nausea and vomiting associated with chemotherapy, the nausea of pregnancy, and postoperative dental pain. (The full report is available by calling 1-800-NIH-CONSENSUS or on the Internet at http://consensus.nih.gov.)

Hesketh (1997) demonstrated that acupuncture treatments administered to stroke patients in addition to rehabilitation speeded their recovery. This study shows the clinical effectiveness of combining eastern and western medicine.

Appiah, et al (1997) used a controlled, randomized prospective study with 33 patients and found that acupuncture was a reasonable alternative for treating patients with primary Raynaud's syndrome.

CON

A problem exists with evaluating negative acupuncture research. Researchers, often nonacupuncturists, perform the acupuncture or they use treatment protocols that an educated acupuncturist would not use. Because the positioning of the needle is of utmost importance, an educated acupuncturist should perform the procedure. The negative research does not mention who conducted the acupuncture.

Taub (1998) suggests that acupuncture had no demonstrable results when used to control nausea and postoperative pain in 100 postoperative patients. Sobel, et al (1997) identified perineal nerve palsy and drop foot that occurred secondary to acupuncture needles. Davies, et al (1998) did not find a statistically significant result in treating nonallergic rhinitis when compared to mock transcutaneous electrical nerve stimulation or sham acupuncture.

Members of the consensus panel (Taub, 1998; Marwick, 1997; & Ernst, 1997) point out "there are also studies that do not find efficacy for acupuncture in pain," and that there is "evidence that acupuncture does not demonstrate efficacy for cessation of smoking and may not be efficacious for other conditions." All suggest caution in the use of acupuncture.

What Is Acupuncture Used to Treat or Improve?

The World Health Organization (WHO) has identified 104 uses for acupuncture, some of which are:

- Eye problems (inflammations, myopia) (Cho, et al, 1998)
- GI disturbance (ulcers)
- Bone and muscle disorders (tennis elbow, tendonitis, myositis, arthritis) (Longworth & McCarthy, 1997)
- Neurologic disorders (trigeminal neuralgia, Meniere's disease, paralysis from cerebrovascular accident [CVA], speech-aphasia, Sciatica)
- Pain, acute and chronic (Farber, et al, 1997)
- Anesthesia
- Addictions (food, alcohol, tobacco)
- Skin conditions (burns, gangrene)
- May reduce the need for surgery in carpel tunnel syndrome and osteoarthritis and thus reduce overall medical costs
- Migraines (Baischer, 1995)
- Sinusitis
- Respiratory conditions (common cold, tonsillitis, asthma)
- Environmentally induced illness (pesticide poisoning, air pollution, radiation disease)
- Skin conditions (psoriasis and eczema; has limited success alone, but is used effectively as an adjunct)
- HIV (supportive and some relief of symptoms)

What Happens During a Visit?

- The acupuncturist takes an extensive history* of problems and symptoms, and explores issues such as the following:
  - What foods do you like and dislike?

*For more information regarding these areas, see the section on Oriental Medicine.

  - What is your family history?
  - What is your lifestyle?
  - A physical examination* is performed:
  - Looking (examining the tongue, fingernails, skin, face, gait, posture, and range of motion)
  - Touching (pulse taking, abdominal and other palpation)
  - Listening and smelling
- Needle insertion: the needles are most commonly made of surgical stainless steel with handles of stainless steel, plastic, silver, or copper. Gold or silver needles are also sometimes used. They range in length from 0.25 to 6 inches and come in gauges from 28 gauge to less than 40 gauge (0.12 mm). Needles are generally disposable, coming presterilized in blister packs, disposed of after use in "sharps" boxes, and subsequently incinerated. Specially made needles may be reused after vigorous procedures to cleanse and resterilize the needles, comparable to those used for surgical instruments. Acupuncturists must learn the proper needle depth for each of the hundreds of acupuncture points.
- The practitioner is seeking to access the patient's Chi flow with the needle. The sensation of accessing the Chi is called "*deqi*" (acquiring the Chi) and can be sensed by the patient and the practitioner. The patient may experience a tingling or a numb sensation at the needle insertion sites and along the line of the meridian. The sensation is different than what one experiences from an injection. The patient can be helpful to the practitioner in advising when the needle has reached the correct point. The experienced practitioner can also develop a subjective sense when deqi is reached.
- Needling techniques
  - Reinforcing technique: to reinforce a deficiency of Chi
  - Reducing technique: to reduce excessive Chi
  - Even technique: to neither reduce nor reinforce Chi

To accomplish these techniques, the needles may be lightly flicked (to enhance the quality of Chi), manipulated (to reinforce Chi), or vigorously rotated (to stir up stagnant Chi). The practitioner may use different techniques on different points. The practitioner must focus the Chi and must always be aware of what he or she is seeking to achieve with the therapy. Acupuncture is an art and a science and takes many years to master.

- Length of time: needles are retained in place for a few minutes to more than an hour, with 20 minutes being average.

---

*For more information regarding these areas, see the section on Oriental Medicine.

ADDITIONAL ACUPUNCTURE TECHNIQUES

- Electroacupuncture. A pair of needles or several pairs are connected to a small D/C charge to stimulate the flow of Chi. The frequency and strength of the electric pulse can be varied. Research by Pomeranz (1996) and others has shown that electroacupuncture stimulates increased release of endorphins, enkephalins, and other neurotransmitters
- Moxibustion. Direct or indirect moxibustion with *moxa*, a dried herb (a variety of mug wort [*Artemisia vulgaris]*) is used. Loose moxa is burned on the handle of the needle or directly on the skin. When lit, moxa burns slowly and provides a penetrating heat that can enter the channels to influence the Chi and blood flow. Moxa burns with a characteristic musky odor and gives off a copious amount of smoke. When applied directly to the skin, the moxa is piled into the shape of a cone. The top of the cone is lit and burns slowly toward the skin. The moxa is extinguished before the skin is burned, although ancient acupuncturists allowed the skin to burn. Moxibustion has been shown to increase white blood cell counts and is used throughout Asia to enhance immune function.
- Cupping. This form of treatment may precede a treatment or be used during a treatment. It is sometimes performed as an alternative to acupuncture. The cups are placed over the acupuncture points but the treatment covers a larger area. Most often glass cups are heated and placed on the skin. A strong vacuum is created in the cup by burning a taper and removing the oxygen. The cup may be left on the skin for a short period of time or up to 1 hour. Cupping draws blood to the external capillaries of the body, which may cause a small weal to be left after treatment.
- Auricular acupuncture. Ear points may be used for a more general acupuncture session. Press needles (needles placed on a small patch of adhesive bandage that acts as a form of mild acupressure) or ear seeds may be left in place for a week or more.

Paul Nogier, MD, a neurosurgeon from France, is considered to be the Father of auricular acupuncture. In 1989, auriculotherapy was officially recognized by the WHO as a viable medical modality. Auriculotherapy is used in the treatment of pain, addictions (Holder, 1991), functional imbalances, dyslexia, and other conditions.

Are There Any Risks Involved With Acupuncture?

There are no acute risks involved with acupuncture, but it should not be used alone to treat severe trauma, cancer, or acute infections.

In addition, there are a few contraindications:

- Hemophilia
- Pregnancy (Certain points and needle manipulations are contraindicated in pregnancy. An educated acupuncturist would understand the contraindications.)
- Psychosis
- Recent intake of psychotropic drugs or alcohol (however, recent research has shown benefit in drug and alcohol addiction)
- Outside temperature exceeds body temperature
- The patient is fasting
- There is a lightning storm
- There is a full moon

(American physicians have discovered independently of one another that people bleed more readily for the 2 days into the full moon and the 2 days out of the full moon. In ancient times the needles were much more course, therefore, the admonition to avoid puncture for those 4 days. In modern times, with much thinner needles, acupuncture is safe on those days although bruising is somewhat more likely.)

What Training Is Required of the Practitioner?

All practitioners should be educated in special schools. The schools may offer a certificate or a doctor of acupuncture degree. There are 34 schools and colleges of acupuncture and Oriental Medicine in the United States that are accredited or for which accreditation is pending. There are also numerous schools of integrated medicine that include acupuncture as a treatment modality. Acupuncture is taught in a few dental schools as an adjunct for pain control during dental procedures. Medical doctors, osteopaths, or dentists who receive acupuncture training may do so with a 250-hour home study program, and chiropractors, a 120-hour home study program. There is no clinical application and no education in pulse taking and tongue diagnosis, which are basic to the practice of acupuncture. These practitioners should offer acute pain treatment only. If the symptoms do not resolve or when there are complex problems, the patient should be referred to an educated acupuncturist.

There are more than 7,000 acupuncturists in the United States and nearly 4,000 physicians who use acupuncture in their practices. Acupuncture research is ongoing at numerous institutions including medical schools and the NIH. As with other forms of alternative health care, the legality of practicing acupuncture varies between states. Thirty-eight states require licensing, whereas some have no licensing requirement and others limit practice to physicians such as medical doctors and chiropractors. In California and a few other states, acupuncturists are considered primary health care professionals and can see any patient without a physician's referral. Where acupuncture is licensed, the acupuncturist must have graduated from an approved college and have passed a state licensing examination or a national board examination administered by the National Commission for the Certification of Acupuncture and Oriental Medicine (NCCAOM). The NCCAOM requires a minimum of 1,800 hours of training. Some health insurance companies will pay for acupuncture (California, Florida, Maine, Montana, Nevada, Oregon, and Washington) and bills are pending in New York and Virginia. (See Chapter 1 for more information regarding insurance coverage.)

Bibliography

Anonymous. Panel makes point about acupuncture. (1997). Journal of the National Cancer Institute. 89, 1751.

Appiah, R., Hiller, S., Caspary, L., Alexander, K., & Creutzig, A. (1997).Treatment of primary Raynaud's syndrome with traditional Chinese acupuncture. Journal of Internal Medicine. 241, 119–124.

Baisher, M. D. (1995). Acupuncture in migraine: long-term outcome and predicting factors. Headache. 35, 472–474.

Becker, R. O. (1990). Cross currents. The promise of electro-medicine. The perils of electropollution. Los Angeles, CA: Jeremy P. Tarcher, Inc.

Becker, R. O, & Selden, G. (1985). The body electric: Electromagnetism and the foundation of life. New York, NY: William Morrow and Company, 235.

Cho, Z. H., Chung, S. C., Jones, J. P., et al. (1998.) New findings of the correlation between acupoints and corresponding brain cortises using functional MRI. Proceedings of the National Academy of Sciences of the United States of America. 95, 2670–2673.

Davies, A., Lewith, G., Goddard, J., & Howarth, P. (1998). The effect of acupuncture on nonallergic rhinitis: A controlled pilot study. Alternative Therapies. 4, 70–74.

Deng, Y., Zeng, T., Zhou, Y., & Guan, X. (1996). The influence of electroacupuncture on the mast cells in the acupoints of the stomach meridian. (Chinese). Chen Tzu Yen Chiu Acupuncture Research. 21, 68–70.

DeSmul, A. (1996.) Very new waves in very old meridians: quantum medical physics of the living. Acupuncture & Electro-Therapeutics Research. 21, 15–20.

De Vernejoul, P., et al. (1985). Study of acupuncture meridians using radioactive tracers. (In French). Bulletin de L; Academie Nationale de Medicine. Oct. 22, 1071–1075.

Ernst, E. (1997). Acupuncture, fools and horses. Journal of Pain & Symptom Management. 14, 325–326.

Farber, P. L., Tachibana, A., & Campiglia, H. M. (1997). Increased pain threshold following electroacupuncture: analgesia is induced mainly in meridian acupuncture points. Acupuncture & Electro-Therapeutics Research. 22, 109–117.

Gerber, R. (1993). Vibrational medicine. Santa Fe: NM: Bear & Company.

Hesketh, T., & Zhu, W. (1997). Health in China: Traditional Chinese medicine: 1 country, 2 systems. British Medical Journal. B15, (7100), 115–117.

Holder, J. (1992). New auricular therapy formula to increase retention of the chemically dependent in residential treatment. National Acupuncture Detoxification Association Newsletter. Dec, 1–6.

Longworth, W. & McCarthy, P. W. (1997). A review of research on acupuncture for the treatment of lumbar disk protrusions and associated neurological symptomatology. Journal of Alternative & Complementary Medicine. 3, 55–76.

Marwick, C. (1997). Acceptance of some acupuncture applications. Journal of the American Medical Association. 278, 1725–1727.

Mitchell, B. B. (1996). Educational and licensing requirements for acupuncturists. Journal of Alternative & Complementary Medicine. 2, (discussion 41-3), 33–35.

Pomeranz, B. (1996). Acupuncture and the raison d'etre for alternative medicine. Alternative Therapies. 2, 85–91.

Sobel, E., Huang, E. Y., & Wieting, C. B. (1997). Drop foot as a complication of acupuncture injury and intragluteal injection. Journal of the American Podiatric Medical Association. 87, 52–59.

Taub, A. (1998). Thumbs down on acupuncture. Science. 279, 5348:159.

Further Reading

Benfield, H. & Krongold, E. (1991) Between heaven and earth: A guide to Chinese medicine. New York, NY: Ballantine Books.

Mitchell, E.R. (1987). Plain talk about acupuncture. New York, NY: Whalehall, Inc.

Moloe, P. (1992). Acupuncture—Energy balancing for body, mind, and spirit. Rockport, MA: Element Books Ltd..

Williams, T. (1996). Chinese medicine. Rockport: MA. Element Books Ltd.

Kaptchuk, T. (1992). The web that has no weaver: Understanding Chinese medicine. New York, NY: Congdon and Week.

RESOURCES

American Association of Acupuncture and Oriental Medicine
4101 Lake Boone Trail, Suite 201
Raleigh, NC 27607
(919) 787-5181

National Commission for the Certification of Acupuncturists
1424 16th Street NW, Suite 601
Washington, DC, 20036
(202) 232-1404

National Accreditation Commission for Schools and Colleges of Acupuncture and Oriental Medicine
1424 16th Street NW, Suite 501
Washington, DC, 20036
This organization provides accreditation.

American Acupuncture Association
4262 Kissena Blvd.
Flushing, NY 11355

Acupuncture Research Institute
313 West Andrix Street
Monterey Park, CA 91754

International Association of Clinical Laser Acupuncturists
10704 Tesshire Drive
St. Louis, MO 63123

National Acupuncture Foundation
1718 M. Street, Suite 195
Washington, DC 20036

COLLEGES OF ACUPUNCTURE

New England School of Acupuncture
30 Common Street
Watertown, MA 02172
(617) 926-1788

Traditional Acupuncture Institute
American City Building, Suite 108
Colombia, MD 21044
(301) 596-3675

American College of Traditional Chinese Medicine
455 Arkansas Street
San Francisco, CA 94107
(415) 282-7600

Midwest Center for the Study of Oriental Medicine
6226 Bankers Road, Suite 5
Racine, WI 53403
(414) 554-2010

Acupuncture Training for Nurses
Tri-State Institute for Traditional Chinese Acupuncture
80 8th Avenue at 14th Street, 4th Floor
New York, NY 10011
(212) 496-7869

INTERNET

Office of Alternative Medicine
http://altmed.od.nig.gov/

Acupressure/Acupuncture
//fox.cs.vt.edu/acu/index.html
www.acupuncture.com

Chinese Medical Journal
www.pavilion.co.uk/jcm/welcome.html

American Academy of Medical Acupuncture
www.medicalacupuncture.org

National Certification Commission for Acupuncture and Oriental Medicine
www.nccaom.org

Oriental Medicine E-mail discussion group
Send "subscribe your email address or Med" to listserv@bkhouse.cts.com

Big Yellow
www.bigyellow.com

AYURVEDIC MEDICINE

What Is Ayurvedic Medicine?

Ayurvedic medicine (science of life and longevity) is a comprehensive system of medicine that combines natural therapies (herbs, diet, exercise, aromatherapy, and massage) with a highly personalized approach to the treatment of disease. The first question an ayurvedic physician asks is not "What disease does my patient have?" but "Who is my patient?" The "who" meaning the constitution of the patient—the health profile, individual strengths, and susceptibilities. Once this identification has occurred, it becomes the foundation for all clinical decision.

Ayurvedic is the art of living in harmony with the laws of nature and encompasses the entire life. The aims and objectives of this science are to maintain the health of a healthy person and to heal the disease of an unhealthy person. Both maintenance and healing are carried out by entirely natural means.

Health is a perfect balance among the body's three fundamental energies or doshas (*vata, pitta, kapha)* (Table 6-1) and an equal balance among body, mind, and soul or consciousness. Body, mind, and soul are in constant interaction and relationship with other people and the environment.

When the sperm and egg join at the time of conception, the *vata*, *pitta*, and *kapha* factors from the parents' bodies are the most active and predominate at that moment; the season, the time, the emotional state, and the quality of their relationships form a new individual with a particular constellation of qualities. From the moment of conception, this constitution is created by the universal energies of Space, Air, Fire, Water, and Earth. The five elements are the most fundamental to ayurvedic science (Table 6-2). The five elements combine into the three

TABLE 6-1 THE THREE DOSHAS

	Vata	Pitta	Kapha
Body build	Thin, delicate body Prominent features and joints Cool, dry skin; rough, cracked nails, hands, and feet	Medium build Fair, thin hair Warm, ruddy, perspiring skin Distinctive eyes	Heavyset Large body frame Thick, wavy hair Cool, thick, pale, oily skin Obesity
Psychological	Hyperactive Moody Vivacious Imaginative Nervous disorders Enthusiastic, infectious energy Intuitive Anxiety Open minded Craves sweets, sour, salty tastes	Orderly, efficient Intense Sharp memory Short temper Lives by the clock Intelligent Warm, loving Passionate Articulate Perfectionist	Relaxed Slow to anger Display attachment to relationships Affectionate Forgiving and tolerant Compassionate Procrastination Loves sitting and doing nothing
Body function	Eats and sleeps at all hours Constipation Cramps	Doesn't miss a meal Ulcers, heartburn Sensitive teeth Hemorrhoids Acne	Slow, graceful Eats slowly Sleeps long, heavily Allergies, sinus High cholesterol Repeated colds, coughs
Other	Loves to travel	Does not tolerate sun Does not tolerate bulk Does not like fried food	Loves to hug Often needs coffee in AM to get awake Strong desire for stress Craves sweets

TABLE 6-2 THE ELEMENTS

	Space	Air	Fire	Water	Earth
Characteristics	Empty, light, omnipresent	Dry, light, clear, mobile	Hot, dry, sharp, penetrating	Fluid, heavy, soft, viscous, cold, dense	Heavy, hard, rough, firm, dense, slow-moving, bulky
Energy	Nuclear	Electrical	Radiant	Chemical	Mechanical/physical
Associated with	Sound, hearing	Touch	Light, vision	Taste	Smell
In body	Mouth, nose, gastrointestinal tract, respiratory tract, abdomen, thorax	Movement of muscles (heart, lungs) Neurotransmission from/to brain	Solar plexus, body temperature metabolism, digestion, absorption	Plasma, cytoplasm, serum, saliva, cerebrospinal fluid, urine, sweat, maintains nutrition	Strength, structure, stamina, bones, teeth, hair, skin
Psychologically	Freedom, peace, expansion of consciousness	Flow of thoughts, desire, will	Intelligence, transformation, attention, comprehension, understanding	Contentment, obesity	Forgiveness, groundedness, growth
Feeling	Love, compassion, isolation, anxiety, fear	Happiness, joy, excitation, anxiety, fear, insecurity	Anger, hatred, envy, ambition, competitiveness	Thirst	Attachment, greed, depression

doshas. Air constitutes *veta*, which is the energy of movement; fire and water constitute *pitta*, the principle of digestion (the transformation of matter into energy); and water and earth make up *kapha*, the energy of structure and lubrication (Fig. 6-2). From this inherited genetic code our individual constitution (*prakroti*) forms, and does not change during life.

Although our prakroti remains our fixed reality, our essential individuality is constantly being bombarded by numerous forces, such as age, environmental changes, feelings, emotions, and the food we eat. Unhealthy living disturbs the balance, thus disease occurs. Healing cannot take place unless all areas of life are improved. Maintaining health and balance requires moment-to-moment awareness, consciousness, and healing.

According to Ayurveda, our life has a purpose. Simply stated, that purpose is to know or realize the Creator (Cosmic Consciousness) and to understand our relationship with That, which will entirely influence our daily living. This great purpose is to be achieved by balancing four fundamental aspects of life: *dharma*, which is duty or right action; *artha*, material success or wealth; *kama*, positive desire; and *moksha*, spiritual

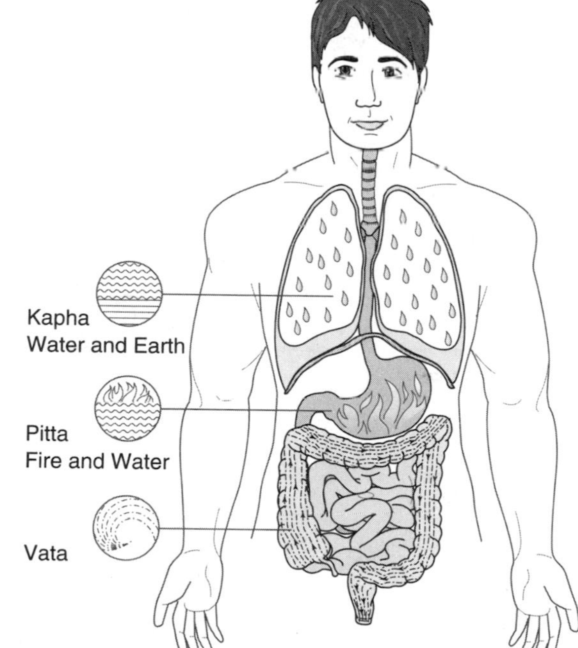

FIGURE 6-2
The Seat of the Three Doshas in the Body.

liberation. These are called the four *purusharthas*, the four great aims or achievements in the life of any individual.

The foundation of all these facets of life is health. To maintain *dharma* and carry out our duties and responsibilities to ourselves and others, we must be healthy. Likewise, to create affluence and achieve success in action, good health is indispensable. To have creative, positive desire, we need a healthy mind and consciousness, a healthy body, and healthy perception. (Desire—*kama*—is sometimes translated as sex and refers to progeny and family life, but it is really the positive energy or force of desire that generates and propels any creative work.) *Moksha*, or spiritual liberation, is perfect harmony of body, mind, and consciousness or soul. Thus the whole possibility of achievement and fulfillment in life rests on good health.

According to ayurvedic medicine, the source of all existence is universal Cosmic Consciousness, which manifests as male (*Purusha)* and female (*Prakruti)* energy (Table 6-3). Whatever is present in the universe is present in human beings. Man is a miniature of nature.

Every cell in the body also has a mind, intelligence, and consciousness, through which it manifests selectivity and choice. From all the possible nutrients in the environment, every cell chooses its own food—the choice is intelligence at work.

Again the five elements combine into the three doshas or metabolic body types. Each is a blueprint of innate tendencies, such as body build, personality, reactions, and food likes and dislikes. The doshas govern our psychobiologic functioning; when in balance, there is health and order, when out of balance, there is disease and disorder. Each person is a reflection of one or more of the doshas, thus each person has a pattern of energy. The characteristics of each dosha is summarized in Table 6-1.

TABLE 6-3 COSMIC CONSCIOUSNESS

Purusha		Prakruti
male		female
choiceless		choiceful
passive		active
pure awareness		
	Both are external, timeless, and immeasurable.	
formless		form
beyond space and time		color
pure existence		attributes
becomes many		
lover		beloved

Understanding one's own constitution has many benefits:

1. Self-understanding is the foundation of life.
2. Helps identify habits and tendencies that directly influence health.
3. Helps anticipate problems and illness that may occur so therapy can be instituted to prevent them from happening.
4. Assists one to understand others so relationships improve.
5. Provides one with knowledge about achieving balance in life.

DEFINITION OF HEALTH

Health is not merely the absence of disease, but a state of balance among body, mind, and consciousness—a state of being totally happy with one's self.

DEFINITION OF DISEASE

Disease is out of balance with nature. The mind, body, and soul are no longer coordinated. Disease is a disruption of the spontaneous flow of nature's intelligence with our physiology. Natural law has been violated. There are seven factors that can disrupt physiologic harmony: genetic causes, congenital causes, internal or external trauma, seasons, natural tendencies or habits, and magnetic or electrical influences.

ENERGY AND THE CHAKRA SYSTEM

In the ayurvedic system, health is seen as a harmonious balance of life energies within us. The life force in Oriental philosophy is Chi; the life force in ayurvedic philosophy is Prana. Chi flows through meridians, Prana through Chakras.

The idea of the seven major chakra centers of the body and the myriad of minor chakras has long been postulated within the Indian spiritual traditions (Fig. 6-3). Ancient Indian texts suggest that the chakras are similar to energy vortices or centers that exist within our subtle energy levels that directly access the cellular structure of the physical body. Chakras may take on the function of "energy transformer," allowing higher-frequency organizational energy fields to function at the relatively lower-frequency levels of the physical body. Each major chakra appears to be associated with a particular gland of the endocrine system giving access to the hormonal flows and changes in the body. It is suggested that the chakras are connected to each other and that they are linked through the body by subtle energetic channels called "nadis."

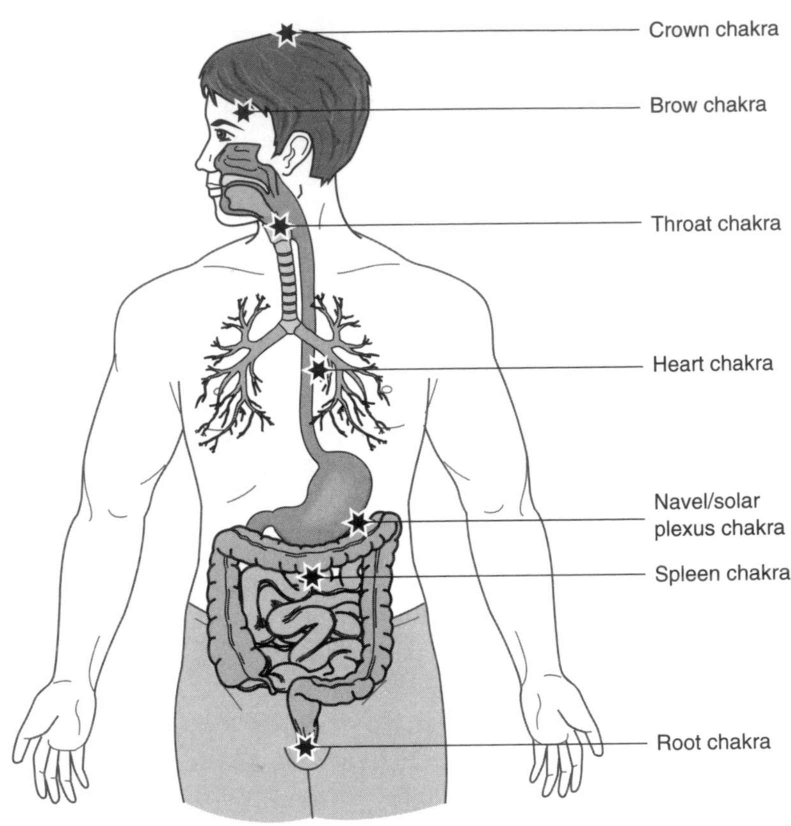

FIGURE 6-3
The Chakras.

What Is the History of Ayurvedic Medicine?

Ayurvedic medicine has been practiced continuously for more than 5,000 years in India. Ayurvedic medicine is an enduring science of life that has never lost its integrity and essential nature. It is a system based on the ayur veda, a sacred text of the ancient Aryans. Approximately 3,000 years ago (900 BC), three great scholars, Charaka, Sushruta, and Vagbhata, wrote down the principles of the already ancient wisdom. Their textbooks are still used by students, practitioners, and teachers.

Ayurvedic medicine is often considered the mother of all healing systems. It has eight principle branches (pediatrics, gynecology and obstetrics, ophthalmology, geriatrics, otolaryngology, toxicology, general medicine, and surgery) that are also branches of traditional Western medicine. Many of the modern healing modalities (massage, diet, herbs, polarity therapy, kinesiology, shiatsu, acupressure and acupuncture, color and gem therapy, and meditation) have roots in ayurvedic philosophy.

The great sage, physician Charaka, said, "A physician, though well versed in the knowledge and treatment of disease, who does not enter into the heart of the patient with the virtue of light and love, will not be able to heal the patient." Maybe we in traditional Western medicine could learn from the past.

What Research Exists?

PRO

Qutab (1996) has demonstrated how most women can have their menopausal signs and changes well-controlled using ayurvedic treatments. Special herbs for strengthening and rejuvenating the female reproductive system, along with herbs to regulate hormones and calm the emotions are used. Devi (1997a) uses herbs and diet to treat and possibly cure breast cancer. The ayurvedic approach stresses the emotional, spiritual, and environmental levels of treatment. Devi (1997b) successfully treats depression by first determining the type of depression (the dosha type) and then develops a treatment of herbs, diet, and lifestyle changes. It is important for the physician to give reassurance that "this too will pass." Multiple research studies were reported by Dahanukar (1997), who investigated the benefit of Ayurvedic herbs. The author concluded that the herbs work by enhancing white blood cell (WBC) production, by preventing neutrophil destruction, by enhancing phagocytosis, and by increasing macrophage activity. Therapy with Ayurvedic herbs appears to decrease mortality in patients with obstructive jaundice, enhance other treatments in patients with TB, and enhance general well-being in patients with breast cancer. All these products are capable of causing adverse effects and self-medication is not encouraged.

CON

Prpic-Majie, et al (1996) studied the connection between lead poisoning and the use of traditional Ayurvedic metal mineral tonics. There is a wide range of lead content in Ayurvedic preparations. It is suggested that the import of these mineral tonics should be strictly controlled and self-medication should be discouraged.

What Is Ayurvedic Medicine Used to Treat or Improve?

Ayurvedic medicine is used to treat or improve everything. It is a total method of health care. In a landmark book in 1990, Dr. Deepak Chopra demonstrates the ayurvedic medicine is a fully articulated model of the quantum-mechanical human body. Several recent reports suggest that Ayurvedic therapy is appropriate for treating coronary artery disease. Ayurvedic medicine can lower cholesterol, increase high density lipoproteins (HDL are protective), and reduce arterial plaque formation in the coronary arteries.

The 1994 report to the NIH entitled *Alternative Medicine: Expanding Medical Horizons* states that because of the potential of Ayurvedic therapies for treating conditions for which modern medicine has few, if any, effective treatments, this is a fertile area for further research. In addition, the National Cancer Institute has included Ayurvedic compounds on its list of potential chemopreventive agents.

What Happens During Ayurvedic Therapy?

Ayurvedic physicians traditionally have relied on observation rather than equipment and costly laboratory results. Treatment is based on observation, questioning of patient and family, palpation, and listening to the heart, lungs, and intestines. Increasingly, ayurvedic medicine is being used concurrently with Western medicine.

The pulse, tongue, eyes, and nails are observed. Each dosha has its own characteristic pulse. A physician can distinguish six pulses (three superficial and three deep) on each wrist. The strength, vitality, and function of the internal organ can be determined through these 12 sites. The tongue is observed closely for discoloration or sensitivity. Areas on the tongue represent organs in the body (Fig. 6-4). A urine examination is always performed, usually on a midmorning sample. The ayurvedic physician observes the color, smell, and clarity.

After a thorough examination, the doshas disorder is determined and treatment begun. Treatment consists of:

a. cleansing and detoxifying (*shodan*)
b. palliation (*shaman*)
c. rejuvenation (*rasayana*)
d. mental hygiene and spiritual healing (*satvajaya*)

Remedies are individual to each person and to each dosha. Thus two people with the same symptoms will be treated differently because of their individual make-up.

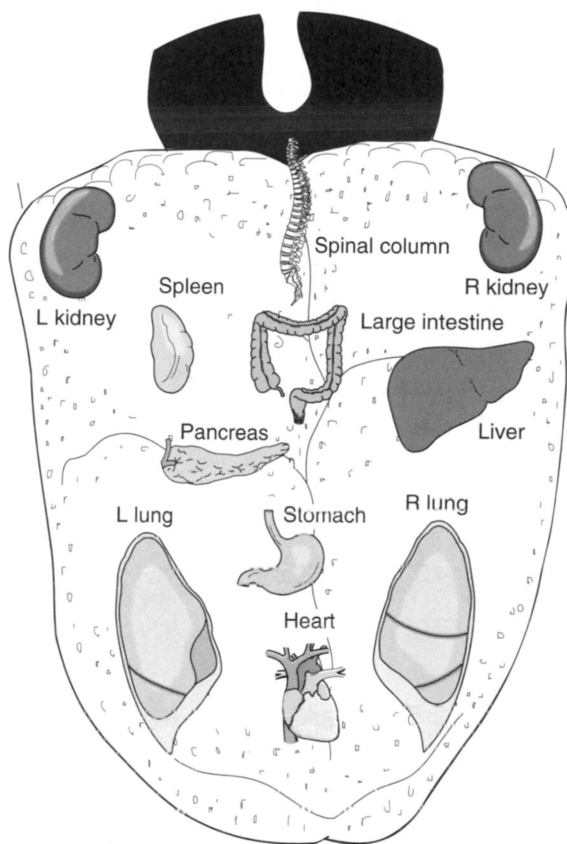

FIGURE 6-4
Tongue Diagnoses.

Remedies are used until the symptoms disappear, which may take several days to a few months. It is important during this time to determine the underlying cause of the condition and to rethink diet, daily routines, exercise, and so on.

CLEANSING AND DETOXIFICATION

Cleansing and detoxification procedures, such as vomiting, bowel purging enemas, blood cleansing, and nasal douching, are used to remove toxins from different areas of the body. Before cleansing is done, herbal oil massage or herbal steam sauna are used to help eliminate toxins and pesticides from the body. The cleansing eliminates vata, pitta, and kapha impurities from the body. After bowel cleansing, preparations of ghee (clarified butter), yogurt, and herbs are used to reestablish intestinal flora. Ghee increases digestive fire and improves absorption. Ghee carries the medicinal properties of herbs to all areas of the body.

PALLIATION

Palliation is used to balance and pacify the body doshas. A combination of herbs, fasting, chanting, yoga stretches, breathing, exercises, meditation, and lying in the sun (for a limited time) are used. These techniques are useful for patients with disease but also are used by healthy people. Development of a daily routine is stressed as it puts us in harmony with nature. A daily routine is said to directly aid digestion, absorption, and assimilation of food, and generate self-esteem, discipline, peace, happiness, and a long life.

REJUVENATION

After the cleansing program, the body is ready for a tune-up. There are three categories of treatment used to rejuvenate and restore the body: special herbs, mineral preparations suited to the particular dosha, and yoga exercises.

MENTAL HYGIENE/SPIRITUAL HEALING

This step attempts to improve the mind to reach a higher level of mental and spiritual functioning. This is accomplished by releasing psychological stress, emotional distress, and unconscious negative beliefs. The techniques used are:

Mantras: sound therapy

Yantras: concentrating on geometric shapes to take the mind out of the everyday world

Tantras: direct energy through the body

Meditation: to alter the state of consciousness

Gems, metals, and crystals: for the subtle, vibratory healing power

What Are the Risks Involved With Ayurvedic Medicine?

There are no risks with ayurvedic medicine when consulting a qualified Ayurvedic practitioner. However, self-treatment may cause adverse effects.

What Training Is Required of the Practitioner?

Ayurvedic medical school is required.

Bibliography

Dahanukar, S. & Thatte, U. (1997).Current status of ayurveda in phytomedicine. Phytomedicine. 4, 359–368.

Devi, A. (1997). A. Ayurvedic specific condition review: breast cancer. The Protocol Journal of Botanical Medicine. 2, 53–56.

Devi, A. (1997). B: Ayurvedic specific condition review: affective mood disorder. The Protocol Journal of Botanical Medicine. 2, 67–71.

Douillard, J. (1996). Ayurvedic specific condition review: benign prostatic hyperplasia. The Protocol Journal of Botanical Medicine. 1, 27–28.

Prpic-Majic, D., Pizent, A., Jurasovic, J., et al. (1996). Lead poisoning associated with the use of Ayurvedic metal-mineral tonics. Journal of Toxicology-Clinical Toxicology. 34, 417–423.

Qutab, A. (1996). Ayurvedic specific condition review: menopause. The Protocol Journal of Botanical Medicine. 1, 104–105.

Sharma, H. M., Triguana, B. D., & Chopra, D. (1991). Maharishi Ayr-veda: modern insights into ancient medicine. Journal of the American Medical Association. 265, 2633, 2634, 2637.

Further Reading

Chopra, D. (1993). Ageless body, timeless mind. New York, NY: Harmony Books.

Chopra, D. (1991). Perfect health. New York, NY: Harmony Books.

Chopra, D. (1990). Quantum healing. New York, NY: Bantam Books.

Frawley, D. (1990). Ayurvedic healing. Salt Lake City, UT: Morson Publishing.

Lad, V. (1998). The complete book of ayurvedic home remedies. New York, NY: Harmony Books.

Lad, V. (1984). Ayurveda. the science of self-healing: a complete guide to all therapies used in ayurvedic medicine. Wilmont, CA: Lotus Light Press.

RESOURCES

American School of Ayurvedic Sciences
10025 NE 4th Street
Bellevue, WA 98004
(206)453-8022

Ayurvedic Institute
11311 Menaul NE, Suite A
Albuquerque, NM 87112
(505) 291-9698

The College of Maharishi Ayur-Veda Health Center
PO Box 282
Fairfield, IA 52556
(515) 472-5866

Invincible Athletics
PO Box 541
Lancaster, MA 01523
(508) 368-1818

The Maharishi Ayur-Veda Health Center
RR #2
Huntsville, Ontario Canada P0A 1K0
(705)635-2234

Sharp Institute for Human Potential and Mind-Body Medicine
8010 Frost Street, Suite 300
San Diego, CA 92123
(800) 82-SHARP

INTERNET

Meditation and Yoga
    http://www.syda.org/glossary.html
    http://www.sivananda.org/meditati.htm
    http://www.diamondway-buddhism.org/meditations/me-e-gy.htm
    http://www.geocities.com/RodeoDrive/1415indexc.htm

DeepakChopra
    http://www.randomhouse.com/chopra

Maharishi University
    http://www.mum.edu/

Office of Alternative Medicine
    http://altmed.od.nig.gov/

HOMEOPATHY

What Is Homeopathy?

Homeopathy is a 200-year-old system of healing based on the laws of similars. Dr. Samuel Hahnemann, the founder of homeopathy, developed the natural law of "like cures like." For example, a person with a rash is given a substance that creates a rash. Homeopathy is not about neutralizing the rash; the treatment addresses the underlying cause of the rash itself.

After much research, Hahnemann formulated the principles of homeopathy:

- Like cures like (Law of Similars)
- The more dilute the remedy, the greater its potency (Law of the Infinitesimal Dose)
- An illness is specific to the individual (Holistic Medical Model)

HOMEOPATHIC DILUTION				
X Dilution				
Original substance	**Successed 10 times with**	**Distilled water or alcohol**	**Yields**	**Resulting solution: x**
1 part	+	9 parts	→	1x
1 part of 1x	+	9 parts	→	2x
1 part of 2x	+	9 parts	→	3x
1 part of 99x	+	9 parts	→	100x
C Dilution				
Original solution	**Successed 10 times with**	**Distilled water or alcohol**	**Yields**	**Resulting solution: c**
1 part	+	99 parts	→	1c
1 part of 1c	+	99 parts	→	2c
1 part of 2c	+	99 parts	→	3c
1 part of 12c	+	99 parts	→	13c (original solution no longer measurable)

LIKE CURES LIKE

"Like cures like" was recognized as far back as Hippocrites (400 BC) and later became the theoretical basis for vaccines by Jenner, Salk, and Pasteur. The law of similars says the same substance that in large doses can produce the symptoms of an illness, in minute doses cures it. There has been much technical research in physics, biology, biochemistry, and other sciences to determine how the law of similars works (Bellavite & Signorine, 1995; VanWijk & Wiegrant, 1994). As a systematic observer of nature and healing, Hahnemann recognized that the body makes amazing and impressive efforts to heal itself, but that it is not always strong enough to complete the healing process. Often, the body needs a catalyst to stimulate its defenses, particularly when battling serious, chronic, or genetic disorders. Using the law of similars, the right catalyst is individualized for the patient, which initiates the body's defenses and begins the healing process.

THE MORE DILUTE THE REMEDY, THE GREATER ITS POTENCY

Homeopathic remedies are prepared by mixing one part of the original substance in nine parts of distilled water or alcohol and then it is "successed" (the vial is forcibly struck 10 times against a leather pad). This dilution is called a 1×; one part of the 1× dilution is mixed with nine parts of diluent and successed 10× = 2× solution; one part of a 2 solution is mixed with nine parts of diluent and successed 10× = 3 solution. This dilution can be continued indefinitely. The signifies that the formula has been diluted to a proportion of 1:9, the c potency means it has been diluted to a 1:99 level. When the medicine gets to a 12 c, there is no longer any measurable original substance. The remedies are taken orally. The action of homeopathic medications cannot be explained in terms of existing pharmacologic concepts because the traditional homeopathic remedy has no active ingredient. So "what" is producing the effect (Widakowich, 1996; Fisher 1995)? Research has found that the original substance leaves its energy pattern or electromagnetic frequency in the diluted solution. The more dilute the solution (200 c), the more powerful the medicine. DelGiudice, et al (1990) and Rubik (1991) have demonstrated that homeopathy remedies give off a measurable electromagnetic signal. These signals show that specific frequencies are dominate in each homeopathic substance. DelGiudice, et al (1990) and Gerber (1988) further suggest that the electromagnetic message in the remedy matches the specific electromagnetic frequency or pattern of the illness to stimulate the body's natural healing response.

THE FDA AND HOMEOPATHIC REMEDIES

The FDA recognizes homeopathic remedies as official drugs and regulates their manufacturing, labeling, and dispensing. Homeopathic remedies also have their own official compendium, the Homeopathy Pharmacopoeia of the United States, first published in 1897. See Table 6-4 for a selected list of homeopathic medicines and their source.

Homeopathic medicines are exceptional because they can greatly enhance deep healing without the harmful side effects so commonly caused by conventional medicines.

ILLNESS IS SPECIFIC TO THE INDIVIDUAL

Homeopathy recognizes that each person expresses disease in an individual way. A headache is not just a headache. Homeopathy recognizesmany symptom patterns associated with headaches and has a corresponding remedy for each. Homeopathic medicine views symptoms as an expression of the body attempting to heal itself. When the body is faced with stress, a person reacts emotionally, physically, and mentally to regain balance. The remedy is based on this totality of symptoms, not just the physical

TABLE 6-4 SOME HOMEOPATHIC MEDICINES AND THEIR SOURCES

Medicine/Remedy	Source
Allium Cepa	Onion
Apis Mellifica	Honey bee
Arsenicum Album	Arsenic
Aurum Metallicum	Gold
Belladonna	Deadly nightshade
Calcarea Carbonica	Oyster shell
Chamomilla	German chamomile
Lachesis	Bushmaster snake
Lycopodium	Crushed club moss spores
Mercurius	Mercury
Rhus Toxiconendron	Poison ivy
Sepia	The ink of a cuttlefish
Spongia Tosta	Roasted sea sponge
Tuberculinum Bovinum	Tuberculous lung of a cow

symptom of the headache. Covering up symptoms only pushes them to a deeper level, causing more serious consequences in the long term.

THE HEALING CRISIS

As the stages of healing occur, the patient may get worse before he gets better. Dr. Constantine Hering, the father of American Homeopathy, developed the "Hering's Law of Cure." Hering suggests that healing progresses from the deepest part of the body to the extremities, from the emotional to the physical, and from the upper body to the lower body. The long-term benefit of homeopathy to the patient is that it not only alleviates the symptoms, but it reestablishes internal order at the deepest levels and thereby provides a lasting and complete cure. The whole principle of homeopathy is to restore health as gently, quickly, and as permanently as possible. Disease is limiting to the person, health is freedom.

What Is the History of Homeopathy?

Homeopathy dates to 1810, the year the founder, Dr. Samuel Christian Hahnemann, published his most important work "Organon of Medicine." Samuel Hahnemann was an esteemed physician and chemist. However, he left the practice of medicine because he felt he was doing more harm than good with the traditional treatments of the day:

bloodletting, poisonous doses of mercury and arsenic, and other dangerous treatments.

To support his family, Hahnemann began translating various medical and literary texts. While translating a work by William Cullen, a leading physiologist of the time, he was startled to learn that the bitter and astringent properties of Peruvian bark (which contains quinine) accounted for its effectiveness in treating malaria. Hahnemann set out to test Cullen's hypothesis. He began taking small doses of Peruvian bark and was surprised to find that he developed symptoms similar to malaria. As time went on, he found that an overdose of the medicine caused symptoms similar to those of the illness for which they were used to treat. Mercury used to treat syphilis, caused syphilis-like ulcers. Arsenic caused fevers and was given to treat fevers. Silver nitrite, used to treat eye inflammation, caused severe irritation when placed in the eye. From this point in time, Hahnemann began to develop the principles of homeopathy (life-suffering).

Hahnemann was the first to recommend giving medicinal drugs to healthy people to assess their physiologic properties. These experiments are called "provings." A person is administered an extremely small dose of a single substances on a daily basis until symptoms are elicited. Careful observations and records are made of the symptoms that occur. Each substance (plant, mineral, or animal), creates a variety of physical, emotional, and mental symptoms unique to that substance. The detailed records of symptoms produced during the provings are compiled in reference books known as *materia media*. Most of the provings were done in the late 1800s and early 1900s, but many organizations including the American Institute of Homeopathy are still conducting provings. Some of the latest medicines to be entered into the *materia media* are plutonium, granite, and neon.

The first homeopathic physician arrived in the United States in 1828. In 1836, the Hahnemann Medical College opened in Philadelphia. The American Institute of Homeopathy was founded in 1844 and became the first national medical society. American homeopaths were more successful than allopaths were in treating the cholera epidemic that swept the United States in the 1840s. This success brought money and prestige to homeopaths.

In 1855, the AMA demanded that all state medical societies accept the code of ethics, requiring them to expel homeopaths or homeopathic members. In the 1860s, the AMA brought charges against physicians who were found to have consulted with homeopaths. By the end of the 19th Century, few homeopaths existed in the United States. Since the 1970s, there has been a resurgence in homeopathic schools and interest in homeopathic medicine.

What Research Exists?

There is considerable amount of research available regarding homeopathy. The following are selected studies.

PRO

Jacobs, et al (1994) studied homeopathic remedies for diarrhea in Nicaraguan children. This double-blind clinical trial demonstrated a statistically significant association between homeopathic treatment and shorter duration of diarrhea. Barnes, et al (1997) performed a meta-analysis on many studies studying the treatment of postoperative ilius. The meta-analysis demonstrated a statistically significant result in favor of homeopathy over placebo to first flatus.

Davidson, et al (1997) concluded that homeopathy may be useful in the treatment of affective and anxiety disorders in patients with mild to severely symptomatic conditions. Rogers (1997) suggests that homeopathy can provide a valid and effective therapy to help clients break the cycle of alcohol dependence.

Sudan (1997) studied the treatment of seborrholic dermatitis with homeopathic remedies and found the condition remised. Sudan suggests that homeopathic remedies may also provide treatment for other allergic and inflammatory disorders. A controlled study (Reilly, et al, 1994) found that homeopathy can benefit patients with allergic asthma. With continued treatment, the number of acute asthma attacks were reduced significantly. Kleijnen, et al (1991) reviewed 107 controlled trials using homeopathy that supported its use in symptom or disease reduction or elimination.

Ludtke (1996) demonstrated that *galphemia glauca* was significantly better in relieving the symptoms of allergy than conventional antihistamines were.

CON

When evaluating negative research, it is always important to verify that the proper remedy was administered. Because each individual is different, they may have the same presenting signs and symptoms, but should receive different remedies. The question is always, "Did they?"

Vickers, et al (1997) designed a double-blind, placebo-controlled trial to study homeopathic remedies to prevent muscle soreness after exercise. This study did not find any benefit to the homeopathic remedy. Whitmarsh, et al (1997) cannot conclude from their study of homeopathy in migraine treatment and prevention that it is without effect; however, they recommend homeopathy for migraine prophylaxis after their double-blind parallel group trial. Linde, et al (1997) performed a meta-analysis on 89 studies to determine if the effect from homeopathy was a placebo effect. From their finding, they suggest there is insufficient evidence from these studies that homeopathy is efficacious for any clinical condition.

Further clinical trials with double-blind groups are indicated to further study homeopathy.

ON-GOING RESEARCH

Several studies involving the effectiveness of homeopathic cures and medicines are on-going around the world. Homeopathy International Research and Development group is studying: basic science of homeopathy, new product research, and applied clinical research. Hanover University in Germany is conducting a 5-year study (to be completed late 1997/early 1998) studying the action of homeopathic medicines. A 12-year study at Utrecht University in Holland is the Law of Similars using cell cultures. The Integrative Primary Care Outcomes Study is studying the effectiveness of homeopathic treatment in six common clinical conditions encountered in primary care. Homeopathy is being studied to relieve the symptoms of premenstrual syndrome. This study should be completed in 1998.

What Is Homeopathy Used to Treat or Improve?

Homeopathy is a complete system of natural medicine that can have a therapeutic effect on almost any disease or health condition. Homeopathy has proven beneficial in treating:

- Headaches, ear infections
- Respiratory infections (asthma, colds)
- Digestive problems (diarrhea, abdominal pain, constipation, hemorrhoids)
- Sprains and general aches and pains
- Postoperative infections
- Low back pain
- Sexually transmitted disease
- Neck stiffness
- Dental pain
- Flu
- Motion sickness
- Childhood diseases (colic, teething, bed-wetting)
- Women's health (vaginitis, PMS, cramps, cystitis, menopausal signs and changes)

- Men's health (bladder infections, prostate problems, testicular problems)
- Allergies (contact dermatitis, hives, eczema)
- Emotional upsets
- Accidents and injuries (bruises, burns, heat exhaustion, animal and insect bites)
- Depression, anxiety, attention deficit disorder (ADD), hyperactivity

What Happens During a Visit?

Five basic steps are followed during a visit:

- Case taking involves collecting complete and accurate information about the illness (Table 6-5), such as contributing causes, onset, character of symptoms, location of a particular symptoms, modality of symptoms, and general symptoms; how has the patient's behavior changed; what makes symptoms better or worse; sleep habits and how they are different; general psychological symptoms; all past illnesses; and information about the person in general (often takes 1 to 2 hours).
- Case analysis involves evaluation of the information about the illness and the person. Homeopathic resources and diagnostic guides are called *repertories* and *materia medicas*. A repertory is a compilation of symptoms matched with the medicines that have been known to cure them. Computer repertories are available that decrease the time necessary to develop a treatment plan. An attempt is made to match the symptoms to the medicine rather than the medicine to the person. During the case analysis, the homeopath determines which symptoms are most limiting to the person's optimal physical and psychological function.
- Select the homeopathic medication that best suits the person and the illness.
- Administer the remedy. Usually one dose is administered in the office. The medicines are inexpensive.
- Observe the reaction to the treatment and decide whether to repeat or change the medication (see example in Table 6-6). No more medication is administered until the previous dose has ceased to act, no matter how long or short a time that may take. There are several points to keep in mind for treating acute and nonchronic conditions:
  - The more severe the person's acute symptoms, the more often the medicine should be repeated or the higher the potency
  - The medicine is continued for no more than 2 or 3 days if there are no results

TABLE 6-5 CASE-TAKING QUESTION FOR COLDS

Character of the symptoms:
- At what stage is the illness: early (within the first 24 hours), late (after a week or so), or in between?
- Which are the more bothersome symptoms: runny or stuffy nose, watery eyes, laryngitis, or cough?
- Do the symptoms alternate?
- Describe the color and consistency of the nasal discharge. Do the tears or discharge irritate the skin?
- Is the patient hoarse? Does the patient have a constant need to clear the throat?
- Is the cough dry, or wet and rattling? Where is the "tickle?" What is the color and consistency of any coughed-up mucus, and is there any blood in it? How hard is it to raise the mucus?
- Describe any pain or other sensations (such as tightness or pressure) in the chest.

Modalities:
- At which time of day is each symptom more or less bothersome?
- How is each symptom affected by external warm or cold, warm or cold drinks, motion, swallowing, or touch?
- Is the cough related to sleep? Does it come on just before or during sleep, or when first awakening? Does it wake the patient from sleep?

Other symptoms:
- Is there a nosebleed? Any skin eruptions? A headache?
- Has the patient lost the sense of smell or taste?
- Is there mental-emotional irritability; does the person want company or solitude? Is the person fearful, happy, whiney, etc.?

(From Cummings S, Ullman D. Everybody's Guide of Homeopathic Medicines. New York: Tarcher/Putman. 1997.)

- Enough time is allowed for the medicine to work before changing to a new remedy
- No more than two or three remedies should be used

Are There Any Risks Involved With Homeopathy?

Homeopathy should not be used when there is a danger of the homeopathic cure not being effective because an acute illness could result. Homeopathy is probably not as effective for emergency care as is allopathy (e.g., a fracture will need to be cared for using traditional allopathic treatments), but the pain associated with the fracture and subsequent healing may be managed well with homeopathy.

TABLE 6-6 REMEDY SUMMARY FOR COLDS

Remedy	Essentials	Confirmatory Symptoms
Allium Cepa	• Clear, burning nasal discharge irritating nostrils and upper lip. • Profuse tearing of the eyes that does not cause irritation of the skin, although the eyes are red and burning	• Symptoms worse in warm rooms, indoors, and in the evening; better in open air • Frequent sneezing better in the open air • Tickling in larynx causing dry, painful cough; person grasps the throat while coughing • Thirst
	• Nonirritating, watery nasal discharge • Copious burning tears • Nasal flow of clear to slightly whitish mucus, thicker than water (may look like raw egg whites or boiled starch)	
	• Dry, tickling, and scraping sensations in the nose • Nose alternately stuffed up and runny; stuffy at night, runny in warm rooms and during the day • Frequent sneezing • Profuse, watery nasal discharge that burns the skin (discharge may become yellow in time) • Nose runs freely but feels stuffed • Irritation and tickling in the nose and frequent, violent sneezing	• Colds developing after exposure to cold or cold, dry weather • Symptoms worse from eating • Throat raw and rough • Tickling in the larynx; teasing, dry cough causing soreness in the chest • Cough worse in the morning (especially on waking), between midnight and daybreak, in cold air, after eating, or after mental work; better after warm drinks
Gelsemium	• Symptoms develop gradually • Nasal discharge watery • Tiredness; body feels heavy	• Chills running up and down the back • Headache above the nape of the neck
Kali Bichromium	• Later stages of a cold with thick, yellow or greenish discharge	
Pulsatilla	• Mental or general symptoms of *Pulsatilla* are pronounced • Nasal discharge thick, yellow-green, nonirritating	• Nose alternately stuffed up and runny; runs more in open air and in the evening, becomes stuffed up in a warm room

[a] *Give the medicine 3 to 4 times a day, less frequently as symptoms improve. Try another medicine if no changes are observed after 48 hours.*

What Training Is Required of the Practitioner?

Naturopathic schools include homeopathy as part of a 4-year training program. There are also numerous schools of homeopathy that require a 3-year course of study after high school. There are also master's and doctorate programs in homeopathy. Additional 1- to 5-day programs are available. Certification is required by some states and insurance companies, and certification bodies exist. A registered homeopathic uses the initials RSHom(NA). The NA being North America, the area in which that registration was issued.

Bibliography

Barnes, J., Resch, K. L., & Ernst, E. (1997). Homeopathy for postoperative ileus? A meta-analysis. Journal of Clinical Gastroenterology. 25, 628–633.

Bellavite, P. & Signorini, A. (1995). Homeopathy: a frontier in medical science. Burkely: N. Atlantic.

Davidson, J. R, Morrison, R. M., Shore, J., Davidson, R. T., & Bedayn, G. (1997). Homeopathic treatment of depression and anxiety. Alternative Therapies in Health and Medicine. 3, 46–49.

DelGiudice, E. & Preparata, G. Superradiance: a new approach to coherent dynamical behaviors of condensed matter. Frontier Perspectives 1. no. 2 (Fall/Winter 1990) Philadelphia: Temple University, Center for Frontier Sciences.

Fisher, P. (1995). The development of research methodology in homeopathy. Complementary Therapies in Nursing & Midwifery. 1, 168–174.

Frye, J. Homeopathy in office practice. Primary Care; Clinics in Office Practice. 24(4):845-65, Dec., 1997.

Gerber, R. (1988). Vibrational medicine. Santa Fe, NM: Bear & Co. 84.

Jacobs, J., Jiminez, L., et al. (1997). Treatment of childhood diarrhea with homeopathic medicines: a randomized clinical trial in Nicaragua. Pediatrics. 93, (5), 719.

Kleijnen, J., Knipschild, P., et al. (1991). Clinical trials of homeopathy. British Medical Journal. 302, (6772), 316.

Leviton, R. (1989). Homeopathy. Yoga Journal. 85, 42–51, 97, 98, 100, 105.

Linde, K., Clausius, N., Ramirez, G., Melchart, D., Eitel, F., Hedges, L. V., & Jonas, W. B. (1997). Are the clinical effects of homeopathy placebo effects? Lancet. 350, (9081), 834–843.

Ludtke, W. (1996). A meta analysis of homeopathic treatment of allergy. Korsch Komplementarmed (German). 3, 230–234.

Reilly, D., Taylor, M., et al. (1994). Is evidence for homeopathy reproducible? Lancet. 344, (8937), 1601.

Rogers, J. (1997). Homeopathy and the treatment of alcohol-related problems. Complementary Therapy in Nursing and Midwifery. 3, (1), 21–28.

Rubik, B. (1991). Frontiers of homeopathic research. Frontier Perspectives. 2, (1), Philadelphia: Temple University, Center for Frontier Sciences.

Skinner, S. (1996). The world according to homeopathy. Journal of Cardiovascular Nursing. 10, (3), 65–77.

Sudan, B. J. (1997). Total abrogation of facial seborrhoeic dermatitis with extremely low-frequency 'imprinted' water is not allergen or hapten dependent: a new visible model for homeopathy. Medical Hypotheses. 48, (6), 477–479.

VanWijk, R. & Wiegrant, F. (1994). Cultured mammalian cells in homeopathy research: the Similia principle. Utrechte, The Netherland: University of Utrecht. 1023.

Vickers, A. J., Fisher, P., Smith, C., Wyllie, S. E., & Lewith, G. T. (1997). Homoeopathy for delayed onset muscle soreness: a randomised double blind placebo controlled trial. British Journal of Sports Medicine. 31, (4), 304–307.

Whitmarsh, T. E., Coleston-Shields, D. M., & Steiner, T. J. (1997). Double-blind randomized placebo-controlled study of homeopathic prophylaxis of migraine. Cephalalgia. 17, (5), 600–604.

Widakowich, J. (1996). Facts and a postulate on the mode of action of potentiated remedies. Medical Hypotheses. 47, (1), 15–17.

Further Reading

Many books are available. This is only a selected list.

Bruning, N. & Weinstein, C. Healing homeopathy remedies. Dell. New York, 1995.

Clover, A. Homeopathic first aid. California: Thorns, 1990.

Cummings, S. & Ullman, D. Everybody's guide to homeopathic medicines. Los Angeles: Jeremy P. Tarcher/Putman, 1997.

Katz, T. (1997). Homeopathic treatment during the menopause. Complementary Therapeutic Nursing and Midwifery. 3, (2), 46–50.

Lockie, A. The family guide to homeopathy: symptoms and natural solutions. New York: Prentice Hall Press, 1993.

Oswal, G. D. (1996). New homeopathic medication in rehabilitation of cerebral palsy and mental retardation. Nursing Journal of India. 87, (11), 242–244, 261–264.

Ullman, D. Discovering homeopathy: your introduction to the science and art of homeopathic medicine. Berkeley, CA: North Atlantic Books, 1991.

Ullman, D. The consumer's guide to homeopathy. New York: Jermany P. Tarcher/Putman. 1996.

Ullman, D. Homeopathic medicine for children and infants. Los Angeles: Jeremy P. Tarcher, 1992.

Wayne, J. & Jacobs, J. Healing with homeopathy. New York: Warner. 1996.

RESOURCES

American Institute of Homeopathy
925 E. 17th Avenue
Denver, CO 80218

British Institute and College of Homeopathy
520 Washington Boulevard, Suite 423
Marina Del Rey, CA 90292
(310) 306-5408

Homeopathic Academy of Naturopathic Physicians
Box 12488
Portland, OR 97212
(503) 795-0579

Homeopathic Education Services
2124 Kittredge Street
Berkeley, CA 94704
(510) 649-0294, (800) 359-9051

International Foundation for Homeopathy
2366 Eastlake Avenue, East, Suite 301
Seattle, WA 98102
(206) 324-8230

National Center for Homeopathy
801 North Fairfax, Suite 306
Alexandria, VA 22314
(703) 548-7790

INTERNET

A link to many homeopathic Web sites throughout the world.
www.dungeon.com/~cam/hemeo.html

Homeopathic Organizations
//antenna.nl/homeoweb/

Homeopathic Veterinarian Care
www.monmouth.com/~altvetmed/

Homeopathic Magazine on-line
www.wolfe.net.com/~enos/ho_web/index.html

Office of Alternative Medicine
http://altmed.od.nig.gov/

E-mail discussion group
Send "subscribe" to homeopathy-request@dungeon.com

National Center for Homeopathy & Homeopathic Education Services
www.homeopathic.org

North American Society of Homeopaths
www.homeopathy.org

NATUROPATHIC MEDICINE

What Is Naturopathic Medicine?

Naturopathic doctors (ND) believe in a state of complete physical, mental, and social well-being, not merely the absence of infirmity. Americans coined the word "Naturopathy." WHO has recommended the integration of naturopathic medicine into conventional health care systems. Naturopathy uses an array of healing practices, such as diet and nutrition, homeopathy, acupuncture and acupressure, herbs, exercise, spine and soft tissue manipulation, counseling, and light therapy. The concept of naturopathy is sometimes referred to as the "natural cure"—assisting nature in the cure of disease. The naturopathic philosophy states that if nature gives the body, mind, and emotions what they need to heal, that healing is the natural course. If the naturopathy can remove the barriers to cure and support the body, the body will heal. Naturopaths believe that the body is designed to maintain health and symptoms of illness are essentially signs that the body is ridding itself of toxins. Cold symptoms are an attempt to restore balance to the body, so rather than suppressing a fever or congestion with medications, naturopaths recommend rest, healthy diet, vitamins, herbs to control the symptoms, and possibly homeopathic remedies.

Principles of naturopathy include:

- Do no harm. All treatments are totally safe.
- Treat the whole person. A multifactorial approach to illness and health is used.
- Nature has healing powers. The body will heal itself if assisted and supported.
- Treat the cause rather than the effect. Avoid suppressing the body's natural response to disease, but determine the underlying causative factors, e.g., stress, diet, lack of exercise, and so on.
- Educate and empower the patient. The physician educates, empowers, and motivates patients to take responsibility for their health.
- Prevention is the best cure.
- Good nutrition is essential.

Naturopathy involves treating the whole person and practicing preventive medicine, which does not mean early detection of a disease; it means teaching people early on that, if they do certain things, they will help prevent chronic degenerative diseases.

What Is the History of Naturopathic Medicine?

Before the 1900s, naturopathy grew out of the alternative healing movement in the 18th and 19th Centuries. The Europeans tradition of "taking the cure" at natural springs and spas gained a foothold in the United States by the middle of the 19th Century. As a formal system of treatment, naturopathy dates back only to 1900, when its founder, Benedict Lust (1872–1945) established the first naturopathic college.

Dr. Lust, a German-born physician, was dissatisfied with the medical practice. He was convinced of the innate healing powers of nature, and he looked for a more natural, less harmful method of treatment. Dr. Lust adopted the philosophy of light, fresh air, herbs, and hydrotherapy as treatment options. Hydrotherapy was used by Father Sebastian Kneipp (1821–1897), who supposedly cured himself from a fatal lung condition by plunging into ice water everyday for months and using herbs.

Early naturopaths attached great importance to a natural, healthy diet. Dr. John Kellogg, a physician and vegetarian, ran a sanitarium that used natural therapies such as hydrotherapy. His brother, Will, built and ran a factory to produce health foods such as shredded wheat and granola biscuits. The Kellogg brothers, along with a former employee, C. W. Post, popularized naturopathy ideas about food and simultaneously founded the cereal companies that still bear their names.

Unlike homeopathy and osteopathy, naturopathic medicine never seriously challenged allopathy by drawing converts from the orthodox ranks. Naturopathy did not develop from a unified doctrine, but emerged slowly and without clear definition. Naturopathy flourished until the 1930s, when the AMA became all powerful and eliminated nearly all natural healing techniques. The last 20 years have brought a resurgence to naturopathic practice.

All naturopaths reject surgery and strong drugs, but otherwise have many different philosophies regarding treatment. Naturopathy offers a refreshing balance to the aggressive, invasive, and unnatural practice of modern medicine.

What Research, Reviews, and Comments Exist?

PRO

Head (1997) suggests that naturopathic remedies are ideal for breast cancer prevention and adjucative treatment along with conventional therapy. Naturopathic treatments alone are inappropriate for treating breast cancer. Wotton (1997) suggests that multiple naturopathic treatments (aromatherapy, nutritional, homeopathic, botanical, and hydrotherapy) are helpful in treating ADD. Costarella (1997) suggests naturopathic treatments such as herbs (St. John's wort, kola, Siberian ginseng, lemon balm, rosemary, ginkgo) offer improvement to persons with depression. In addition, the source of depression is explored, such as nutritional deficiencies, food sensitivities, parasites, nutritional influences, heavy metal intoxication, stress, prolonged anxiety, or amino acid disorders. Hobbs (1996) has demonstrated a relief of symptoms with naturopathic treatments in patients with prostatic hypertrophy. Hudson (1996) suggests that naturopathic treatments such as herbs are as successful as traditional hormone replacement therapy for controlling the signs and changes occurring in menopause.

CON

Flora, et al (1996) evaluated naturopathic remedies for chronic liver disease. When using a biochemical marker or histology examinations, the researchers were unable to find any objective evidence of improvement. No adverse effects from therapy have been identified. More than half of the patients in the study reported they felt better.

What Is Naturopathic Medicine Used to Treat or Improve?

- All health conditions and diseases can be treated. Acute conditions, trauma, or others requiring surgery are best treated with allopathic medicine, but the recovery phase and rehabilitation is treated well with naturopathy.
- Acute infections, such as ear infections, colds, and flu, can be treated with naturopathic medicine. Herbs and other therapies are used to reduce symptoms and then a care plan is designed to reduce or eliminate all the precipitating factors that may have contributed to the condition. If symptoms are severe or are present for more than 10 days, traditional medicine may be added.
- Chronic conditions are treated by attempting to find and eliminate the precipitating cause through a healthy living program., e.g., the naturopath addresses a chronic urinary tract infection by looking at the possible cause, i.e., emotional factors caused by long-standing sexual abuse.
- Naturopathic medicine focuses on the person, not the disease.
- Adjunctive treatments for illnesses such as cancer and heart disease (along with traditional treatment) to support the patient and decrease the symptoms are part of naturopathic medicine.
- Naturopathic medicine works well with "undoing" the ill effects of our environment and toxic medical treatments such as the overuse of antibiotics and the side effects of chemotherapy.

What Happens During a Visit?

- A detailed history of past illness, health history of parents and grandparents, genetic tendencies, diet history, level of exercise and stress, what drugs (vitamins or herbs) are being taken, and what has

been used in the past with what results is obtained (usually takes 1 to 1.5 hour).
- Blood tests or lab tests may be ordered
- Patient education and counseling about healthy living is discussed
- A treatment program and a health promotional plan are developed between the patient and ND. This plan is modified until the patient is able to "live" the program.
- A naturopath is likely to make home visits to instruct on healthier living and holistic nutrition

Are There Any Risks Involved With Naturopathic Medicine?

- Minimal risks, but naturopathy is possibly not as effective for acute conditions because treatments often take days or weeks to be effective, e.g., acute trauma is best treated with allopathic medicine, but the recovery phase can be handled well with naturopathic medicine.
- Treatments are generally safe and noninvasive.
- Because most NDs do not have hospital privileges, it may be necessary to have a traditional family practitioner.

What Training Is Required of the Practitioner?

- There are several accredited schools of naturopathy in the United States and Canada (see listing of schools). These programs provide the same type of basic education obtained in medical school. The difference is their approach to treatment focusing on natural therapies, such as botanical medicine, homeopathy, manipulation, Chinese medicine, and clinical nutrition, instead of surgery or pharmaceuticals.
- Educational programs may also be home study, for example, 4 years after high school or in a college setting. Master's and PhD programs are available.
- Twelve states and several Canadian provinces require a licensing examination, but most do not. Licensor is through the American Academy of Naturopathic Physicians.

Bibliography

Costarella, L. (1997). Naturopathic specific condition review: Depression. The Protocol Journal of Botanical Medicine. 2, (1), 62–66.

Flora, K. D., Rosen, H. R., & Benner, K. G. (1996). The use of naturopathic remedies for chronic liver disease. American Journal of Gastroenterology. 91, (12), 2654–2655.

Head, K. (1997). Naturopathic specific condition review: Breast cancer. The Protocol Journal of Botanical Medicine. 2, (3), 47–52.

Healy, H. (1997). The naturopath's perspective. Creative Nursing. 3, (3), 10–13.

Hobbs, C. (1996). Naturopathic specific condition review: Therapeutic botanical protocol for prostatic hyperplasia and a comparison with modern medicine. The Protocol Journal of Botanical Medicine. 1, (3), 22–26.

Hudson, T. (1996). Naturopathic specific condition review: Menopause. The Protocol Journal of Botanical Medicine. 1, (4), 99–103.

Wotton, E. (1997). Naturopathic specific condition review: attention deficit/hyperactivity disorder. The Protocol Journal of Botanical Medicine. 2, (1), 29–31.

Further Reading

Healy, H. (1997). The naturopath's perspective (interview by Mary Jo Kreitzer). Creative Nursing. 3, (3), 10–13.

Murray, M. & Pizzorno, J. Encyclopedia of natural medicine. Rocklin, CA: Prima Publishing, 1991.

Murray, M. & Pizzorno, J. Textbook of natural medicine, vols. 1–2. Seattle, WA: John Bastry College Publications, 1989.

RESOURCES

American Association of Naturopathic Physicians
2366 Eastlake Avenue, Suite 322
Seattle, WA 98102
(206) 298-0126

The Institute for Naturopathic Medicine
66½ North State Street
Concord, NH 03301-4330
(603) 225-8844

Schools of Naturopathy
*Bastyr University
144 NE 54th
Seattle, WA 98105
(206) 523-9585

*National College of Naturopathic Medicine
11231 SE Market Street
Portland, OR 97216
(503) 255-4860

**Southwest College
6535 E. Osborn Road
Scottsdale, AZ 85251
(602) 990-7424

---

*Accredited.
**Applying for accreditation.

Canadian College of Naturopathic Medicine
60 Berl Avenue
Etobicoke, Ontario, Canada M8Y 3C7
(416) 251-5261

INTERNET

Office of Alternative Medicine
http://altmed.od.nig.gov/

Natural Medicine
www.amrta.org/~amrta

Herbalgram
www.herbalgram.org/

American Association of Naturopathic Physicians
www.naturopathic.org

Marietta Naturopathic Health Services
www.actionco.com/mnhs

Alternative Medicine Homepage
www.pitt.edu/~cbw/altm.html

Task Force—Complementary Therapy
www.ahc.umn.edu/tf/cc.html

Organization of Naturopathic Physicians
www.infinite.org/naturopathic physician

Alternative Practitioners
www.teleport.com/~mattlmt/index

Bastyr University
www.bastyr.edu

ORIENTAL MEDICINE

What Is Oriental Medicine?

Isn't it interesting, that we in the West, call Oriental/Chinese Medicine complementary? Oriental Medicine began more than 3,000 years ago, and it has developed into a true science that peaked between the 10th and 13th Centuries, then declined, and is now in a resurgence. A fourth of the world's population uses traditional oriental medicine.

Oriental medicine's primary goal is to cultivate people's capacities and to correct whatever underlying disturbances are causing distress. To achieve this goal, it is useful to investigate how a disorder arises so the process can be disassembled and reorganized, not merely masked. In oriental medicine, everything is linked with everything. Health and illness coexist and arise out of the same conditions. Disease does not come from nowhere, it emerges from a lived life. Oriental medicine not only focuses on the disease, but on the person who has it. Oriental medicine is a method of restoration and recovery.

The philosophy that forms the basis of oriental medicine is Taoism, Confucianism, and Buddhism. All share a fundamental proposition that there is not an isolatable, immutable self that is wholly separate from the world. All have no limits. In Taoism, Confucianism, and Buddism, health is the harmony of heaven and universe, attained by a proper balance of internal and external forces. All believe in a basic universal energy that flows into and through the human body. This universal energy is referred to as Chi (Ch'i or Qi) (Fig. 6-5).

Chi is consciousness, the fundamental reality. Chi is everything that moves or changes. Chi is the motivating force, and anything that has to do with actualization, movement, and change. Chi exists along a continuum—mind is one end of the spectrum, whereas the universe is the other. Using an analogy of water: at one end of the spectrum, water is frigid, hard, and dense (ice), at the other end it is vapor, but it is still H_2O.

Energy is transferable from nature to man. Nature gives food and air to man. When these meet in the body, vital energy or human Chi is created. Chi is nourishing and protective. As the Chinese say, "When Chi gathers, so the physical body is formed; when Chi disperses, so the body dies." Chi can be built up and restored by proper nutrition, exercise, and leading a balanced lifestyle. Chi can be depleted by inappropriate living habits: excesses of alcohol, food, stress, drugs, and the like. Chi is often referred to as water. A useful analogy that is often used to describe Chi flow is that of a river. A river has a source, and it follows its course ultimately toward the ocean. As it flows, it will vary from shallow to deep, quick-flowing to deep, quiet flowing to slow flowing, while always following the most "natural"

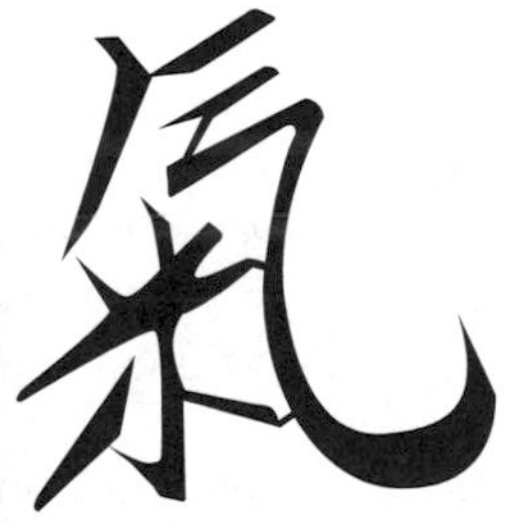

FIGURE 6-5
The Chinese Character for Chi.

path. Chi energy from the universe enters the body and connects the physical body with the universe. When disharmony or disease appears in the body, it will first manifest itself at the universal level. Physical illness comes at the end of a chain of energy connections. The challenge of the next century will be to explore this nontangible universal energy.

Oriental medical philosophy believes:

- Each person is unique
- Illnesses are manifested differently
- Treat the person, not only the disease

Oriental medicine stresses prevention through education—diet, exercise, stress management, rest, and relaxation. Oriental medicine tries to detect and treat "invisible disease." It does not wait until there are full-blown symptoms and "visible disease." An analogy that is used is that waiting for and treating visible disease is like "digging a well after you are thirsty." The concept of treating invisible disease makes oriental medicine a wonderful complement to traditional Western medicine because Western medicine is better at treating visible disease and has difficulty treating invisible disease.

WHAT IS HEALTH AND DISEASE?

Health is a state of harmony; therefore, disease is a state of disharmony. Causes of disharmony may be internal, external, or miscellaneous. The major internal causes of disharmony are considered psychological in nature and are termed the seven emotions (anger, joy, sadness, grief, pensiveness, fear, and fright). External causes pertain to climatic conditions known as the six pernicious influences or the six outside evils (wind, fire, heat, cold, dryness, damp, and summer heat). The miscellaneous causes of disharmony include constitutional factors, lifestyle factors, work, exercise, diet, sexual activity, and unforeseen events such as accidents and injuries. The Asians believe that disease will only attack organs that are weakened.

In nature, extreme wind, dampness, dryness, heat, and cold wreak havoc in the world. These same forces derange balance within the human body, weakening or obstructing the movement of Chi in the organs. As wind shakes trees, scattering leaves, internal wind manifests as vertigo, unsteady movement, and trembling. As saturated earth generates swamps, so dampness becomes edema and phlegm. As aridity withers vegetation, so dryness causes chapping or cracking of mucous membranes. Just as ice inhibits the rush of winter water in a stream, so internal cold retards circulation and depresses metabolism. And just as fire scorches the earth, so internal heat may inflame tissue or generate fever.

These internal and external pathogenic agents also contribute to the congestion or depletion of body constituents. Chinese medicine identifies five pernicious body climates as cold, heat, wind, dampness, and dryness. When fire burns the skin, it causes redness, swelling, and pain. According to correspondence logic, when these symptoms arise spontaneously, they are caused by the pathogenic influence of internal fire, or heat. The source of this fire cannot necessarily be seen, but its effects can be observed. Because heat produces inflammation and agitation, such symptoms are referred to as signs of heat.

Similarly, a person exposed to icy weather shivers and becomes lethargic, dull, and unresponsive. When these symptoms arise regardless of the external temperature, the person is manifesting the condition of cold. Coldness is associated with decreased metabolic activity, depressed mental function, retarded circulation, weakness, and malaise.

Jerky movement, dizziness, incoordination, or discomfort that migrates from one region to another, appearing and disappearing suddenly, suggests the presence of wind. External wind manifests as soreness, tightness, itching, and sensitivity of the skin and muscles. The common cold is an example when symptoms include dizziness, migratory pain in the joints, muscles, and head. Internal wind is characterized by labile emotions, vertigo, spasm, and emotional instability. Chills, body ache, and clear, runny secretions are indicative of wind-cold; fever, thirst, stuffy nose, sore throat, and yellow secretions indicate wind-heat. Wind-damp produces neurologic disorders such as clumsiness, numbness, paralysis, disequilibrium, headache, vertigo, joint pain, and muddled thinking.

Dampness appears as swelling and a sense of fullness, heaviness, or indolence. It can appear on the surface of the body as oily skin, sticky perspiration, and subcutaneous edema, or as joint swelling, cloudy urine, and malodorous vaginal discharges.

Congealed moisture becomes phlegm, recognized by heaviness of the head and limbs, dull pains, abundant sputum, fall or kidney stones, mental illness, epilepsy, or nodular deformities and cysts. Dampness and phlegm are similar, but dampness tends to affect the lower body, whereas phlegm invades the upper body. Signs of damp-heat are signaled by red, painful swelling, thick discharge, blisters as in herpes, and inflammations such as prostatitis, jaundice, dysentery, and bronchitis.

Dryness damages fluids and is manifested by symptoms of dehydration such as brittle hair and nails, wrinkled, cracked skin or mucous membranes, irritated eyes, dry stool or constipation, lack of perspiration, thirst, and scant urine. Dryness can generate irritation, inflammation, and heat caused by lack of lubrication and secretions; heat may lead to dryness.

Supplementing moisture will relieve dryness, just as eliminating moisture will counteract dampness. The principle of complementarity applies: for cold, warm; for heat, cool; for congested Chi, moisture, or blood, encourage movement; for depletion, nourish; for internal wind, subdue; for external wind, relieve surface congestion; and for phlegm, dissolve (Beinfeld, H. & Korngold, E. [1995]. Chinese traditional medicine: an introductory overview. Alternative Therapies. 1, 1, 48–49.)

Yin Yang Forces

Oriental philosophy believes in opposing forces—two opposite and complementary qualities to all aspects, called yin and yang (Table 6-7). This is a system of interdependence and interrelatedness. Each cannot exist alone; they must exist together. Both are complementary aspects of the

TABLE 6-7 YIN VERSUS YANG

tissue organ	activity of an organ
internal, lower	external, upper
front of body	back of body
blood	energy Chi
innate instincts	learned skills
negative	positive
contractive	expansive
female	male
dark, small	light, big, bright
night	day
right side	left side
interior of object	surface of object
cold, stillness	warmth, activity
metal, water	wood, fire
descends	ascends
heart	small intestine
spleen	stomach
lung	large intestine
kidney	bladder
liver	gallbladder
passive	functional
solid	hollow
If Deficient	
Organ does not have enough raw material to function.	Organ doesn't function adequately when needed.
TSM = thyroid function	

[a]superior and stronger-like water, which is all powerful and can wear away rock

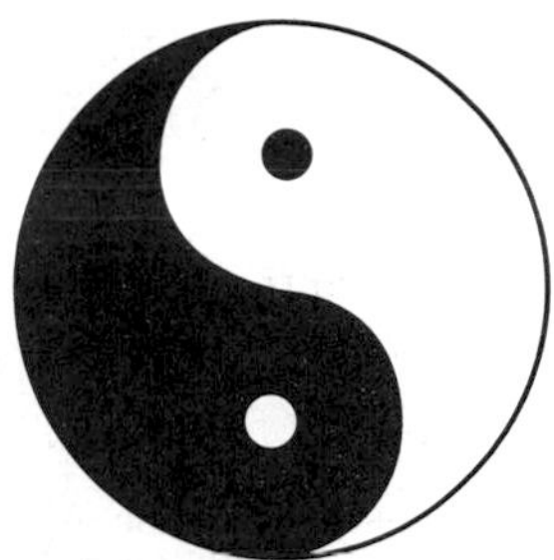

FIGURE 6-6
Yin and Yang. The elements of female (yin) and male (yang) separate, but always come back together. Note that in the dark (female, negative) side, there is a small spot of light and conversely, in the light (male, positive) side, there is a small spot of dark. Thus, there is always some feminine in the masculine and vice versa. This concept make possible the balancing of Chi.

whole. Yin and yang work as interactive opposites. This wholeness is dynamic and moving with one essence flowing into the other continuously. All substances, objects, times, places, organs, foods, and all other aspects of life and creation are mixtures of these qualities. Proper classification enables the Chinese to combine them in ways that promote general balance. For example, an overly yin person should eat more yang foods to promote health.

Oriental medicine views the body in terms of yin and yang aspects. A dynamic balance between yin and yang is characterized by a health state, and by implication, an unhealthy state is indicative of some imbalance between them. The yin and yang symbol is in Figure 6-6. Yin and yang is a way of thinking about the world.

Twelve Organs

The Chinese identify 12 organs, or "networks" (Zangfu) (Fig. 6-7); however, they do not always correlate to the name used in Western medicine. The Chinese term tsang (organ) means "sphere of function." For example, when there is an excess of Chi in the liver, the Chinese are not talking about the liver as we know it, but the sphere of bodily functions that may include all or part of the liver function. Two of the twelve Chinese organs have no anatomic correspondence: the triple heater referring to the opening of the stomach, small intestine, and bladder and the energy system that processes food and fluid; and the "circulation-sex" refers to the pericardium.

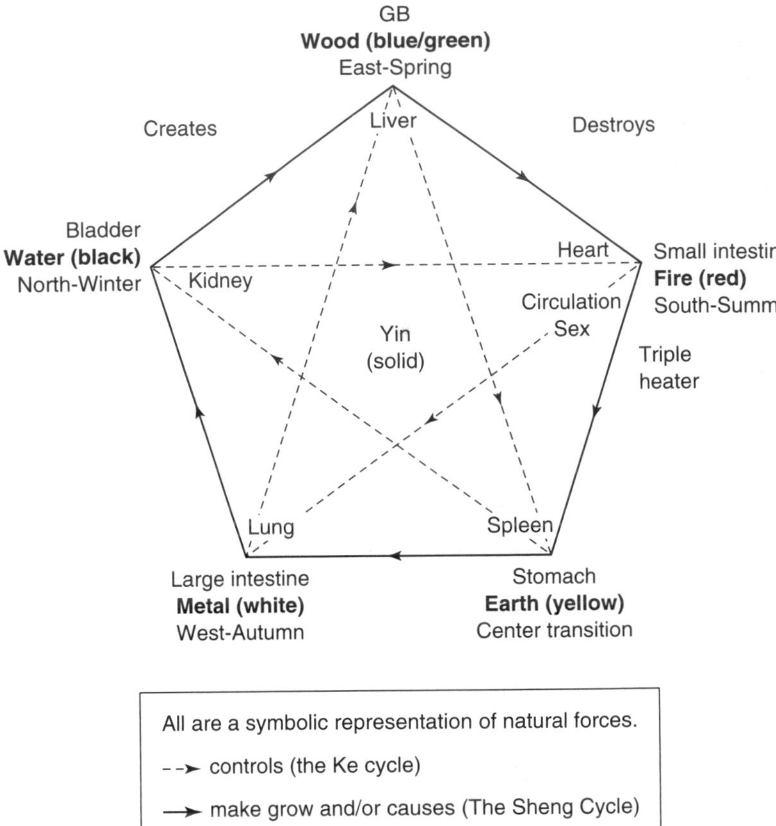

FIGURE 6-7
The Five Elements and Twelve Organs of Oriental Medicine.

Chinese custom prohibited autopsy in the past, so Chinese doctors had to proceed without detailed knowledge of anatomy and physiology. Surgery was rarely embraced as a therapeutic method. (The first recorded successful removal of a brain tumor in 150 AD was performed using acupuncture, wire, and hemp.) Because they were unable to assess pathologic changes in the internal body, they learned to recognize and correct imbalances of body function. Organs are also classified as hollow or yang (gallbladder, small intestine, large intestine, stomach, and bladder), and solid or yin (liver, heart, spleen, lung, kidney, circulation-sex).

The organs are arranged into a system that places each in one of five categories: fire, earth, metal, water, and wood (Fig. 6-7). This system, called the Five Phase Theory, or the Five Elements, is based on the premise that each organ nourishes or inhibits the proper functioning of another organ.

The Five Phases

The Five Phases is a fascinating circular model that beautifully represents the world of traditional oriental medicine and plays an important part in diagnosing illness. The Five Phases are used to observe natural progresses that occur and change with the seasons of the year. Each phase is representative of the natural world during a given season. Spring, for instance, is represented by wood, the birth process, and the color green. The summer season is fire and creative growth, the color red, sharp, sometimes bitter tastes, but also joyousness. Fall, by contrast, is metal, dryness, the color white, pungent tastes, and pensive moods (Fig. 6-7). Each phase demonstrates the cyclical nature of all life and the strong influences that these forces have on our health.

The Sheng Cycle (solid lines and arrows of Fig. 6-7) represents the matter in which the elements (and also the organ systems) support and promote each other, e.g., water nourishes the growth of wood, wood generates fire, fire burns to create earth, earth compresses to become metal, and metal generates water. The same concept applies to organs.

The Ke cycle (the broken lines on Fig. 6-7) demonstrates how the five elements control each other. Fire controls metal because fire will melt metal. Water will control fire. Metal can cut wood and wood will become earth. This concept also applies to the organs. The Chinese believe that the liver controls the spleen and is controlled by the lung. The relationship indicates the direction of the flow of Chi energy from one organ to another (Fig. 6-7).

Chi flows through each organ along meridians (Jinglue). The meridians begin and end at the fingers and toes where the polarity of Chi is said to change. There are a total of 59 meridians in the body, of which 12—the main meridians—dominate the others (see Fig. 6-1). Each of the main meridians represents a biologic energy system centered around one of the twelve organs. Chi flows from one meridian to another in a certain order until the entire network is covered, delivering vital energy to every part of the body. Chi completely flows around the body once a day. In addition, there are eight "ancestral," twelve "muscle," and fifteen "connecting" meridians. All are branches of the 12 main meridians, and serve to distribute Chi to those areas not covered by them. Stimulating one of the main meridians with acupuncture or herbs has a specific effect on the connected organ, as well as a general effect on the entire system.

What Is the History of Oriental Medicine?

Oriental medicine had its beginnings more than 5,000 years ago. Oriental medicine became a profession approximately 2,000 years ago. By that time, a widespread system of orderly government had been established, which has survived as such today. The philosophy that forms the basis of oriental medicine is a combination of Confucianism, Buddhism, and Taoism, which deal with the theory of a cosmic law and structure and man's place within the structure. It follows then that if physical health became an integral part of the whole body of law of Chinese spiritual and social life, the same principles of correlation and balance of forces also applied to diet and medicine. Food and medicine became interrelated: foods were chosen as much for their therapeutic qualities as for nourishment and taste.

Herbal tonics of garlic, ginseng, ginger, tofu, fennel, and arrowroot were used to treat disease and were being written about as early as 1500 BC. These products still exist in the oriental pharmacy.

China's first doctor lived from 407 to 310 BC, practiced medicine and acupuncture, and introduced the first gynecologic and pediatric treatments. The pharmacopoeia of herbal products probably dates to this period in time. Oriental medicine continued to flourish until the 1920s. At that time, many Chinese were being educated abroad, and on their return to China, instituted Western medicine and banned herbal therapy. In 1931, the League of Nations in Geneva created a committee to undertake research into the effectiveness of Chinese medicine. Today, oriental medicine and Western medicine are practiced side by side in China.

What Research, Reviews, and Comments Exist?

PRO

Specific oriental herbs have been studied for their anticarcinogenic effect (Kurashige, 1998). A preparation of eight Chinese herbs, called shikaron, has been found to have anticarcinogenic effects by activating natural killer and LAK cells, and cytokine production of T lymphocytes.

Chi, et al (1997) found that oriental medicine plays a significant role in Taiwan's ambulatory health care system. The oriental medicine practiced in Taiwan is considered highly professional, with a formal system of education, training, licensure, and regulation.

Xu (1996) reviews several patient case studies that were helped with Chinese medicine. Each patient had the Western diagnoses of senile dementia, but each had a different presentation in Oriental medicine, thus each was treated differently. Wang (1996) also reviews several case studies of epilepsy. Again each case had a different presentation, so each was treated differently with herbs and acupuncture. Most patients showed improvement.

CON

Sadler (1996) reported on a new treatment for severe atopic eczema in children—Chinese herbs. The eczema was found to improve in 60% of the children. The drawbacks to this treatment are twofold: the herbs often consist of leaves, bark, and small twigs, and when brewed into a tea are unpalatable; and the preparation often contains 10 to 25 ingredients often mixed with fungi, animal materials, and minerals to enhance their action, but which also carry the risk of serious side effects, including cardiotoxicity and renal and liver damage.

What Is Oriental Medicine Used to Treat or Improve?

Oriental medicine is practiced as a complete method of diagnosing and treating all acute and chronic conditions.

What Happens With Oriental Medicine?

Some practitioners will approach their understanding of a patient's difficulties from the perspective of the Five Elements and determine their interventions according to these principles. Other practitioners use yin and yang to understand the patient's problems in relationship to excess or deficient energy patterns. If five patients sought medical care from Western physicians because of symptoms of an ulcer, they would all be given the same standard treatment. If those same five persons went to a Chinese doctor, the doctor would look at their response to the disease, which is different for each, and would thus provide different treatments to each of them.

DIAGNOSIS

Oriental medicine is ultimately concerned with diagnosing the location and nature of the energy imbalance and the organs affected and determining if there are deficiencies or excesses of energy. Treatment is a matter of correcting the problem by drawing Chi away from organs of excess and bringing more Chi to the organs of deficiency.

The Chinese doctor makes a diagnosis by:

- Inspection of the complexion, general demeanor, body language, and tongue
- Questioning the patient about symptoms, medical history, diet, lifestyle, history of the present complaint, and any previous or concurrent therapies received
- Listening to the tone and strength of the voice
- Smelling any body excretions, the breath, or the body odor
- Palpation (or feeling with the fingers) of the pulse at the radial arteries of both wrists (pulse diagnosis), the abdomen, the musculature, and the meridians or acupuncture points

Chinese pulse diagnosis is a highly refined, difficult-to-master art, requiring years of attentive practice and careful correlation with symptoms. It is recognized that there are approximately 28 different pulse qualities that can be felt on three different positions and three different depths on the wrist of each hand (Fig. 6-8). The practice of pulse taking considers the position, depth, rate, width, strength, quality, and rhythm (Table 6-8).

Inspection of the tongue—observing its size, shape, and texture as well as the quality of its fur—reveals the severity, nature, and location of

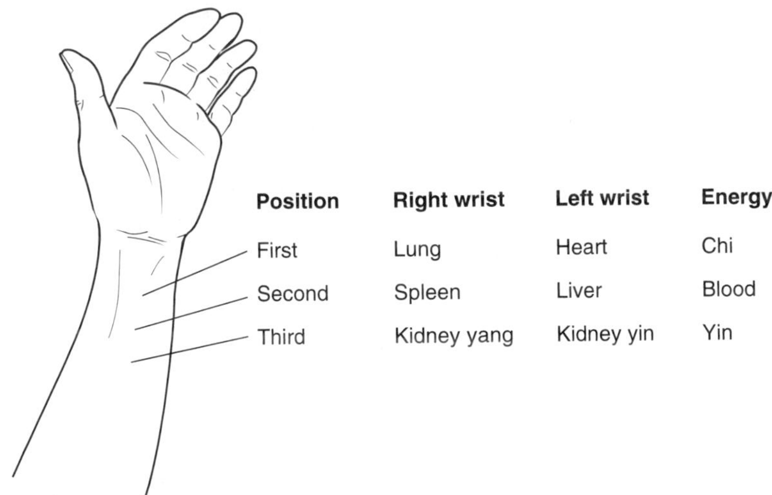

FIGURE 6-8
The pulse is taken at three depths and in three positions on the left and right wrists.

TABLE 6-8 PULSE CHARACTERISTICS

Pulse	Characteristic	Significance
choppy	feels uneven; like fingers bobbing on surface of sea	blood deficiency
deep	more apparent at deep level; lacking at surface and superficial levels	internal disharmony
empty	feels similar to a large pulse; but lacks the distinctness	blood and Qi deficiency
floating or superficial	more apparent at surface; lacking at middle and deep levels	invasion by external factor—Cold, Wind, etc.
full	feels similar to a large pulse; powerful at all levels	excess condition
intermittent	skips beat regularly	heart disharmony (serious)
irregular/knotted	slow; may skip a beat on an intermittent basis	heart-blood disharmony
large/big	feels broad but distinct under the fingers	excess condition
rapid	fast pulse, significantly above average	internal heat
slippery	"slips" along under the fingers; like a viscous fluid	internal damp; spleen disharmony
slow	slow pulse, significantly below average	internal cold
thready/thin	feels like a fine thread under the fingers; distinct	blood deficiency
tight	similar to wiry pulse but feels like a vibrating cord	excess condition; stagnation
wiry	feels taut and distinct beneath fingers; like guitar string	liver disharmony

illness. A pale tongue with white fur indicates the presence of cold, whereas a red tongue with yellow fur indicates heat. A flabby or thin tongue indicates deficiency of Chi and blood, whereas a tense or swollen tongue suggests congestion of these constituents. A quivering or rigid tongue indicates the presence of wind.

Feeling the temperature, tone, and moisture of the skin and muscles, testing the flexibility of the joints, and probing the sensitivity of the acupuncture points and channels provides further information about the state of the organ networks and the presence of pathologic conditions (From Beinfeld, H. & Korngold, E. [1995]. Chinese traditional medicine: an introductory overview. *Alternative Therapies*. 1, (1), 49–50.)

TREATMENT

The primary treatment modalities used in oriental medicine include acupuncture, herbal medicine, moxibustion, cupping, acupressure massage, Qigong (all discussed in other parts of the book), diet, and general lifestyle factors. Oriental medicine is not about changing people, it is about helping them to live better and be who they are. Usually, strengths are linked to weaknesses. There is always duality at work—yin and yang.

In oriental medicine, a crude drug or herb is rarely used alone, but rather is used as an ingredient in a composite medical preparation, usually prepared as a tea, broth, fermentation, or pill.

Some herbs often used are:

astragalus *(Astragalus membranaceus)*

echinacea *(Echinacea angustfolia, echinacea purpurea)*

licorice *(Glycyrrhizae radix)*

ginger *(Zingiberis rhizoma)*

peony root *(Paeoniae radix)*

dong quai *(Angelica sinensis)*

purple loco weed *(Astragalus molissimus)*

ma haung *(Ephedra equisetina)*

Asian ginseng *(Panax ginseng)*

Oriental medicine tends not to use a single treatment for a single disease because the body itself is complex, the oriental approach is multimodal to match that complexity. Herbs are usually used in synergistic combination rather than as specific agents. From the oriental medicine point of view, echinacea is a cold, dry, detoxifying herb that counters inflammation and swelling, whereas astragalus is a warm, nutritive herb that strengthens resistance by invigorating the body. Echinacea is used in time of illness, whereas astragalus, like ginseng, is an adaptogen that restores the body's capacity not only to resist illness, but to work, reproduce, and store energy.

Are There Any Risks Involved With Oriental Medicine?

As with western medicine, oriental medicine should only be prescribed by those properly trained in oriental medicine diagnosis and treatment. When so administered, it is relatively safe.

What Training Is Required of the Practitioner?

Oriental medical school is 4 years long, and is entered after high school. Many years of apprenticeship are required. In addition, in the United States, oriental medicine, including acupuncture, is offered as integrated programs in acupuncture colleges as postgraduate degrees.

Bibliography

Anastasi, J. K., Dawes, N. C., & Li, Y. M. (1997). Diarrhea and human immunodeficiency virus: Western and Eastern perspectives. Journal of Alternative and Complementary Medicine. 3, (2), 163–168.

Beinfield, H. & Korngold, E. (1998). Eastern medicine for western people. Alternative Therapies in Health and Medicine. 4, (3), 80–88.

Beinfield, H. & Korngold, E. (1995). Chinese traditional medicine: an introductory overview. Alternative Therapies in Health and Medicine. 1, (1), 44–52.

Chi, C., Lee, J., Lai, J., Chen, S., Chen, C., & Chang, S. (1997). Utilization of Chinese medicine in Taiwan. Alternative Therapies in Health Medicine. 3, (4), 40–53.

Fahey, C. (1998). Medical decisions. Energy Times. 49–53.

Hikino, H. (1985). Recent research on oriental medicinal plants. Economic and Medicinal Plant Research. Academic Press. London.

Kurashige, S., Jin, R., Akuzawa, Y., & Endo, F. (1998). Anticarcinogenic effects of shikaron, a preparation of eight Chinese herbs in mice treated with a carcinogen, N-butyl-N'-butanolnitrosoamine. Cancer Investigation. 16, (3), 166–169.

Null, G. (1998) Natural healing. Kensington Books. NY.

Sadler, C. (1996). Chinese herbs for eczema: risks and benefits. Community Nurse. 2, (5), 21–22.

Wang, Q. (1996). Advances in treatment of epilepsy with traditional Chinese medicine. Journal of Traditional Chinese Medicine. 16, (3), 230–237.

Williams, T. (1996). Chinese medicine. Rockport, MA: Element

Xu, J. (1996). Experience in treating senile dementia according to differentiation of syndromes. Journal of Traditional Chinese Medicine. 16, (3), 176–181.

Further Reading

Geinfield, H. & Korngold, E. (1991). Between heaven and earth: a guide to Chinese medicine. NY: Ballantine Books.

Ni, H-C. (1993). Tao: the subtle universal law and the integral way of life. Santa Monica, CA: Seven Star Communications, 1993.

Ni, M. & McNease, C. (1993). Tao of nutrition. Santa Monica, CA: Seven Star Communications.

RESOURCES

American Association of Acupuncture and
Oriental Medicine
4101 Lake Boone Trail, Suite 201
Raleigh, NC 27607
(919) 787-5181

INTERNET

Office of Alternative Medicine
http://altmed.od.nig.gov/

Chinese Medical Journal
http://www.pavilion.co.uk.jcm/selcome.html

Alternative Medicine Network
www.sonic.net/nexus/links.html

Chinese Medicine, Schools, list of practitioners, products for sale
www.acupuncture.com/

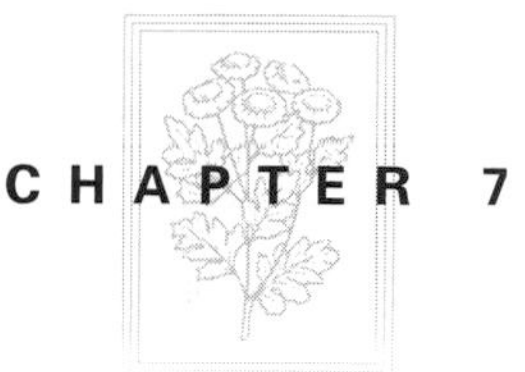

CHAPTER 7

MANUAL HEALING

ACUPRESSURE

What Is Acupressure?

Acupressure is a system that involves working on the Chi (see Oriental Medicine) by pressing the fingers and thumbs on specific points that are located along the meridians. These pressure points are the places where the channels come near the body's surface. By manipulating the points, it is possible to strengthen, disperse, or calm the Chi, helping it to flow more smoothly in the body and to bring harmonious relationship between body and mind, relieving any symptoms (Fig. 7-1).

What Is the History of Acupressure?

Acupressure dates back to ancient times and the discovery of meridians (see Oriental Medicine and Acupuncture sections for more information).

What Research, Reviews, and Comments Exist?

PRO

Bottaci, et al (1997) used the point Pericardium 6 (Chinese meridian point) during surgery and for 6 hours during the postoperative period after colorectal surgery. Patients having this point stimulated had a significant reduction in postoperative nausea and vomiting; therefore, the authors strongly recommend this point be used in patients with major

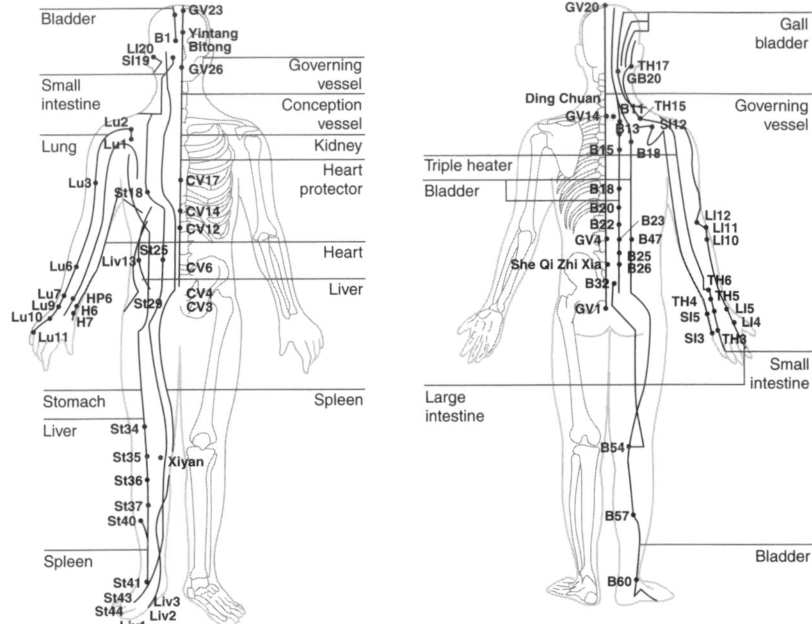

FIGURE 7-1
The Channels and Pressure Points.

abdominal surgery. Felhandler (1996) also used acupressure to decrease postoperative pain with great success. Hir, et al (1995) also used the same point to control the symptoms of visually induced motion sickness and gastric tachyarrhythmia with great success.

CON

No con research was found in a Medline search.

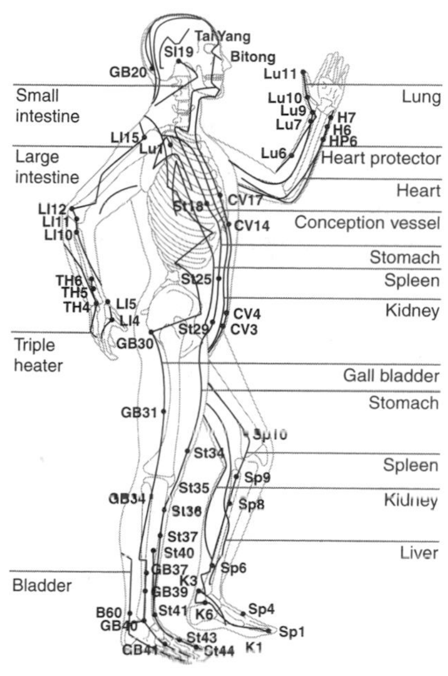

FIGURE 7-1
Continued.

Numbering the points
Each Channel is either more Yin or more Yang (see p.21). The numbering of points on the Yin Channels starts from the feet and works upward, since Yin Energy comes from the earth. The points on the Yang Channels are numbered from the head downward, since Yang Energy comes from the sun.

Each Channel has a wider network of connections with other Channels. The treatments in Part Two take account of this network and recommend treating the points that bring most benefit because of their internal connections within the Channel network.

Location of points
To locate each acupressure point, first read the description of how to find it on the treatment plan. Then use the illustrations on pages 24–27 to build up a clearer idea of the bone structure, and the Summary on pages 88–91, with its anatomical illustrations, to become familiar with the skeleton as a whole.

Horary rhythm
The order of the Channels in the Key represents the order in which Qi is thought to flow through the Channels during a 24-hour cycle. Qi flows most strongly through the Lung Channel between 3am and 5am, and during the course of the day flows for two-hour periods in each Channel in turn, surging through them in the order shown.

Key		
	Lu	Lung
	LI	Large Intestine
	St	Stomach
	Sp	Spleen
	H	Heart
	SI	Small Intestine
	B	Bladder
	K	Kidney
	HP	Heart Protector
	TH	Triple Heater
	GB	Gall Bladder
	Liv	Liver
	CV	Conception Vessel
	GV	Governing Vessel

What is Acupressure Used to Treat or Improve?

Acupressure can be used to treat many conditions:

- Fatigue
- Headaches
- Depression
- Sleeping disorders
- Chronic fatigue syndrome
- Respiratory conditions (colds, coughs, flu, sinusitis, asthma, bronchitis)
- Gastrointestinal (GI) disturbances, to improve appetite, reduce acidity, constipation, diarrhea

- Cerebrovascular (CV) conditions
- Reproductive disorders (menstrual pain, premenstrual syndrome [PMS], heavy menstruation, menopausal symptoms)
- Orthopaedic disorders (pain of arthritis, stress, muscle pain)
- Sensory organs (earache, sore eye, headache)

What Happens During Acupressure?

Acupressure is a versatile form of treatment that can be administered whenever and wherever it is convenient. The equipment is simple—a pair of hands. Traditional treatment is administered when the patient is lying down, but it can be done in any position and even by the patient. It is best if the recipient wears a thin layer of clothing to avoid the practitioner having his or her attention drawn to the feel and texture of the skin.

The practitioner and recipient should be relaxed. There are three techniques for stimulating pressure points:

- Tonify: disperse blocked or stagnant Chi and calm overactive Chi. Apply stationary pressure with thumb or finger tip, perpendicular to the point and hold for 2 minutes.
- Disperse Chi: apply moving pressure with thumb or fingertip in nine circular movements or “pump” in and out on the point for approximately 2 minutes. This technique encourages the smooth flow of Chi along the channels.
- Calming: use the palm to cover the point, or apply light moving pressure (gentle stroking) for 2 minutes.

For chronic, long-term conditions, the points are treated every other day. For acute short-term conditions, the points are treated two times daily. The treatments are continued until the symptoms disappear.

Are There Any Risks Involved With Acupressure?

Acupressure is a gentle form of therapy and no risks exist. However, if acupressure is used in an attempt to rid the body of a long-term, chronic complaint, the body may rid itself of toxins; and the patient may experience physical symptoms such as headache, GI complaints, or skin rashes, or experience emotional reactions such as depression, crying, or melancholy. Usually, these reactions are short-term.

Acupressure should not be applied to an open wound, or where acute inflammation or swelling is present. There are also some acupressure points that should not be used during pregnancy (Fig. 7-2).

What Training Is Required of the Practitioner?

Acupressure can be self-taught or taught by a teacher.

Bibliography

Bottaci, L., Drew, P. J., Hartley, J. E., et al. (1997). Artificial neural networks applied to acupressure treatment for prevention of postoperative nausea and vomiting. Anesthesia and Analgesia. 84, 821–825.

Felhendler, D. & Lisander, B. (1996).Pressure on acupoints decreases postoperative pain. Clinical Journal of Pain. 12, 326–329.

Hir, S., Ronda Stritzel, R., Chandler, A., Stern, R. M. (1995). P6 acupressure reduces symptoms of vection induced motion sickness. Aviation Space and Environmental Medicine. 66, 631–634.

Further Reading

Hova-Kramer, D. (1996). Healing touch: a resource. Albany, NY: Delmar Publishers.

Hu, K. (1994). Chinese massage and acupressure. (5th ed). New York, NY: Bergh.

Jarmey, C. & Tindall, J. (1991). Acupressure for common ailments. New York, NY: Fireside Books.

Maxwell, J. (1997). The gentle power of acupressure. RN:53-56. April.

RESOURCES

Acupressure Institute
1533 Shattuck Avenue
Berkeley, CA 94709
(800) 442-2232

INTERNET

http://www.acupunctureplus.com/plans.html
http://www.seirin.net/uk/acu/geschich.htm
http://www.meriden.lib.ct.us/acupunc.htm
http://www.science.uts.edu.au/depts/hs/clinic/faq.htm
http://falcon.cc.ukans.edu/~moriarty/acupressure/acuguide.html
http://www.hightouchnet.com/p4.html
http://www.rowantree.co.uk/reflexology/reflexology.htm

Office of Alternative Medicine
http://altmed.od.nig.gov/

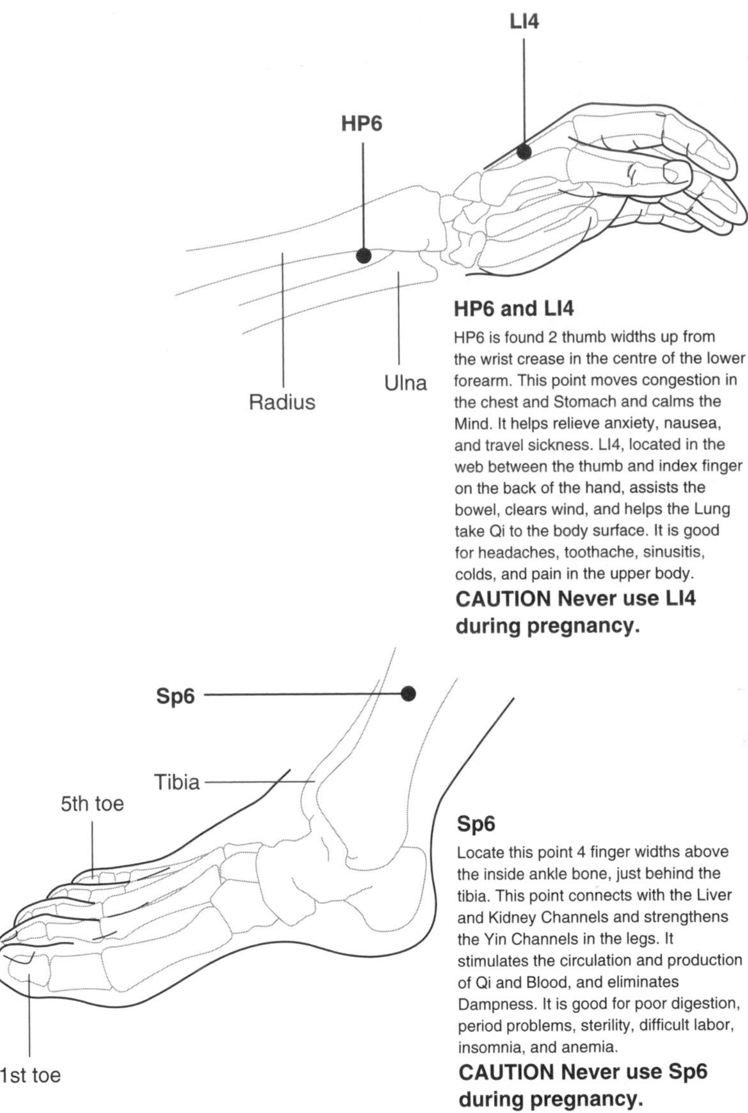

FIGURE 7-2
Acupressure Points Not To Be Used During Pregnancy.

APPLIED KINESIOLOGY

What Is Applied Kinesiology?

Applied kinesiology:

- Meshes energy and meridian-based therapy
- Sees a relationship between muscle reaction and disease in the body
- Tests muscles to balance mechanically opposed muscles
- Believes in a triad of health: nutrition, body structure, and psychological
  - Nutrition: how food nourishes the body and what foods are contraindicated in certain conditions; also drugs, both prescription and over the counter, and their effect on health
  - Body structure: concerns all the body's skeletal, muscle, and organ systems and how they function together
  - Psychological: emotions and mental attitudes
- Purports to determine health imbalances in the body's organs and glands by identifying weaknesses in specific muscles. By stimulating or relaxing these key muscles, the practitioner can diagnose and resolve a variety of health problems.

What Is the History of Applied Kinesiology?

Applied Kinesiology was founded by a Michigan chiropractor, G. J. Goodhart, Jr., in 1964. Dr. Goodhart claimed to have corrected a patient's chronic winged scapula by pressing on the nodules found near the origins and insertion of the involved serratus anterior muscle. Later, influenced by the writings of F. Mann, MD, Goodhart incorporated acupuncture meridian therapy into Applied Kinesiology. In addition, the vertebral challenge method and therapy localization technique, both based on Dr. L Truscott, DC, were added to Applied Kinesiology.

What Research, Reviews, and Comments Exist?

PRO

No pro research was identified in a Medline search.

CON

Lawson and Calderon (1997) studied interexaminer agreement for Applied Kinesiology on manual muscle testing. The clinicians with 10 years or more experience had agreement on piriformis and pectoralis muscles, but no agreement on hamstrings or tensor fascia lata muscles.

Klinkoski and Leboeuf (1990) attempted to establish a research basis for Applied Kinesiology by reviewing all research articles regarding Applied Kinesiology performed from 1981 to 1987. There were no articles that included all of the traditional research modalities; therefore, no valid conclusion could be drawn concerning the effectiveness of Applied Kinesiology. Kenney, et al (1988) found that Applied Kinesiology was no more useful than random guessing to evaluate nutrient status.

What Is Applied Kinesiology Used to Treat or Improve?

Persons who practice Applied Kinesiology say that it:

- Improves function of the entire body
- Is particularly helpful to diagnose problems for persons with diseases of the bones, joints, and muscles
- Controls pain, both acute and chronic
- Helps decrease migraine headaches
- Can identify allergies to foods, vitamins, and other substances

What Happens During a Visit to an Applied Kinesiologist?

- Patient history is obtained (diet, lifestyle).
- Muscle testing, which includes raising an arm to one side of the body and having the kinesiologist push down as resistance, is offered. Foods, drugs, or vitamins may be taken orally and the same muscles tested again to assess improvement or worsening of the muscle strength. If muscle strength worsens, an allergy to that substance is suggested.
- Results of testing may indicate the need for altered nutrition, stimulation of acupressure points, spinal adjustments, or traditional blood tests.
- Sessions last 20 to 60 minutes.

Are There Any Risks Involved With Applied Kinesiology?

There are no risks with this therapy. If symptoms continue, traditional medicine should be consulted. This therapy should not be used as the only therapy.

What Training Is Required of the Practitioner?

The practitioner is a chiropractor, osteopath, or other health care provider certified in kinesiology. To be certified, a health professional must possess a license to diagnose in his or her own specialty and then have training through the International College of Applied Kinesiology.

Bibliography

Kenney, J. J., Clemens, R., & Forsythe, K. D. (1988). Applied kinesiology unreliable for assessing nutrient status. Journal of the American Dietetic Association. 88, 698–704.

Klinkoski, B. & Leboeuf, C. (1990). A review of the research papers published by the International College of Applied Kinesiology from 1981 to 1987. Journal of Manipulative Physiological Therapy. 13, 190–194.

Lawson, A., Calderon, L. (1997). Interexaminer agreement for applied kinesiology manual muscle testing. Perception Motor Skills. 84, 539–546.

Further Reading

Goodhart D. C., Jr. (1997). George Goodhart Jr., D. C. and a history of applied kinesiology. Journal of Manipulative & Physiological Therapeutics. 20, 331–337.

Goodhart, D. C., Jr. (1989). You'll be better, the story of applied kinesiology. Geneva, OH: AK Printing.

Maffertone, P. (1990). Everyone is an athlete. Mahopac, NY: David Barmore Productions.

Valentine, T. C. (1989). Applied kinesiology: muscle response in diagnosis, therapy and preventive medicine. Rochester, VT: Inner Traditions.

RESOURCES

International College of Applied Kinesiology
PO Box 905
Lawrence, KS 66044-0905
(785) 542-1801

Touch for Health Foundation
1174 North Lake Avenue
Pasadena, CA 91104
(310) 827-7781

CHIROPRACTICS

What Is Chiropractics?

Chiropractics is a drugless, nonsurgical therapy that uses manipulation. Chiropractors consider themselves to be a healing profession that uses manual and physiologic approaches to healing. Vertebral subluxation (an incomplete dislocation; although a relationship is altered, contact between joint surfaces remains and may affect proper nerve function) is at the core of chiropractic theory, and its detection and correction are at the heart of chiropractic practice. Because of inhibition of the neural impulses there is impingement on the nerve root. Thus chiropractors see the proper exiting of the nerve roots from the spinal column as essential to the control of bodily functions, such as digestion, glandular, circulation, movement, respiratory, and so on.

Chiropractors suggest that chiropractics should be classified as a "complete" system for complementary health care, rather than as a therapeutic modality. Chiropractors often use acupressure, massage, mineral supplements, and herbs in their practice. Most of these techniques are taught in chiropractic school. In 1994, chiropractics was approved for the treatment of low back pain. Today, many insurance companies will pay for chiropractic adjustments.

Contemporary chiropractic theory is divided into two schools. The orthodox ("straights") school keeps to the founders' notion that vertebral subluxation is the fundamental cause of disease and treatment should be restricted to adjustments of the spine. The unorthodox ("mixers") school has expanded the scope of chiropractics to include any treatment (such as physical therapy, nutrition, vitamins) that enhances the natural healing mechanisms of the body. A popular technique used by the unorthodox group involves muscle testing called applied kinesiology (see appropriate section for more information). Applied kinesiology synthesizes chiropractic theory with the energy-meridian theory of classic Chinese acupuncture.

What Is the History of Chiropractics?

Chiropractics dates from 1895 when the developer Daniel David Palmer (1845–1913) discovered what he believed to be the universal cause of all disease and its cure. Palmer was a self-educated beekeeper, fish peddler, and grocer from Iowa. Before developing the chiropractic method, he was involved in lay healing for 9 years using "animal magnetism." Throughout this time period he studied numerous books regarding anatomy and physiology, with his focus being the human spine and spinal nerves.

Palmer performed his first spinal adjustment on a janitor who said he experienced a "give" in his back 17 years earlier and since that time could not hear. After the adjustment by Palmer, the man could hear. Popularity of Palmer's work spread quickly and he established the Palmer Infirmary and Chiropractic School in Davenport, IA, in 1897. This is the most prestigious chiropractic school in existence and is still administered by the Palmer family.

Palmer believed, as did the Asian philosophers, in an "innate intelligence" within all living matter, which governs its existence. He considered the nervous system to be, physiologically, the "control system" over the body's and mind's function.

What Research, Reviews, and Comments Exist?

Much of the earlier research regarding the effectiveness of chiropractics was performed in a nonscientific way, which did not permit replication. Early results of studies were enthusiastically interpreted as indisputable proof of the investigators prior assumption about the effectiveness of chiropractic methods. It has only been recently that more scientific methods have been used to collect data.

PRO

Hawk, et al (1997) studied chiropractic flexion/distraction and trigger point technique to relieve chronic pelvic pain in women. Only 19 women completed the study, but the technique had positive short-term results. A randomized larger clinical trial is under investigation. Stano and Smith (1996) examined the cost-effectiveness, favorable patient satisfaction, and medical outcomes of treating low back pain with chiropractics versus traditional medical care. Chiropractics was considerably less expensive but equally as effective when 6,000 patient cases were examined. Verhoef, et al (1997) examined the changes in pain experience, changes in functional ability, and degree of patient satisfaction with chiropractic care. Three hundred sixty-nine patients were studied with statistically significant positive findings.

CON

Shekelle, et al (1998) found that 25% of patients treated with chiropractic manipulations were treated for indications that were judged inappropriate. The conclusion in this research was that inappropriate spinal manipulations should decrease. Assendelft, et al (1996) attempted a systematic review of the chiropractic research literature between 1969 and 1998 to determine its effectiveness in treating low back pain. Of the many studies performed, all had serious design flaws, executing and reporting. Therefore, no convincing evidence could be found that supported chiropractic manipulation in the effective treatment of low back pain. Koes, et al (1996) also attempted a review of the research literature examining the effectiveness of chiropractic manipulation on low back pain. Their finding was that efficacy for spinal manipulation for patients with acute and chronic low back pain has not been demonstrated in sound, randomized clinical trials.

What Is Chiropractics Used to Treat or Improve?

Many conditions can be treated by chiropractics:

- Muscle strains, joint sprains
- Arthritis, tendonitis, bursitis, fasciatis
- Peripheral neuritis
- Scoliosis, kyphosis
- Carpal tunnel syndrome
- Traumatic injuries such as whiplash
- Headaches
- Respiratory disorders
- Hyperactivity
- Acute and chronic pain syndrome

What Happens During a Visit to a Chiropractor?

A chiropractor will always take an extensive history and then perform a complete physical examination (including testing of mobility, agility, and reflexes). Radiographs and blood and urine examinations may be performed as needed. The physical examination often takes place on a treatment table, which is adjustable and contoured to accommodate spinal adjustment. Some chiropractors use a heated pad to warm the muscles before they begin the manipulation.

There are more than 100 distinct chiropractic treatments available to the practitioner. Most commonly, the manipulation emphasizes a quick thrust of the specific subluxated vertebrae (Fig. 7-3) or pressure, traction, and stretching of the soft tissue that attach to the bony skeleton. Most people report feeling immediate relief after the first adjustment. In many cases the pain returns and may even be worse than before the treatment. However, this is considered part of the "healing," and relief should last longer as treatments continue. Usually exercises are prescribed after the treatment to assist with healing. Rarely is one treatment enough and chiropractors routinely suggest many visits to treat the underlying condition.

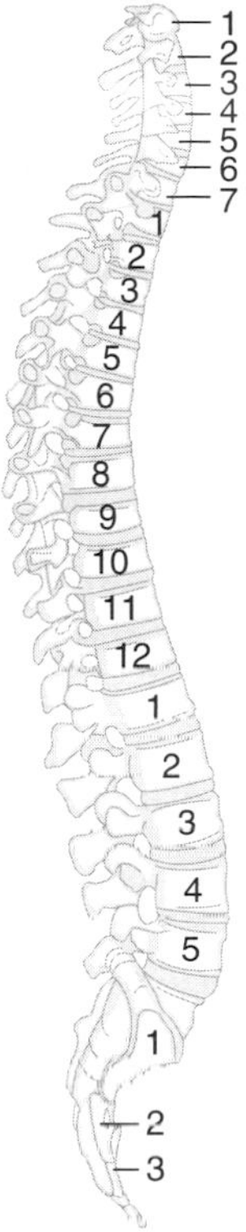

Vertebrae Names of the vertebra and nerves in the spine	Areas Areas known to receive nerve fibers from these nerves	Chiropractic treatments for
1C	Blood supply to the head, the pituitary gland, the scalp, bones of the face, the brain itself, inner and middle ear, the sympathetic nervous system.	Headache
2C	Eyes, optic nerve, auditory nerve, sinuses, mastoid bones, tongue, forehead.	Sinuses
3C	Cheeks, outer ear, face bones, teeth, trifacial nerve.	Neuralgia
4C	Nose, lips, mouth, eustachian tube.	Hayfever
5C	Vocal cords, neck glands, pharynx.	Sore throat
6C	Neck muscles, shoulders, tonsils.	Stiff neck
7C	Thyroid gland, bursa in the shoulders, the elbows.	Thyroid condition
1T	Arms from the elbows down, including the hands, wrists and fingers, also the esophagus and trachea.	Asthma
2T	Heart including its valves, and covering, also coronary arteries.	Heart conditions
3T	Lungs, bronchial tubes, pleura, chest, breast, nipples.	Lung conditions
4T	Gallbladder and common duct.	Gallbladder conditions
5T	Liver, solar plexus, blood.	Liver conditions
6T	Stomach	Stomach problems
7T	Pancreas, islands of Langerhans, duodenum.	Diabetes
8T	Spleen, diaphragm.	Leukemia
9T	Adrenals or supra-renals.	Allergies
10T	Kidneys	Kidney problems
11T	Kidneys, ureters.	Kidney problems
12T	Small intestines, Fallopian tubes, lymph circulation.	Gas pains
1L	Large intestines or colon, inguinal rings.	Constipation
2L	Appendix, abdomen, upper leg, cecum.	Cramps
3L	Sex organs, ovaries or testicles, uterus, bladder, knee.	Knee pains
4L	Prostate gland, muscles of the lower back, sciatic nerve.	Lower back pain
5L	Lower legs, ankle, feet, toes, arches.	Poor circulation in legs
Sacrum	Hip bones, buttocks.	Spinal problems
Coccyx	Rectum, anus.	Hemorrhoids

FIGURE 7-3
Chiropractic Treatment Areas.

The North American Spine Society and other chiropractic organizations have attempted to define reasonable and customary number of visits with relation to particular conditions. For example, the recommendation for acute low back pain is two to five treatments/week for the first 2 weeks, then one to two treatments/week for a month, with a maximum of 2 to 4 months. The rationale for multiple treatments is that soft tissue injury accompanying the problem may result in adhesions, deformation of certain tissues, and tearing or rupture of tissue. As the joint function returns to normal, time must be given to the soft tissue to heal. During the healing process, multiple visits are required to evaluate changes and to intervene and aid the structures during recovery.

Are There Any Risks Involved With Chiropractics?

Several risks and discomforts are identified with chiropractics. Women and patients with long-lasting problems are most likely to report treatment reactions (Leboeuf, et al, 1997).

- Overexposure to x-rays because of over use
- Spinal injury
- CVA (does not happen often but chiropractics should not be used as the first technique to treat upper cervical neck rotation) (Klougart, et al, 1996).
- Local discomfort, headache, tiredness, radiating discomfort (Senstad, et al, 1996; Senstad, et al, 1997).

If acute problems do not resolve within a reasonable time period, traditional treatment should be used.

What Training Is Required of the Practitioner?

Chiropractic training is offered in 16 chiropractic colleges in the United States, with approximately 4,800 hours of class time required to graduate. Approximately 13,000 students are enrolled. The education consists of 3 years of classroom study and 1 year of residency. The technique of chiropractics is also taught to other complementary practitioners in their educational programs, such as naturopathy, osteopathy, and in integrative medical school programs.

Chiropractics is practiced in more than 65 countries. Licensing requirements are required in the entire United States and many foreign countries. The United States and Canada require passing a local examination to be licensed.

Bibliography

Assendelft, W. J., Koes, B. W., van der Heijden, G. J., & Bouter, L. M. (1996). The effectiveness of chiropractic for treatment of low back pain: an update and attempt at statistical pooling. Journal of Manipulative and Physiological Therapeutics. 19, 499–507.

Hawk, C., Long, C., & Azad, A. (1997). Chiropractic care for women with chronic pelvic pain: a prospective single-group intervention study. Journal of Manipulative and Physiological Therapeutics. 20, 73–79.

Keating, J. C., Jr., Green, B. N., & Johnson, C. D. (1996). "Research" and "science" in the first half of the chiropractic century. Journal of Manipulative and Physiological Therapeutics. 18, 357–377.

Klougart, N., Leboeuf-Yde, C., et al. (1996). Safety in chiropractic practice, Part I; The occurrence of cerebrovascular accidents after manipulation to the neck in Denmark from 1978-1988. Journal of Manipulative and Physiological Therapeutics. 19, 371–377.

Koes, B. S., Assendelft, W. J. J., et al. (1996). Spinal manipulation for low back pain: an updated systematic review of randomized clinical trials. Spine. 21, 2860–2871.

Leboeuf-Yde, C., Hennius, B., et al. (1997). Side effects of chiropractic treatment: a prospective study. Journal of Manipulative & Physiological Therapeutics. 20, 511–515.

Senstad, O., Leboeuf-Yde, C., & Borchgrevink, C. (1997). Frequency and characteristics of side effects of spinal manipulative therapy. Spine. 22, (discussion 440-1). 435–440.

Senstad, O., Leboeuf-Yde, C., Borchgrevink, C. (1996). Predictors of side effects to spinal manipulative therapy. Journal of Manipulative and Physiological Therapeutics. 19, 441–445.

Shekelle, P. G., Coulter, I., et al. (1998). Congruence between decisions to initiate chiropractic spinal manipulation for low back pain and appropriateness criteria in North America. Annals of Internal Medicine. 129, 9–17.

Stano, M. & Smith, M. (1996). Chiropractic and medical costs of low back care. Medical Care. 34, 191–204.

Verhoef, M. J., Page, S. A., & Waddell, S. C. (1997). The chiropractic outcome study: pain, functional ability and satisfaction with care. Journal of Manipulative and Physiological Therapeutics. 20, 235–240.

Further Reading

Palmer, D. D. (1910). The science, art of philosophy of chiropractics. Portland, OR: Portland Printing House.

Lawrence, D. (Ed). (1996). Advances in chiropractics. St. Louis, MO: CV Mosby.

Wardwell, W. (1992). Chiropractic history and evolution of a new profession. St. Louis, MO: CV Mosby.

Gatterman, M. I. (1995). Foundations of chiropractics - subluxation. St. Louis, MO: CV Mosby.

Redwood D (ed): Contemporary Chiropractics. Churchill Livingstone New York NY, 1997.

RESOURCES

American Chiropractic Association
1701 Clarendon Boulevard
Arlington, VA 22209
(703) 276-8800

International Chiropractors Association
1110 North Glebe Road, Suite 1000
Arlington, VA 22201
(703) 528-5000

Association for Network Chiropractic Spinal Analysis
PO Box 7682
Longmont, CO 80501
(303) 678-8086

INTERNET

Office of Alternative Medicine
http://altmed.od.nig.gov/

Chiropractics Association
www.amerchiro.org/aca

Chiropractics
www.mbnet.mb.ca/~jwiens/chiro.html

Chiropractics Resource Center
www.chiro.org/

Osteopathic manipulation
www.aao.medguide.net

MASSAGE THERAPY

What Is Massage Therapy?

Massage is a systematic and scientific manipulation of the soft tissue of the body. Techniques used include gliding, stroking, percussion, shaking, compressing, friction, kneading, and vibration. Every language has a word for massage. The origins of the word massage are unclear. It may come from:

Arabic, *mash*, meaning to press softly

Greek, *massein*, meaning to knead

French, *masser*, meaning to shampoo

Massage has many benefits. It improves blood flow to muscles, removes waste products from cells, provides deep cell cleansing; enhances flow of lymph particularly where lymphatic flow has been impaired by surgery (postmastectomy), reduces stress and enhances body/mind connection, and provides many other benefits.

There are more than 80 different types of massage therapy and body work. Many are variations on each other. Most varieties can be divided into five broad categories.

TRADITIONAL EUROPEAN MASSAGE

Based on the knowledge of anatomy and physiology and soft tissue manipulation including:

- *Effleurage:* gliding strokes toward the heart
- *Petrissage:* strokes that lift, roll, or knead tissue
- *Friction:* circular strokes
- *Vibration*
- *Tapotement:* percussion or tapping

Swedish Massage

Swedish massage uses all of the previously mentioned strokes to enhance circulation of blood through the soft tissues. Oil or talcum powder can be used to facilitate the movements.

CONTEMPORARY WESTERN

Massage therapy uses the knowledge of anatomy and physiology, and a variety of techniques to enhance personal growth, emotional release, and to balance the mind-body spirit. Most of these techniques have developed since the 1960s.

Esalen

- Developed at Esalen Institute, Big Sur, CA
- Creates a deep state of relaxation and general well-being
- Uses more slow, rhythmic, hypnotic techniques
- Focuses on the mind and body as a whole

Neuromuscular Therapy

- Soft-tissue manipulation to relieve pain and dysfunction by balancing the nervous system with the musculoskeletal system.

Deep Tissue Massage

- Releases chronic patterns of muscular tension
- Movements are directed across the grain of muscles
- Uses fingers, thumbs, and elbows with greater pressure than in Swedish massage

Sports Massage

- Massage and stretching to enhance athletic performance
- Removes lactic acid and increases range of motion
- Part of athlete's training regime
- Promotes healing from injury
- Uses three major strokes, compression, trigger point or direct pressure, and cross fiber friction
- National certification in sports massage offered by the American Massage Therapy Association.

Manual Lymphatic Drainage

- Light, slow, repetitive strokes to boost circulation of lymphatic system
- Facilitates removal of excess water, wastes, and toxins

STRUCTURAL/FUNCTIONAL/MOVEMENT INTEGRATION

These techniques organize and integrate the body in relation to gravity and assist with balancing the body and nervous system. These techniques work on body structure and how it moves and some do not involve touching.

Hellerwork

- Founded by J. Heller 1979 (one of Ida Rolf's first students and first president of the Rolf Institute.)
- Movement re-education process with exercises that teach stress-free body movements for everyday activities, such as walking, bending, and sitting; includes interactive dialogue between practitioner and client
- Includes video feedback
- Has 11 sessions

Rolfing

- Developed by Dr. Ida Rolf in 1920
- Deep tissue work for reordering the body so as to bring its major segments (head, shoulders, thorax, pelvis, and legs) into alignment
- Loosens or releases adhesions in fascia (for more information see section on Rolfing)

Structural Integration

- Encompasses modalities such as Rolf treatments, Hellerwork, and Aston-Patterning
- Aligns the body through the myofascial system and retraining through movement

Movement Therapy

- Encompasses modalities such as the Alexander Technique and the Feldenkrais Method
- Use of movement to re-educate the body and mind

Rosen Method

- Founded by Marion Rosen in 1972
- Sees the body's tensions as unexpressed, repressed, or suppressed feelings
- Induces relaxation and prevents illness through gentle touch and verbal support
- Enhances awareness, which allows tension to be released
- Work is about transformation from the person we think we are to the person we really are

Trager

- Developed by Dr. Milton Trager
- Sessions are 1.5 hours long
- Nonintrusive, pain-free, hands-on touch and exercises to release deep-seated psychophysiologic areas of holding
- Moves trunk and limbs
- Client is given sets of movements to recreate at home what is done in therapy, called "mentastics" (short for mental gymnastics) mindfulness in motion

Feldenkrais Method

- Developed by Moshe Feldenkrais, a Russian-born Israeli physicist
- May be self-taught, but is usually taught by practitioners accredited by the Feldenkrais Guild. Training lasts 4 years with 200 hours/year of education
- Increases range of motion and improves flexibility and coordination (particularly beneficial in chronic diseases such as multiple sclerosis, cerebral palsy, Parkinson's disease, and posttraumatic disorders)
- Patient develops a better and more direct relationship with interior and exterior worlds
- Stresses how the body is used and misused in daily life
- Focuses on relearning and reprogramming basic movements to allow a person to walk, speak, and act in more comfortable and productive ways
- Improves self-image and increases awareness and health
- Sessions usually last 30 minutes (may be group or one-on-one functional integration classes)

- Often starts with stretching and flexing exercises performed on the floor
- Practitioner uses gentle touch to improve and reorganize posture and self-image

Alexander Technique

(Awareness through movement)

- Developed by an Australian actor, Frederick Alexander
- A 3-year course of study is required
- Uses posture and balance
- Rebalances the body through awareness, movement, and touch
- Stresses improvement in alignment of spine, head, body, neck, and torso
- 30-minute to 1-hour sessions
- Techniques allow for a restoration of natural balance and responsiveness during movement
- Client may be given instructions such as, "Let your head move forward and up to allow your torso to lengthen and widen." While saying this, the practitioner gently prevents the old habit and encourages a new improved response of the head/neck/back relationship. During this time, the client is instructed to "do nothing"; the patient thinks the instruction given by the practitioner. Eventually, the patient constructs a new body image, and by doing so retrains and reorganizes the way he or she moves.

Ortho-Bionomy

- Developed by Arthur Lincoln Pauls, DO, in the 1970s
- Enhances balance and well-being through gentle, noninvasive touch, dialogue, and movement education
- No force or pressure is used
- Attempts to restore structure, alignment, and balance

ORIENTAL METHODS

- Based on principles of energy (Chi) flow
- Often used concurrently with herbs and acupuncture

Jin Shin Jyutsu

- Comes from an ancient Japanese healing tradition
- Sessions last 1 hour
- Practitioner uses pulse diagnosis (see Oriental Medicine section) to identify energy blockages

- Gentle application of the hands along energy pathways to promote well-being

Shiatsu

- Balances the body through applying pressure to specific acupressure points with fingers (means "finger pressure")
- Stretching and movement are also used

ENERGETIC METHODS, NON-ORIENTAL

Therapeutic Touch

- Developed by Dr. Delores Krieger in the early 1970s
- Corrects imbalances by modulating the energy field that surrounds the body (see Therapeutic Touch section for more information)

Polarity Therapy

- Developed by R. Stone, DO, DC, ND
- Certification is required by the American Polarity Therapy Association
- Therapy is built on Eastern concept that illness originates from blockages in energy
- Polarity bodywork is invigorating and rejuvenating, and can result in positive changes on the physical, mental, and emotional levels
- Releases energy blockages and restores energy
- Practitioners place their hands on the patient, enabling energy flow to be balanced and strengthened
- Polarity hands-on techniques include manipulation of pressure points and joints, massage, breathing techniques, hydrotherapy, exercise, reflexology, and holding pressure points on the body. Both hands are used (one is positive, the other negative) to release energy blockages in the body and help to restore a natural flow.
- The return of energy calms nerves and reinvigorates the body and spirit
- Enhances understanding of self
- Treats most conditions, acute and chronic.
- May also give counseling on diet and nutrition, and emphasizes importance of positive thinking.

Reiki

- Ancient oriental approach to healing (see Reiki section for more information)

- Uses universal life force energy
- Balances and amplifies energy through light hands-on touch and visualization

OTHER APPROACHES

There are a few techniques that combine approaches and can be called integrative massage.

Reflexology

- Improves circulation, eases pain, and increases relaxation through the manipulation of reflex areas in the feet and hands (for more information see Reflexology section)

Craniosacral Therapy

- Named by Drs. Upledger and Retzlaff in 1977
- Gentle, noninvasive pressure to the bones and soft tissue of the skull and pelvis to release tension and create balance
- Reports suggest the Craniosacral therapy can be used to treat depression, migraines, dyslexia, spasticity of cerebral palsy, Meniere's syndrome, and many other disorders

Bonnie Prudden Myotherapy

- Relieves pain and dysfunction through pressure to trigger points and corrective exercise

Bioenergetics

- Combination of psychotherapy, breathing, and bodywork to free trapped energy and relieve tension
- Developed by Dr. Alexander Lowen and Dr. John Pierakos, based on work of psychiatrist Wilhelm Reich

Zero Balancing

- Developed by Fritz Smith, MD (courses offered at the Upledger Institute)
- Painless, hands-on therapy to align body energy with body structure
- Particularly helpful in restoring function after trauma or injury
- Attempts to bridge the gap between methods that work with structure and those that work with energy

What Is the History of Massage?

Massage probably began as soon as cave dwellers rubbed their bruises. In 8000 BC, there are notations about massage in Veda books of India. From 3000 to 2000 BC there are references to massage in Egyptian, Persian, and Japanese cultures. Hippocrates and Asclepiades, another eminent Greek physician, learned massage. Asclepiades claimed that massage effected a cure by restoring to the nutritive fluids their natural free movement. He also discovered that sleep might be induced by gentle stroking. The Grecks prescribed massage for their patients and their athletes. The Greeks established elaborate bath houses where exercises, massage, and baths were available.

During the middle ages massage was almost forgotten. Finally, Pes Henrick Ling of Sweden (1776–1839), a fencing master and gymnast, began studying massage to cure his own ills. Ling based his technique (The Ling System or "the Swedish movement treatment") on his knowledge of physiology, which was then emerging as a science. In 1813, the first college to include massage was established.

From 1854 to 1918, the practice of massage developed and the profession of physical therapy (PT) began. (PTs rarely use massage because they do not have the time to spend at least 30 minutes with each patient, the minimum time required for massage treatment.)

In 1900, A. Hoffa published a book *Technique of Massage* in Germany. This book is still the most basic of all texts regarding massage, giving the clearest description of how to execute the strokes and advocating the procedures that underlie all modern techniques.

In modern Germany, massage therapy is covered by national health insurance. In China it is fully integrated into the health care system, in which the hospitals have massage wards. In one Shanghai hospital the massage department covers two floors.

In the United States, the medical use of massage began to diminish in the early part of this century with the evolution of pharmaceutical, surgical, and technologic medicine. It reached a nadir between the 1930s and 1950s because it was considered too time intensive for the modern physician. Massage therapy duties were gradually handed over to aides, who eventually became the physical therapists of the modern era.

The professionalization of massage therapy in the United States began in 1943 when the graduating class of the College of Swedish Massage in Chicago decided to band together and form an association with 29 charter members. What they created was destined to become the American Massage Therapy Association (AMTA).

In the 1960s, while modern medicine continued toward higher technology and drugs and away from physician contact with patients, such concepts as holistic health, self-improvement, and optimal health experienced a rebirth. The 1970s brought even greater interest in health promotion and a new openness to massage. This was followed by explosive growth in the variety of massage and bodywork available, and currently there are more than 80 different varieties. The term "bodywork" evolved as a generic term for referring to this broadening field. It is now loosely used to incorporate massage and other forms of manipulation.

In the survey of alternative medicine that was published in *The New England Journal of Medicine* in 1993, massage therapy ranked third among the most frequently used forms of alternative health care. According to Elliott Greene, president of the AMTA, there are approximately 50,000 massage therapists of various kinds in the United States, and the AMTA may be the fastest-growing organization of health care providers in the country.

There remains a lingering false impression that connects therapeutic massage to what usually takes place in "massage parlors" or "body rub shops." There is no connection. True therapeutic massage has become an integral part of health care.

What Research, Reviews, and Comments Exist?

Much research has been published regarding massage. The Office of Alternative Medicine has recently funded four studies regarding massage: to enhance immune function in patients who are HIV positive, to reduce depression and anxiety in patients having a bone marrow transplant, to reduce anxiety and need for follow-up care in women undergoing surgery for uterine cancer, and to enhance growth and cognitive development in premature infants born to mothers who are HIV positive. The following are a few of those research articles available on a Medline search.

PRO

Field, et al (1997) found that massage during labor decreased anxiety and pain, shortened labor, and shortened hospital stay. Cady and Jones (1997) found that a 15-minute massage at work significantly decreased systolic and diastolic blood pressure. Nixon, et al (1997) found there was a significant reduction of perceived pain after surgery in the group who received massage. Richards (1998) found that patients in the intensive care unit administered a 6-minute back massage slept 1 hour longer than the control group and experienced less pain.

CON

Con articles were not found on a Medline search.

What Is Massage Therapy Used to Treat or Improve?

Numerous research studies indicate that massage:

- Has a sedative effect on the nervous system and promotes voluntary muscle relaxation
- Releases endorphins and enkelphans, the bodies own natural narcotic substances to relieve pain (tension in the muscles and soft tissues results in a deficient supply of nutrients and inadequate removal of waste or toxins)
- Restores healthy structure and function particularly after injury or trauma.
- Is effective in promoting recovery from fatigue and soreness produced by exercise
- Can help break up scar tissue and lessen fibrosis and adhesions that develop as a result of injury and immobilization
- Provides effective treatment of chronic inflammatory conditions by increasing lymphatic circulation
- Helps reduce swelling from fractures
- Enhances circulation through the capillaries, veins, and arteries, and increases blood flow through the muscles, which improves healing
- Can loosen mucus and promote drainage of sinus fluids from the lungs by using percussive and vibratory techniques
- Can increase peristaltic action (muscular contractions that move waste through the system) in the intestines to promote fecal elimination
- Reduces stress and anxiety and enhances relaxation
- Improves muscle and skin tone
- Strengthens immune system
- Increases flexibility and mobility
- Alleviates general aches and pain
- Increases mental clarity, energy, and performance
- Facilitates detoxification
- Relieves headaches
- Releases muscle spasms that cause pain or tingling
- Prevents new injuries
- Alleviates chronic pain (e.g., arthritis, fibromyalgia, scoliosis)
- Stimulates production of natural joint lubrication

- Improves posture and coordination
- Relieves pain and prevents pressure sores from immobilization
- Reduces swelling and fluid retention
- Alleviates insomnia
- Relieves itchy, dry skin
- Enhances breathing
- Slows progress of varicose veins
- Promotes vitality and energy
- Improves overall health

What Happens During a Visit?

- Sessions last 30 to 60 minutes
- Therapist may use cream and oils to massage each body part
- A complete medical history and current drug and herb intake information is obtained
- In a warm, relaxing atmosphere, patient is positioned on a treatment table and covered
- Soft music may be playing or incense may be burning
- Only the "part" being massaged is undraped
- Techniques vary from gentle massage to deep muscle work, depending on what the massage therapist thinks is appropriate for the patient
- A rest period of several minutes is usually recommended after the massage, before the person is allowed to dress and leave

Are There Any Risks Involved With Massage Therapy?

There are no contraindications, but there are several cautions. A licensed massage therapist would not perform massage on:

- Patients with circulatory problems such as phlebitis or varicose veins
- Patients with fever
- Patients with acute infectious disease
- Some types of cancer (over the site of a tumor)
- Inflammatory skin conditions and fractures (over the inflamed skin or fracture)
- The abdomen in pregnant women
- Over recent scars or operations

Massage may increase pain and discomfort in persons with arthritis so care is taken.

A list of drugs and herbs that the person is taking should be obtained. Drugs such as coumadin may change the type of massage technique that is used (e.g., the massage therapist would not use acupressure or shiatsu because these techniques may cause tissue injury that could bleed).

What Training Is Required of the Practitioner?

- *Certification or licensure* varies in each state. Twenty-seven states and the District of Columbia require licensure, but all have different requirements.
- *Certification* is essentially the process of publicly attesting that a specified quality or standard has been achieved or exceeded. The credibility and integrity of the certifying agency determines whether the agency's certification means anything to the public, and therefore, its value. Professional certification is a voluntary process by which a nongovernmental professional organization grants recognition to an individual who has met certain qualifications. It is a credential that attests that the individual has demonstrated a certain level of mastery of a specific body of knowledge and skills within the relevant field of practice. Certification should not be confused with licensing or accreditation. The national certifying examination for massage therapist is administered by the National Certification Board for Therapeutic Massage and Body Work (NCBTMB).
- *Licensure* is a nonvoluntary process by which an agency of government regulates a profession. It grants permission to an individual to engage in an occupation if it finds that the applicant has attained the degree of competency required to ensure that public health, safety, and welfare will be reasonably protected. Licensing it always based on the action of a legislative body. Once a licensing law has been passed it becomes illegal for anyone to engage in that occupation unless he or she has a license. The health care professions are typically licensed at the state or local level, but not usually at the federal level.
- Massage schools vary from 9 months to 2 years (usually a minimum of 500 hours of study).

Bibliography

Cady-Jones, G. E. (1997). Massage therapy as a workplace intervention for reduction of stress. Perceptual and Motor Skills 84, 157–158.

Collinge, M. (1996). The American Holistic Health Associations Complete Guide to Alternative Medicine. New York: Warner Books.

Field, T., Hernandez-Reif, M., Taylor, S., Quintino, O., & Burman, I. (1997). Labor pain is reduced by massage therapy. Journal of Psychosomatic Obstetrics & Gynaecology. 18, 286–291.

Nixon, M., Teschendorff, J., et al. (1997). Expanding the nursing repertoire: the effect of massage on post-operative pain. Australian Journal of Advanced Nursing. 14, 21–26.

Richards, K. C. (1998). Effect of a back massage and relaxation intervention on sleep in critically ill patients. American Journal of Critical Care. 7, 288–298.

Further Reading

Barlow, W. (1991). The Alexander technique. New York: Alfred A. Knopf.

Editors. (1989). Prevention Magazine Health Books, Hands-On-Healing Massage Remedies for Hundreds of Health Problems. 1989, Emmaus, PA: Rodale Press.

Feldenkrais, Moshe, Kimmey, M. (1992). The potent self: a guide to spontaneity. San Francisco, CA: Harper & Row.

Gray, J. (1991). The Alexander Technique. New York: St. Martin's Press.

Hudson, C. (1988). The complete book of massage. New York: Random House.

Laumer, U., Bauer, M., Fichter, M., & Milz, H. (1997). Therapeutic effects of the Feldenkrais method "awareness through movement" in patients with eating disorders. (German). Psychotherapie, psychosomatick, medizinische psychologie. 47, 170–180.

McIntyre, M. (1992). Unlock the trunk. Reprinted from Skiing. Oct.

Reese, M. (1992). Feldenkrais method bibliography. For the Feldenkrais Guild.

Seidman, M. (1991). A guide to polarity therapy: the gentle art of hands-on healing. Boulder, CO: Elan Press.

Stone, R. (1987). Polarity therapy: the complete and collected works. Vols 1–2. Sebastopol, CA: CRCS Publications.

RESOURCES

American Massage Therapy Association
820 Davis Street, Suite 100
Evanston, IL 60201
(312) 761-2682, (708) 864-0123

Massage Magazine
PO Box 1500
Davis, CA 95617
(916) 757-6033

Esalen Institute
Big Sur, CA 93920
(408) 667-3000

The Amma Institute of Skilled Touch
1881 Post Street
San Francisco, CA 94115
(415) 564-1103

Polarity Wellness Center
10 Leonard Street, Suite A
New York, NY 10013
(212) 334-8392

The Feldenkrais Guild
524 Ellsworth Street, PO Box 489
Albany, OR 97321
(503) 926-0981

American Polarity Therapy Association
2888 Bluff Street, Suite 149
Boulder, CO 80301
(303) 545-2080, Fax (303) 545-2161

The Alexander Journal
STAT, 20 London House
266 Fulham Road
London, SW 10 9EL, England

North American Society of Teachers of the Alexander Technique
PO Box 517
Urbana, IL 61901
(800) 473-0620

INTERNET

Touch Research Institute, University of Miami
http//:www.unmiami.edu.touch

Health World on Line
http//:www.healthworld.com

American Massage Association
http//:www.amtamassage.org

Office of Alternative Medicine
http://altmed.od.nig.gov/

People crave laughter as if it were an essential amino acid.

—PATCH ADAMS, MD

If we consider the frequent relief we receive from laughter, and how often it breaks the gloom which is apt to depress the mind, one would take care not to grow too wise for so great a pleasure of life.

—JOSEPH ADDISON

REFLEXOLOGY

What Is Reflexology?

Reflexology is a gentle art and a form of holistic healing. Reflexology should not be confused with foot or hand massage; reflexology is specific pressure therapy. Reflexology is an ancient technique based on the premise that there are reflex points on the feet and hands that correspond to every muscle, nerve, organ, gland, and bone in the body. Pressing on these points breaks up congestion and helps the nerves to relax. This, in turn, reduces vascular constriction so that the blood and nerves flow more freely. As circulation improves, toxins are released.

When the body becomes imbalanced through the course of daily living, nerve impulses can become blocked anywhere in the body. This means that nerve impulses to the muscles, organs, and glands of the body are impeded to some extent. Reflexology works to unblock the channels and improves nerve communication. Reflexology also promotes endorphin release, enhancing one's sense of well-being.

Reflexology is performed most frequently on the foot, but is also performed on the hand. There are roughly 7,200 nerves in each foot. The foot contains 26 small bones, 114 ligaments, and 20 muscles, which are joined together by connective tissue, blood vessels, and nerves, and covered by skin. This finely tuned, intricate structure is balanced on two main arches—one, from the heal to the base of the little toe, the other from the heal to the big toe. The heel (calcaneous) bears the brunt of our weight. It is insulated with protective layers of fat to cushion the impact of each foot step. The hand, which contains 27 bones, may also be used in reflexology (the hands and feet make up half the bones in the body).

Oriental medicine, acupressure, and acupuncture understand that life's vital energy or Chi (see Oriental Medicine) flows through the meridians (energy pathways) (see Oriental Medicine and Acupuncture for further explanation and figures). Six of the twelve meridians can be found in the foot.

Reflexologists believe that the feet are macrocosms or a mini-map of the whole body and all of the organs and body parts are reflected on the feet. The arrangement of the body parts on the feet are similar to the arrangement on the body (Fig. 7-4). The reflexes are found on the soles, tops, and along the inside and outside of the feet.

It is estimated that approximately 80% of adults will develop foot disorders, even though most people are born with healthy feet. Foot problems such as corns, calluses, bunions, and the like are often blamed on ill-fitting shoes, but are only part of the problem. Reflexologists believe that problems of the feet relate to problem within the body.

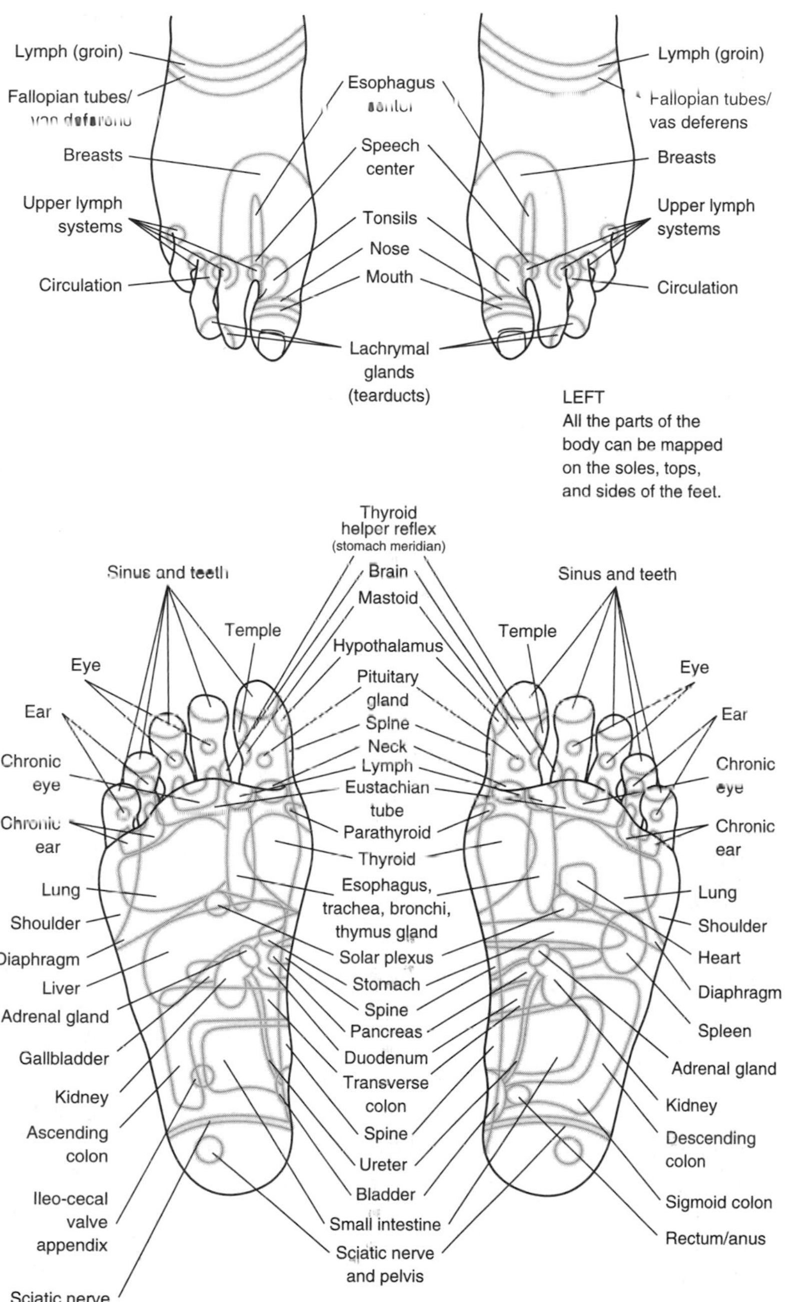

FIGURE 7-4
Mapping the Body on the Soles, Tops, and Sides of the Feet.

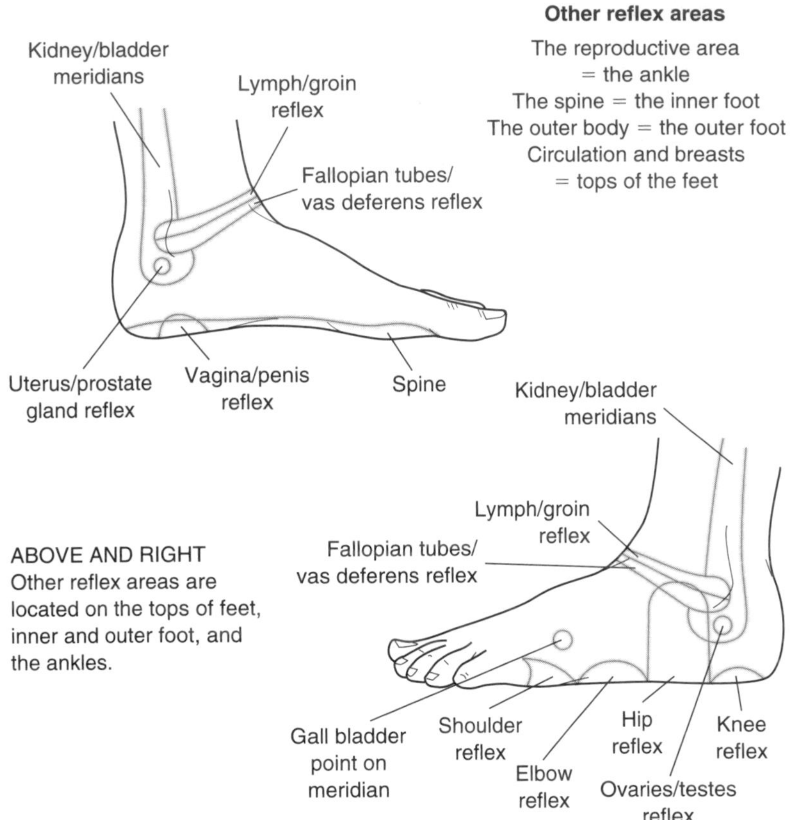

FIGURE 7-4
Continued.

What Is the History of Reflexology?

There are several theories of the origins of reflexology. Reflexology may have its origins in:

- Oriental medicine dating 5,000 years ago that links reflexology with acupressure and acupuncture following the meridians (see Acupuncture and Oriental Medicine sections for more information)
- Egypt dating 2500 to 2330 BC. A pictograph showing reflexology dating to this period has been found in a tomb of an Egyptian physician, Ankahor.
- Native Americans, particularly the Cherokee, believe this technique was handed down by the Incas. The Cherokee believe "the feet walk

upon the earth, and through this, your spirit is connected to the universe."

Wherever the beginnings, reflexology continued to be developed in Europe and the United States. Harry Bond, in his book, "Zone Therapy" in 1582, discussed the practice of reflexology, particularly on the royalty and upper class. Sir H. Head, in the 1890s, discovered zones on the skin that became hypersensitive to pressure when an organ connected by nerves to this skin region was diseased. Dr. Ivan Pavlou (1849–1936) used reflexology as a basis for his own famous research-conditioned reflexes. Dr. A. Cornelius, a German, in 1902, discovered that his own pain from an infection was lessened after foot pressure. He continued to research foot pressure in his medical practice.

In the United States, Dr. William Fitzgerald, in the early 1900s, demonstrated that he could perform minor surgical procedures without patient discomfort by applying pressure to the hands. Dr. J. Riley, in 1919, published a book *Zone Therapy Simplified*, in which he published detailed diagrams and drawings of the reflex points located in the feet. Eunice Ingham (1879–1974) is called the mother of modern reflexology. She used the previously published works regarding zone therapy in her work. She evolved the "map" of the entire body on the feet. Her legacy continues under the direction of her nephew, Dwight Byers, who runs the International Institute of Reflexology in St. Petersburg, FL.

What Research Exists?

While there are descriptive articles that include anecdotal evidence, there is a paucity of research reports published in independent journals to enable health care professionals to make an informed decision regarding the effectiveness of reflexology. A few studies have been performed abroad, but English translations of the full research reports are not readily available to allow critical analysis of their methodology. In addition, studies reported in the "grey literature" suggest that reflexology may be an effective treatment, but these are small-scale studies that provide inadequate details of methodology.

The issue of research methodology suitable for determining the effectiveness of reflexology needs to be addressed. Collaboration between reflexologists and experienced researchers needs to be encouraged because good quality studies are required to determine the effectiveness of reflexology. The Research Consul for Complementary Medicine, set up in 1983, provides advice, funding, and support to complementary therapists who are undertaking research. A research ethos should be developed within reflexology, with education in research methodology provided through reflexology courses. Above all, there needs to be improved dissemination of the results of research studies with encouragement to publish research findings within the journals more readily accessible to health care professionals. It is suggested by Lynn (1996) that Reflexology is difficult to study in double-blind trials because of the personal psychosomatic element that is so individualized.

PRO

Oleson and Flacco (1993) reported a placebo-controlled trial to investigate reflexology's ability to reduce premenstrual distress. At the conclusion of the study, the 35 participants showed a significantly greater reduction in premenstrual symptoms than in the control group, and the results remained for the 2-month follow-up. This study was later criticized by Vickers (1996) for its methodologic quality.

Kovaks, et al (1993) performed a double-blind trial using reflexology to treat low back pain. The authors reported statistically significant improvements in pain, muscular contraction, and mobility in the treatment group, enabling most to discontinue their prescribed pain medication and remain symptom free during the study period.

Dobbs (1985) describes the use of reflexology in caring for seven terminally ill patients with cancer. Self-reports indicate that all the patients felt their quality of life improved with reflexology. This improvement could have been a result of the increase in touch and communication with the reflexologist and not solely a result of reflexology.

Motha and McGrath (1994) performed a study on 64 pregnant women to determine the effect of reflexology on labor. Results suggested that reflexology treatment resulted in a reduction in labor time and in physical symptoms experienced by the expectant mother. This study, although with positive results, was not published in a peer-reviewed journal and used no control group.

CON

Sorenson and Ibsen (1993) expressed concern about patients with diabetes being treated for ulceration and foot infection. They reported a case study of a woman being treated with reflexology who later had to have the foot amputated. There could have been many extenuating circumstances with this woman, but this brings up the concern of using reflexology as the only treatment for individuals with a chronic disease.

What Is Reflexology Used to Treat or Improve?

Reflexologists can treat all age groups from infants to the elderly. Reflexology can be used to balance the entire body rather than "cure" specific disorders, but by its proper application, reflexology can actualize the body's own healing power. Practitioners of reflexology suggest that weekly reflexology treatments can stop most problems early and enhance a quick recovery. Reflexology increases circulation to areas of the body that enhances nutrient absorption and waste elimination. Reflexology also:

- Balances all 11 body systems, so the body can heal itself
- Stimulates underactive areas of the body and mind and calms the overactive areas
- Enhances a positive mental outlook (Health is a harmonious interplay of energies within the body. Negative thoughts and emotions restrict the free flow of these energies, causing congestion that ultimately manifests as disease if not corrected.)
- Expels the suppressed emotions of stress, relaxing the body and attitude to life (Reflexologists believe that 85% of all disease today is in some way stress related)
- Relaxes the body
- Increases endorphin release to help pain control
- Enhances the function of the immune system and improves lymphatic flow
- Maintains a healthy body in balance
- Improves concentration levels
- Improves blood and nerve circulation
- Releases areas of congestion, typically felt as pain

Possible reactions that may occur after a treatment include:

- Increased urination because the kidneys are stimulated to produce more urine that may be darker and stronger-smelling because of the toxic content
- Flatulence and more frequent bowel movements
- Aggravated skin condition, particularly in conditions that have been suppressed; increased perspiration as toxins are released through the pores of the feet.
- Improved skin tone and tissue texture caused by improved circulation
- Increased secretions of the mucous membranes in the nose, mouth, and bronchi

- Change in sleep patterns, deeper or more disturbed sleep
- Dizziness or nausea
- A temporary outbreak of a disease that has been suppressed as the body begins the healing process
- Increased vaginal discharge
- Feverishness
- Tiredness or increased energy
- Headaches
- Depression, overwhelming desire to weep

These reactions are considered part of the treatment and often demonstrate that the body is healing and clearing toxins.

What Happens During a Visit?

Reflexologists are not allowed to practice medicine or diagnose disease.

- A detailed case history including chief complaint, medications (including vitamins and herbs), duration of complaint, basic health history, and whether the patient is under medical treatment.
- Patient is seated comfortably in a chair or recliner and the foot is positioned in front of the practitioner.
- All tight clothing on the lower extremities is loosened, but not removed.
- Shoes, socks, or stockings are removed.
- The feet are wiped with an antiseptic cloth, bathed with absorbent cotton, soaked in disinfectant, or a foot spa with a mild disinfectant is used. The feet are dried completely.
- The feet are examined for temperature, color, blemishes, muscle tone, skin condition, and other pathologies.
- Using thumbs and forefingers, the foot is reflexed. The entire foot is first worked and then areas of specific concern are concentrated on. The pressure releases blockages of energy that inhibit energy flow and cause pain and disease. If the problem is internal, the reflex area and the relevant meridians are particularly sensitive to excess pressure and friction. The areas where corns, calluses, and the like occur are particularly significant to the reflexologist.
- Session lasts 30 to 60 minutes.

Reflexology activates the body's own healing power, so some of the reactions are inevitable as the body rids itself of toxins. This is referred to as a "healing crisis," and is a cleansing process. The severity of the reaction depends on the degree of imbalance.

- Course of therapy is usually 1 to 12 weeks, depending on the condition and length of time it has been present. A single treatment will not correct problems that have developed over years.

Are There Risks Involved With Reflexology?

- No risks exist, but if the symptoms are serious or prolonged, a doctor should be consulted.
- Contraindications include injury to the foot (work hands instead) and contagious pathologic conditions of the foot.
- Cautions should be taken with thrombotic disease of the lower extremities and with diabetes.
- Acute infections could be worsened as a result of increasing the circulation. Caution is advised.

What Training Is Required of the Practitioner?

Classes are usually required and are held all over the United States. Certification is available. Some states require licensing. For that listing, contact the Reflexation Association of America or Reflex Certification Board.

Bibliography

Lynn, J. (1997). Using complementary therapies: reflexology. Professional Nurse. 11, 321–322.

Mackereth, P. (1997). Clinical supervision for 'potent' practice. Complementary Therapies in Nursing and Midwifery. 3, 38–41.

Further Reading

Botting, D. (1997). Review of literature on the effectiveness of reflexology. Complementary Therapies in Nursing & Midwifery. 3, 123–130.

Byers, D. (1987). Better health with foot reflexology. St. Petersburg, FL: Ingham Publishing.

Clark, C. C. (1997). Reflexology: a complementary therapy. Nursing Spectrum. 7, 8.

Dobbs, B. Z. (1985). Oncology nursing: alternative health approaches - reflexology part 6. Nursing Mirror. 160, 41–42.

Douglas, I. & Ellis, S. (1996). Reflexology. Rockport, MA: Element Books Inc.

Douglas, I. & Ellis, S. (1998). The art of reflexology. Rockport, MA: Element Books Inc.

Dougans, I. (1997). The complete illustrated guide to reflexology. Rockport, MA: Element Books Inc.

Gillanders, A. (1995). The joy of reflexology. Boston, MA: Little, Brown and Co.

Ingham, E. (1938). Stories the feet can tell through reflexology. St. Petersburg, FL: Ingham Publishing.

Ingham, E. (1951). Stories the feet have told through reflexology. St. Petersburg, FL: Ingham Publishing..

Kovaks, F. M., et al. (1993). Neuro-reflexology intervention in the treatment of non-specified low back pain. Association of Reflexologists 1994. Reflexology research reports, 2nd ed. London: Association of Reflexologists.

Motha, G. & McGrath, J. (1994). The effects of reflexology on labor outcome. Association of Reflexologists. Reflexology research reports, 2nd ed. London: Association of Reflexologists.

Oleson, T. & Flocco, W. (1993). Randomised controlled study of premenstrual symptoms treated with ear, hand and foot reflexology. Obstetrics & Gynecology. 82, 906–911.

Sorensen, L., Ibsen, K. E. (1993). Purulent myofascitis in a patient with diabetes treated with a vacuum boot by a zone therapist. Ugeskrift For Laeger. 155, 2150–2152.

Vickers, A. (1996). Massage and aromatherapy-a guide for helth professionals. London: Chapman & Hall.

RESOURCES

American Reflexology Certification Board
PO Box 620607
Littleton, CO 81062
(303) 933-6021

International Institute of Reflexology
PO Box 12462
St. Petersburg, FL 33733
(813) 343-4811

The International School of Reflexology and Meridian Therapy
2222 Kilkare Parkway
Mt. Pleasant, NJ 08742
(908) 802-7566

Reflexology Association of American (RAA)
4012 S. Rainbow Blvd.
Box K 585
Las Vegas, NV 89103-2059

INTERNET

Office of Alternative Medicine
http://altmed.od.nig.gov/

Aging Implications
http://www.reflexology-research.com/aging.htm

Chinese Study
http://www.reflexology-research.com/CHINAs_1.HTM

Diabetic abstracts
http://www.reflexology-research.com/diabetes.html

Meeting Emotional Needs
http://www.reflexology-research.com/emotions.html

REIKI (THE RADIANCE TECHNIQUE)

What is Reiki?

Reiki is a Japanese word for "universal life force." In the universe and in nature there are several kinds of energy: transcendental, inner light, cosmic, radiant, and universal (see Fig. 7-5). The inherent purpose of Reiki

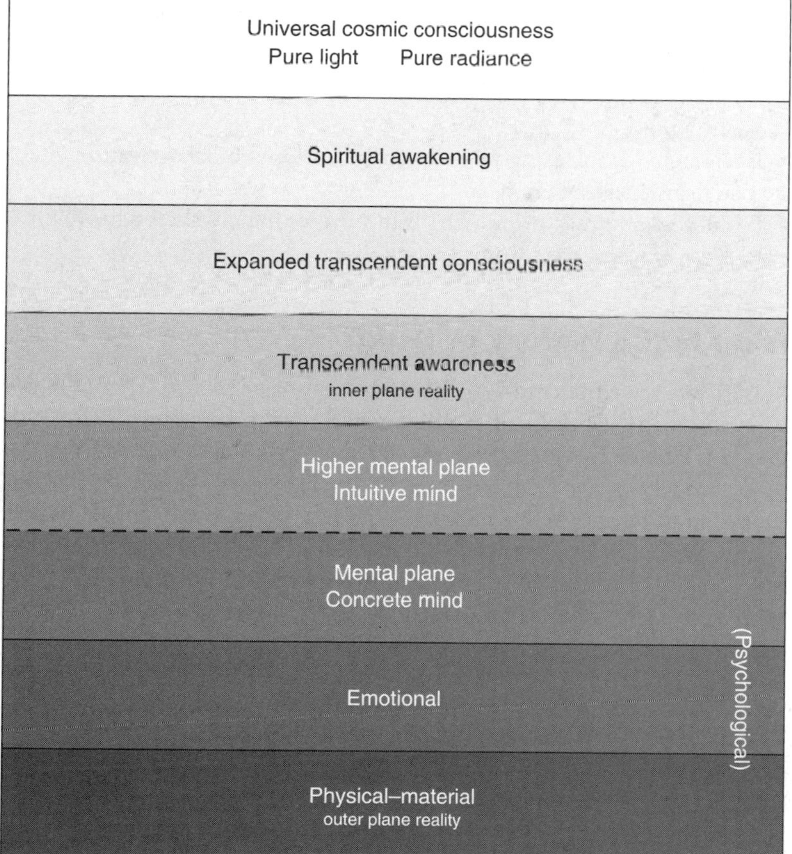

FIGURE 7-5
Energy Model.

is to give the body direct access to transcendental, universal, radiant, and light energy. When properly "attuned" to the inner processes, universal energy can be accessed and used by the practitioner to balance and release energy. The resulting energy movement helps the body to come into a natural state of balance and to begin to heal.

An "attunement" is performed only by a Reiki master (discussed later) and is an initiation ceremony that is supposed to open an inner healing channel within the student and allow (or attune) the student to the flow of Reiki energy. Usually the four upper chakra (energy centers) (see Ayuvedic Medicine section for description of chakras) are opened, so energy can be channeled. The energy provides the strength, harmony, and balance to help heal maladies and reduce stress.

Reiki works on the principle that the body recognizes this universal life energy and uses it to promote balance and total health. Reiki also:

- Is a nonreligious healing practice
- Is based on the belief that life force is in all of us and that energy is a healing power
- Is a system for releasing physical and emotional blockages and increasing internal energy
- Promotes total relaxation, which in turn, enhances the body's ability to recover from stress, injuries, and disease.

What Is the History of Reiki?

Reiki is an ancient hands-on Buddhist healing modality, originally developed by the Tibetans and rediscovered by the Japanese in the 19th Century. The technique was rediscovered by Dr. Usui of Japan and eventually brought to the United States by Ms. Hawaya Takata, where it was passed on in its entirety to Barbara Ray, PhD. There has been splintering from the main body of knowledge with several different forms of Reiki existing. The true, original intact form from Dr. Usui is referred to as the "Radiance technique" or the "official Reiki program." The other, more common form, is referred to as Reiki.

What Research, Reviews, and Comments Exist?

PRO

Wirth, et al (1993) used Reiki to relieve pain of dental extractions. In a double-blind, randomized clinical trial, researchers found that the patients receiving Reiki had significantly less postoperative pain than those in the control group. Wirth, et al (1996) studied several healing modalities in the treatment of full thickness burns. Wirth found a statistical significance result when therapeutic touch and Reiki were used together. Bullock (1997) used Reiki to enhance the end-of-life journey and quality of life in a patient with aggressive cancer. The patient had a greater relief of pain, anxiety, dyspnea, and edema after Reiki than he had had with traditional treatments.

CON

No negative research, reviews, or comments could be found in a Medline search.

What Is Reiki Used to Treat or Improve?

Reiki is used to treat or improve all acute and chronic health problems. It is used to:

- Hasten relaxation
- Reduce pain
- Enhance emotional release
- Provide an overall feeling of well-being

What Happens During Reiki?

- Sessions last 1 hour
- The patient lays on the table with clothes on
- The Reiki practitioner holds hands in 12 basic positions on head, chest, and back (Fig. 7-6)
- No massage or manipulation takes place
- Other hand positions may be used to treat specific conditions such as hiccups, transmandibular joint (TMJ) disease, earache, nose bleeds, chest or breast pain, and so on

Are There Any Risks Involved With Reiki?

There are no risks with Reiki. However, Reiki should not be used to treat undiagnosed pain, broken bones, or bleeding. It also should not be used in place of traditional treatment. The light energy facilitates the body's own ability to heal.

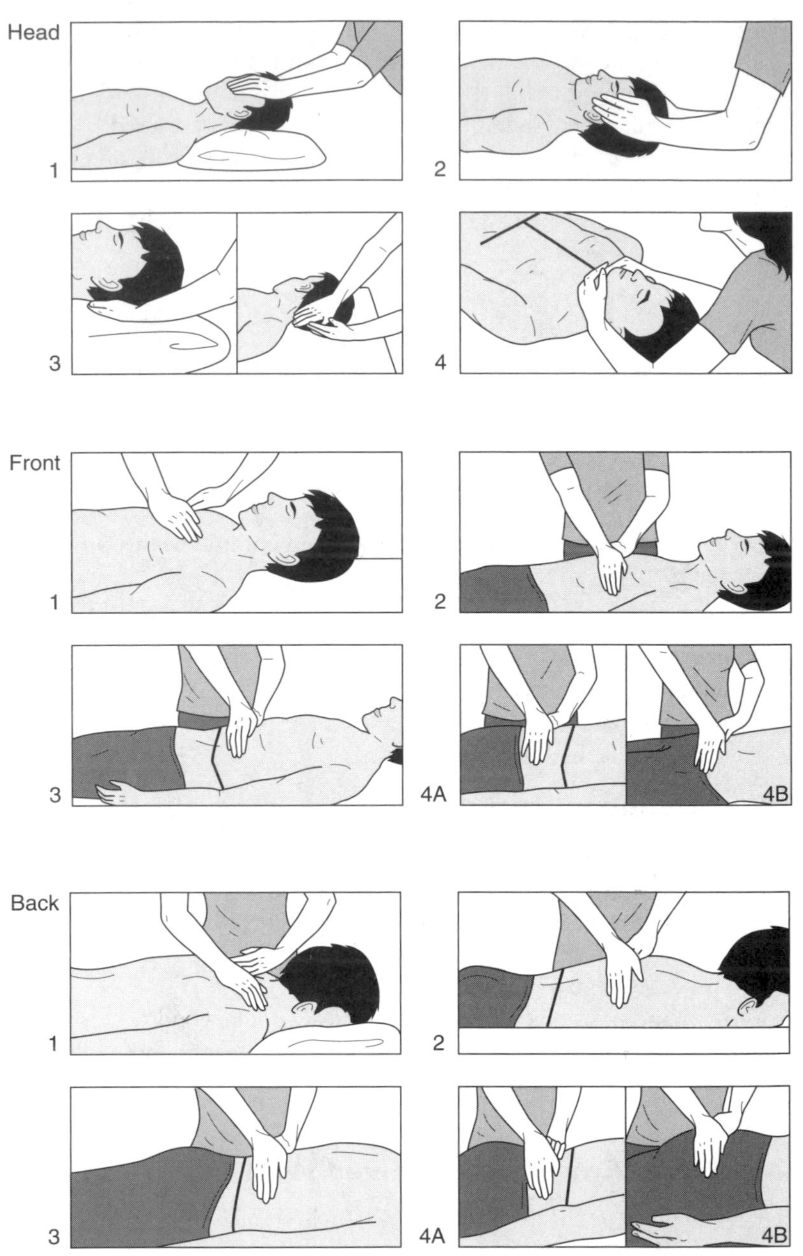

FIGURE 7-6
Positions.

What Training Is Required of the Practitioner?

Reiki must be taught by a Reiki master. There are seven levels of practice with each degree being distinguished by different attunement for that degree (Table 7-1). Most of the degrees can be taught in a 2-day program. Each of the degrees is a subsystem within a whole and each of the Attunement Processes of each degree is connected directly to the whole, not part to part. The subsystems of Attunements and symbols are simultaneously interconnected with each other and with the whole. The

TABLE 7-1

The Degree	Appropriate Attunements	Purpose
1.00	4.00	• opens the gateway to using universal energy • learn the 12 positions for balancing energy on self and others
2.00	1.00	• deepens inner understanding • learn symbols of healing • expands harmony of the emotional and mental planes of energy • learns precise technique for directing universal energy
3.00	1 (with interior processes)	2 parts—3A and 3B 3A • allows for more personal growth • increases capacity to transform and cocreate on multidimensional levels • offerred only by Radiance Stress Management, Inc., not by individual teachers 3B—Reiki Master • prepares a Reiki Master who can teach and do attunements • student completes the Official Teacher Training Program • to be a Reiki master and teach Reiki, a mentorship relationship with a master is established, and the person will devote years to additional study and training.
4.00 5.00 6.00 7.00	1.00 1.00 1.00 3.00	Special advanced seminars taught only by Radiance Seminars, Inc. and Dr. Barbara Ray. Only someone knowing the whole can attune others.

whole and the purpose of the whole is greater than (more than) any individual part or the sum of those individual parts. The inner dynamics of this science is a process of wholes, not parts.

To attune a person to the actual degree the following must be completed:

- The person doing the attuning would have to be already attuned to the proper level (Degree 3B is a Reiki teacher)
- The Attunement Process would have to be connected to the whole system from within.

Bibliography

Bullock, M. (1997).Reiki: a complementary therapy for life. American Journal of Hospital Palliatative Care. 14, 31–33.

Ray, B. (1996). The official handbook of radiance technique. San Francisco, CA: Radiance Technique Association, Inc.

Van Sell, S. (1996). Reiki: an ancient tough therapy. RN. 96, 57–59.

Wirth, D. P., Richardson, J. T., & Eidelman, W. S. (1996). Wound healing and complementary therapies: a review. Journal of Alternative Complementary Medicine. 2, 493–502.

Wirth, D. P., Brenlan, D. R., et al. (1993). The effect of complementary healing therapy on postoperative pain after surgical removal of impacted molar teeth. Complementary Therapies in Medicine. 1, 133.

Further Reading

Baginski, B. J., Sharamon, S. (1988). Reiki: universal life. Mendocino, CA: Life Rhythm Press.

Ray, B. (1996). The expanded reference manual of radiance technique. Miami, FL: Radiance Association of Florida.

Sawyer, J. (1998). The first Reiki practitioner in our OR. AORNJ. 67, 674–677.

Van Sell, S. (1996). Reiki: an ancient touch therapy. RN. 96, 57–59.

Whitsitt, T. (1998). Reiki therapy. Journal of Christ Nursing. 15, 12–13.

Wright, F. (1987). The radiance technique: on the job. Florida Radiance Association.

RESOURCES

Reiki Alliance
PO Box 41
Cataldo, ID 83810
(208) 682-3535, Fax (208) 682-4848

INTERNET

Reikialliance@compuserve.com

ROLFING

What Is Rolfing?

The human body is like a house. It is structured so that each part has its proper place, and each piece interlocks to balance the load of the others. As in the well-built house whose every post and beam is in place, the well-used (more than well-built) body functions efficiently. Because gravity pulls down on everything, out-of-place body parts—beams out of alignment and unsupported by a post—are pulled into painfully unnatural positions. What the Rolfer seeks is a return of the construction to its original blueprint specifications. This is often compared to, first, grabbing the patient by the hair and lifting the patient straight up until he or she is hanging in a perfectly vertical position and then setting the patient down. Putting one "out-of-whack" piece back into place is usually not enough. Everything should be right before a house can stand or a body can work smoothly. This kind of arrangement, in turn, produces "the gospel of Rolfing: when the body is working properly, the force of gravity can flow through it. Then spontaneously, the body heals itself" (Fig. 7-7) (from Mixter, 1983).

Rolfing recognizes that gravity is the basic shaper of the body. We have to balance our bodies somehow within the pull of gravity. From birth to death, gravity is always working on the body, and thus, deviations in the muscle-bone system are never merely local. Gravity's influence spreads them throughout the body. If the natural balance of the body is disturbed—if it does not follow the best geometry of the skeleton—then the whole body will gradually change form to adapt to the deviation. For example, a child falls from a bicycle and injures a knee. To avoid pain, the child tightens the muscles around that knee. Because the body must work against the tug of gravity, the entire muscle and fascial system gradually shifts to compensate for the first change. Movement through the pelvis is influenced, as is the pattern of breathing and the set of the head. Because muscles alone cannot carry the additional tension, the fasciae shorten to support the new movement, and, in time, the shape and function of the whole body alters with them (Mixter, 1983).

The state of balance or imbalance in our bodies—their relationship to the field of gravity—is reflected in feeling states because emotion is intimately involved with muscular tonus. Balance may be thought of in a healthy organism as a resting state, a capacity and a preparedness for responses of all kinds depending on the nature of the stimulus. Imbalance, then, is the response itself (the movement, or impulse to movement), which completes itself by a return to balance when the response has spent itself (Mixter, 1983).

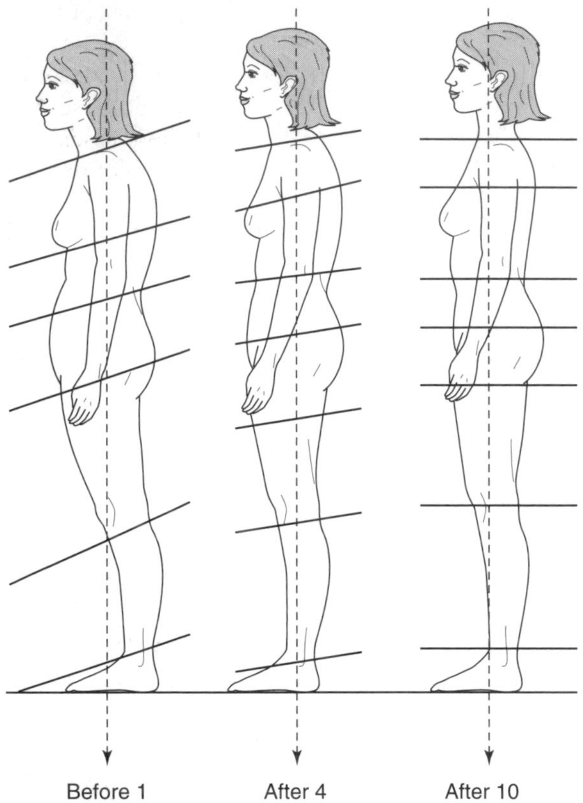

FIGURE 7-7
The Rolfing Method.

The muscular tension and the emotion are two aspects of the same organic pattern. Chronic muscular tension is a permanent shortening of fascial structures; to the extent to which they are no longer capable of lengthening; they have built into the person not only a way of moving but a way of feeling, so that one particular kind of emotion characterizes a person's response to a wide range of stimuli. This programming marks a loss in the ability to respond with full appropriateness to the current situation. So Rolfing:

- Is deep manipulation of the connective tissues of the body. Reaching down to the collagen that cements the cells together to move the supportive tissue of the body's frame to a looser and more fluid state.
- Works with soft tissue and fascia at the surface and at deep levels.

- Believes that human function is improved when the segments of the body are properly aligned.
- Works on the premise that people lose symmetry between the right and left, and back and front planes of their bodies, and that these discrepancies get worse with time and result in dysfunction. Fascia is collagen tissue, and once injured, does not lose the memory of the injury even after the injury has healed.
- Rebalances the fascial network by taking advantage of its tendency to hold the shape induced by applied force.
- Balances the effects of gravity on the body.

As a group, Rolfers are highly diverse and vary in practice. However, all Rolfers have the common goal to improve the human structure, have it balanced, and have it with the appropriate length between its segments all within the field of gravity.

What Is the History of Rolfing?

Rolfing was developed more than 20 years by Ida Rolf (1896–1979). Dr. Rolf was a biologic chemist who became interested in structure and function in the body and their relationship with each other because of her own health problems. Rolf was convinced that the entire structural order of the body needed to be realigned and balanced with the gravitational forces for permanent "changes" to occur. She saw soft tissue manipulation of the osteopath or bony manipulation of the chiropractor as merely shifting the physical strain to another area of the body. Fascia connective tissue is the organ of structure. Fascial layers comprise the layers of structure, the organs that hold the body in the three-dimensional world. The fascia, an organ of structure, is resilient and plastic. It can be changed by adding energy. During Rolfing the actual matrix of the collagen can be changed. Dr. Rolf also connected the structure of the fasica with the role of the autonomic nervous system. As Dr. Rolf developed her technique, she studied the postural positions of Hatha Yoga (see Yoga section for more information). Some of her early work emphasized yoga positions, breathing, and stretching. Dr. Rolf also studied the energetic models of the chakras (energy centers, see Ayurvedic Medicine) and the meridians (energy pathways, see Oriental Medicine). This entire study is incorporated in the Rolfing techniques. Dr. Rolf emphasizes that Rolfers are not practitioners curing disease, but practitioners invoking health.

Rolf taught her technique to osteopaths, chiropractors, and other therapists. In the 1960s, Dr. Rolf was discovered at the Esalan Institute in Big Sur, CA, by Dr. Fritz Perls, a famous psychologist. Dr. Perls' health improved greatly after experiencing Dr. Rolf's body work techniques. In 1970, the Rolf Institute of Structural Integration was established in Boulder, CO. In 1977, Rolf published her book, Rolfing: The Integration of Human Structure.

What Research Exists?

PRO

Research on Rolfing has begun to give objective quantitative data about its effects. Dr. Valerie Hunt, director of the Movement Behavior Laboratory at UCLA and Dr. Julian Silverman, Research Specialist of the California Department of Mental Hygiene, have conducted experiments at Agnews State Hospital in which subjects were tested before and after Rolfing for changes in neurologic control of the muscles, for variation in responses to stimuli, and for biochemical changes. Their findings indicate that after Rolfing there is more efficient use of the muscles, conserved energy, increased refinement of response, and a tendency for motor control to shift toward the more reflexive spinal centers. Other research is planned or in progress (supplied by the Rolf Institute.)

CON

No con research was found in a Medline search.

What Is Rolfing Used to Treat or Improve?

Rolfing does not cure disease, but it:

- Realigns and rebalances the major segments of body weight
- Reduces chronic stress
- Enhances neurologic function
- Improves normal back anatomy
- Relieves muscle spasm, tension, and pain
- Provides improvement in structural integration
- Improves energy level
- Increases range of motion and flexibility, particularly after trauma
- Works to correct structures so that walking, standing, and moving become more comfortable and efficient
- Improves circulation and lymph flow
- Relaxes all structures in the body
- Immunologic conditions (multiple sclerosis [MS], lupus, chronic fatigue syndrome) and cancer may show improvement

What Happens During a Visit?

- Requires 10 sessions usually every 4 to 8 weeks (some people may take months between sessions), each session taking 60 to 90 minutes; then a yearly "tune up"
- A health questionnaire is completed, and what the patient hopes to gain from Rolfing is discussed.
- The patient is asked to undress down to his or her underwear and pose for session 1 photographs. The body is usually viewed in a mirror as the Rolfer points out areas of disorganization.
- The patient lies down on a cushioned table and the work is started.
- Rolfers use pressure applied with the fingers, knuckles, and elbows to release adhesion, which helps to reorganize the tissue back to its proper geometric planes by lifting, lengthening, and balancing the body segments.
  - Session 1 involves superficial releasing of fascial sheath that lies just below the skin's surface. Work done lengthens the trunk up and out of the pelvis, separating rib cage from trunk, and lengthening the spine and lower back. Often, "homework" is assigned to reinforce the session's results.
  - Session 2 centers on the feet and legs, insuring that the foot plant equally distributes weight to all parts of the foot.
  - Session 3 ties sessions 1 and 2 together. The head, shoulders, hips, and ankles are aligned. The rib cage is differentiated from the shoulder girdle and pelvis, each is given its own space with no crowding.
  - Session 4 establishes improved support for the structures that make up the pelvic floor. The core of the body is strengthened and straightened. This is the first section that begins to work more deeply in the body.
  - Session 5 continues the 4th session and should follow within 2 weeks. This session lenghtens and separates the outer structures of the pelvis (rectus abdominis) to allow room for the inner structures to reassert themselves.
  - Session 6 works on the pelvis through the deep rotating muscles under the buttocks. By this time, the pelvis is feeling more symmetrical and organized around a vertical line. Patients with chronic back pain often point to this session as pivotal in their progress.
  - Session 7 balances the head and neck on the spine, opens the connective tissue around the skull and face, and helps improve breathing.

- Session 8, 9, and 10 focuses on putting the body back together again. The body is now poised on a narrow base and can move in any direction with equal ease.

After the initial 10 sessions, it is recommened that the patient avoid more deep structural work for 6 months to 1 year. The changes initiated in these sessions will continue for months, even years after the series is complete.

Patients are encouraged to return once a year for a "tune up." An advanced series of four to six sessions is also available. The advanced sessions concentrate on ways of balanced movement in gravity using the organization established by the original 10 sessions.

Are There Any Risks Involved With Rolfing?

Rolfing is not for everyone.

- Severe arthritis may not be helped
- Should not be performed if person has the flu (virus can render the connective tissue unresponsive)
- Should be performed cautiously on anyone who has had previous exposure to toxic substances
- Should not be done on someone who is severely, clinically dehydrated because connective tissue will be unresponsive
- Caution is advised during pregnancy. Several sessions may be conducted, but not all 10
- Care is used when patient has diagnosed osteoporosis
- Care is used when the practitioner suspects undiagnosed injury. The Rolfer may recommend a visit to the doctor, radiographs, and so on to diagnose previous injuries

What Training Is Required of the Practitioner?

Prerequisites:

- A massage therapist or college courses in the biologic and behavioral sciences (now offered at the Rolf Institute)
- A 4-year college degree

  The education consists of:
  - A 2-year program
  - 20 to 25 weeks of additional training and 18 weeks of clinical practice

  Certification and Licensure:
  - Some states require certification

- Some states require a massage certification or license
- To use the title, "Rolfer," persons must be members in good standing of the Rolf Institute, the sole certifying agency for Rolfers. There are more than 1,000 certified Rolfers around the world.

Bibliography

Mixter, J. (1983). Rolfing. Newark, NJ: Rolf Press.

Further Reading

Rolf, I. (1977). Rolfing: the integration of human structures. New York: Harper and Row.
Rolf, I. (1989). Rolfing. Inner traditions. Rochester, VT.

RESOURCES

International Rolf Institute
PO Box 1868
Boulder, CO 80306
(303) 449-5903

INTERNET

Rolf Institute
www.rolf.org

THERAPEUTIC TOUCH

What Is Therapeutic Touch?

The simplest definition of therapeutic touch (TT) is that it is the use of the hands on or near the body with the intent to help or heal. The practitioner is completely focused in what we assume to be a meditative state, on the intention to help or heal. The consciousness of the practitioner is all important. TT is a contemporary interpretation of an ancient healing practice.

The practitioner acts as a human energy support system until the recipient's own immunologic support system is robust enough to take over. TT can be practiced effectively by health professionals and lay people who are committed to helping or healing persons. Additional qualities required of the practitioner are:

- Compassion with sensitive, balanced receptivity to the unstated and often unrecognized nonphysical needs of the recipient

- Discipline to attune oneself to the messages coming from the farthest reaches of consciousness
- The ability to recognize own limitations

The practitioner does not drain his or her own strengths and resources during the treatment. Rather, the practitioner is a conduit for the universal life energy, or higher power. If the practitioner feels drained, it is a good indication that he or she has not connected to the higher energy source, but used his or her own ego power.

Therapeutic touch recognizes that we as human beings are multidimensional fields of energy (Fig. 7-8). Interaction between persons can be viewed as exchanges of energy between two interacting fields. Each person is surrounded by at least four layers of energy:

- Etheric field is the vital layer most closely associated with the physical body. It interfaces with the emotional dimension. It extends 2 to 12 inches from the skin and is most associated with energy-balancing healing work.
- Emotional field, often referred to as the aura, extends further than the etheric field and comprises affective and feeling energy.
- Casual field, or mental layer, is our thinking patterns and our ability to visualize.
- Astral body, or intuitive layer, is outside of all others and is our spiritual dimension.

By looking at the energy fields, when there is dysfunction at the spiritual or intuitive layer, it impacts on all other layers. Dysfunction at this level is experienced as a loss of purpose or sense of hope in one's life. Dysfunction in the casual field or mental layer results in faulty thought patterns and self-doubt. Dysfunction at the emotional field relates to a constricting affect, such as despair and depression. Dysfunction at the etheric level results in physical symptoms and disease. Therefore, this understanding leads us to believe that physical disease is at the end of the continuum. Physical disease may be manifested quickly by traumatic injury or surgery.

Along with the concept of energy fields, therapeutic touch also looks at the chakras (centers of energy, see Ayurveda Medicine for discussion). The chakras are wheels of light that protrude through the energy fields. There is a complex interrelationship between the chakras and the energy fields.

Therapeutic touch has gained cross-cultural popularity because research has suggested that there are multiple realities. Therefore, illness can have different connotations. Several views of reality do not perceive illness as bad, but rather as an individual's reaction to circumstances. Illness can therefore be helped or healed by the individual.

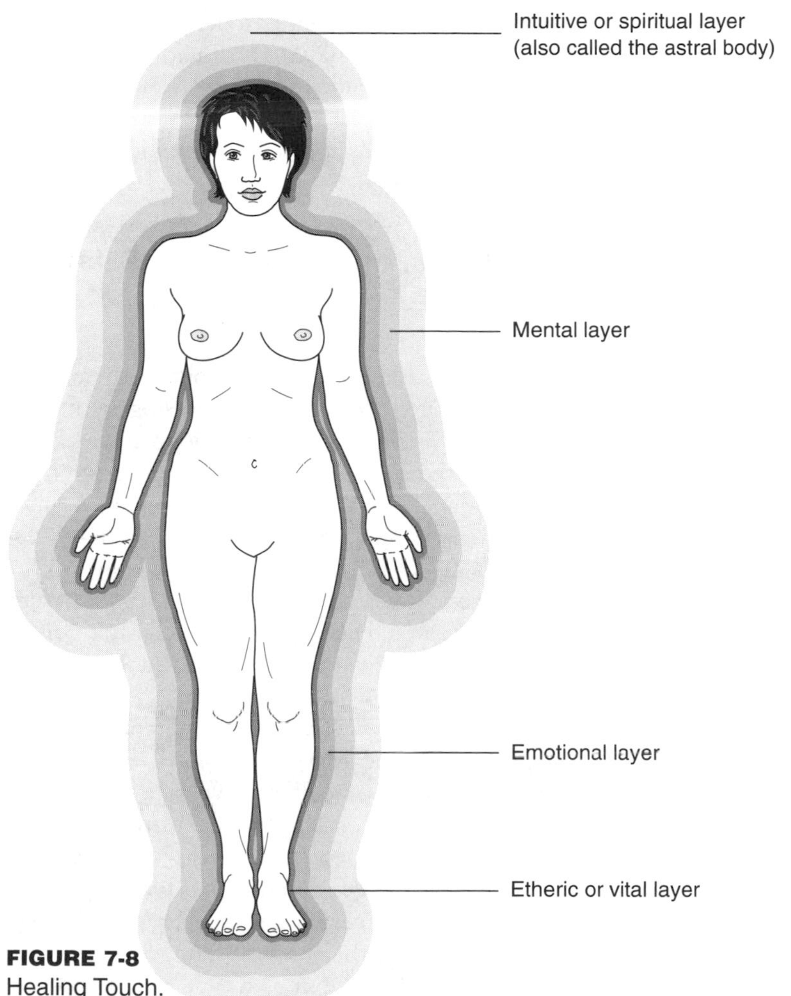

FIGURE 7-8
Healing Touch.

What Is the History of Therapeutic Touch?

Therapeutic touch was founded by Dora Kunz, who derived the techniques for therapeutic touch from the ancient practice of laying-on of hands, "energy transfer" and the inner healer, and Delores Krieger, RN, PhD. In 1972, Dr. Krieger initiated the teaching of therapeutic touch as part of the graduate program in nursing at New York University. The organization that supports practitioners of therapeutic touch is the Nurse Healers Professional Association, Inc.

Because Dr. Krieger developed therapeutic touch, its theoretical framework is drawn from Rogerian Nursing theory, Quantum Field and Systems theory. In Roger's view, therapeutic touch is an example of how professionals practice to strength the coherence and integrity of human and environmental fields for the realization of optimum well-being (Bronstein, 1996).

What Research, Reviews, and Comments Exist?

PRO

There have been hundreds of research articles supporting therapeutic touch since 1975. Easter investigated therapeutic touch using an integrative review of the literature. Using specific methodology, research explores the question, "What is the state of development of research regarding therapeutic touch?" by analyzing primary research reports from 23 articles in 14 referenced journals. The findings of the review indicate positive regard for the use of Therapeutic Touch. All research points to the need for further study in this area. Research methods used are satisfactory, but more rigorous methodologies would promote a more scientific contribution to the body of literature regarding therapeutic touch. The following are a few examples.

The first studies that verified the effectiveness of therapeutic touch were published by Kreiger in 1975 and 1976. Research demonstrated a significantly greater increase in mean hemoglobin level of a group of patients who received therapeutic touch compared to a control group.

Quinn (1982) found that patients who received therapeutic touch had a greater reduction in anxiety than the those in the placebo group. Leller and Bzdek (1986) found the patients receiving therapeutic touch rated their headache pain 70% less, whereas the control group with mimicked therapeutic touch had only a 37% decrease in pain.

Wirth (1991) studied therapeutic touch in wound healing. The study group had a wound 10 times smaller than the control group after 8 days of therapeutic touch. By the end of the treatment period, all patients in the therapeutic touch group had total wound healing, whereas no one in the control group did. Daley (1997) evaluated five studies of cutaneous wound healing using therapeutic touch. The data from the five studies indicated a statistically significant accelerated rate of wound healing for the treatment group in the initial two experiments, and insignificant and reverse significant effects for the remaining three studies. Although experimentally, these results are far from impressive, clinically, the significant results of the first two experiments should be enough to encourage the nurse clinician to explore and use a similar noninvasive therapeutic touch treatment method for patients with dermal lacerations.

Olson, et al (1997) studied therapeutic touch to evaluate its effectiveness in reducing adverse immunologic effects of stress. The therapeutic touch group had a higher IgG level, but it was not significantly different than that of the control group; but apoptoses (programmed cell death) was significantly higher in the therapeutic touch group. This was only a small pilot study, and the researchers recommend replication with at least 90 people.

CON

Rosa, et al (1998) states that although proponents of therapeutic touch refer to voluminous bodies of valid research studies, few have been well designed and controlled. The method, credibility, and significance of most studies are questioned. Twenty-one experienced therapeutic touch practitioners were unable to detect the investigator's "energy field." Their failure to substantiate the most fundamental claim of therapeutic touch is unrefuted evidence that the claims of therapeutic touch are groundless and that further professional use is unjustified. Mulloney and Wells-Federman (1996) advise caution in administering therapeutic touch to psychiatric patients who have been physically abused. These patients seem sensitive to human touch and may feel threatened and become upset.

Peck (1997) evaluated therapeutic touch and progressive muscle relaxation (PMR) for reducing pain in elders with degenerative arthritis. The pain and distress scores were lower for PMR than for TT. Peck suggested that both techniques should be offered together to reduce pain and distress.

Glickman and Burns (1996) invited a practitioner of therapeutic touch to a presentation. They proposed an experiment. They wanted her to assess the energy of several people including an elderly man with a history of heart disease and two healthy girls. After her assessment, she would pick the person whose energy she felt most comfortable identifying. From these people, a subject would be covered with blankets and she would be asked to identify which person was hidden. They would randomly repeat the process several times to see whether she could consistently do this without any visual cues. She declined. She said that "a lot of people would flunk that test." However, she recommended that the group take her therapeutic touch course for $125 to learn how to feel a field. Glickman and Burns have joined forces with a private group that is prepared to offer $700,000 to any therapeutic touch practitioner who can prove that it is possible to feel an energy field.

What Is Therapeutic Touch Used to Treat or Improve?

- All diseases may benefit (through symptom relief or improved healing)
- Increases healing
- Reduces stress and anxiety
- Pain relief (chronic, low back, postoperative, headache, PMS)
- To reduce or control cardiac arrhythmias
- Anxiety relief in pregnancy
- Arthritis
- Nausea control in patients with cancer
- Stress reduction in children
- Blood pressure control
- Breast cancer
- Spinal cord injury (increases vitality, uplifting psychologically, helps focus on daily activities)
- Pregnancy (to enhance relaxation, to promote sleep, reduce discomfort, support during labor)
- Newborns (reduce irritability, increase sleep)
- Lethargy, fatigue (to increase energy)

What Happens During a Visit?

- Patient sits or lays comfortably.
- Five-step process occurs:

Centering. The practitioner begins by sensing his or her own energy field, taking deep breaths, imaging, and relaxing.

Assessing the energy field. The practitioner is able to sense and identify the recipient's energy field without judgment or preconceived notions. Areas of high or low energy are determined.

Soothing or unruffling the field. Hands are placed 1 to 6 inches above the recipient's skin in the etheric layer of the energy field. The hands are held open with the flat surface of the palm brushing down and away from above to below the identified problem site. This unruffling motion may be exaggerated as needed, particularly if the energy or pain "feels stuck." The purpose in this step is to unlock the stagnant energy and to reestablish a normal flow.

Modulating or transferring energy. The hands are placed directly on the selected area of the body and held still for 3 to 5 minutes to allow a transfer or modulation of energy. The goal is to bring balance and harmony to the areas of the field that have been blocked or congested. The practitioner usually can determine when the transfer has taken place because there is a change in feeling (e.g., the hands were cool and are now warm, or vice versa, or tingling or vibration is felt).

Closure. Soothing and modulating may be done several times. It is time to close when there is a sense of balance and symmetry to the recipient's energy field. The recipients may also change their color, breathing rate or depth, or demonstrate other signs of relaxation.

- A feeling of warmth or pleasant vibration may be experienced by the recipient.
- A rest or quiet period should follow to allow the change in energy field to integrate throughout its layers.
- An entire treatment takes 15 to 20 minutes.
- The recipient should experience a:
  - Generalized relaxation response within 5 minutes of the start of therapeutic touch
  - Reduction or cessation of painful symptoms throughout therapeutic touch that often lasts after therapeutic touch is completed
  - Acceleration of the healing process

Are There Any Risks Involved With Therapeutic Touch?

Therapeutic touch is noninvasive and risks are minimal. Side effects of therapeutic touch are most often seen as increased agitation and most likely will occur in the elderly, infants, children, and in persons with psychiatric illness. These persons need to be treated gently with therapeutic touch.

What Training Is Required of the Practitioner?

Therapeutic touch was developed by Kurz and Kruger, and their supporting organization is the Nurse Healers Professional Organization, Inc. Nurse Healers provide a three-step process: Beginning, Intermediate, and Advanced. The focus is on practice and feel. The Nurse Healers Association does not have certification and believes that anyone can provide therapeutic touch.

The Holistic Nursing Association also uses therapeutic touch but refers to it as healing touch. The certification process to become a certified healing touch practitioner through the Holistic Nursing Association is as follows:

The purpose for awarding certification as a Healing Touch Practitioner is to document the collected experiences of the individual, to acknowledge competent and experienced practice based on an established educational program, to identify and acknowledge the new professional, and to communicate with the public by recognizing this educational preparation. The certificate ensures that the participant in the program has achieved a level of skill and personal growth that is comparable to others at the same level of expertise.

The following criteria must be met for certification:

1. Completion of all coursework for the Healing Touch Practitioner: Level I (therapeutic touch is taught with many other body works techniques in Level AA classes), Level II-A, Level II-B, Level III-A, and Level III-B.
2. Evidence of receiving 10 different healing modalities with professionals; evidence of giving 100 Healing Touch sessions of which the 10 best are documented in paragraph form.
3. Development of a professional profile notebook that includes a comprehensive resume, articles written by or about the individual, and a detailed listing of conferences and educational experiences related to professional practice.
4. A brief resume of all education, licenses, and experience, including Healing Touch workshops, dates, places, and instructors.
5. Mentorship with a certified Healing Touch practitioner for 1 year or more, documented by a written evaluation of the experience by the mentor and a self-report from the individual.
6. Evidence of ongoing reading and related educational experiences described in paragraph form (15 to 20 books, tapes studied, conferences attended, and so on).
7. A descriptive case study of work in depth with one patient to demonstrate a minimum of three to five sessions including intake, assessment, treatment planning, implementation, evaluation, referrals, and discharge planning.
8. A self-study describing personal development throughout the educational program, plans for continued personal and spiritual growth, and development of the practice of Healing Touch in the community and in the world as a whole. (Presented with permission from the Certification Board of the American Holistic Nurses' Association, copyright 1994.)

Bibliography

Bronstein, M. (1996). Healing hands. Canadian Nurse. 92, 32–34, 36.

Daley, B. (1997). Therapeutic Touch, nursing practice and contemporary cutaneous wound healing research. Journal of Advanced Nursing. 25, 1123–1132.

Easter, A. (1997). The state of research on the effects of therapeutic touch. Journal of Holistic Nursing. 15, 158–175.

Gehlhaart, C. (1995). Therapeutic touch as adjuvant therapy for cancer pain management. Cancer Pain Update. 35, 5–6.

Glickman, R. & Burns, J. (1996). Speak up! If therapeutic touch works, prove it! RN. 59, 76.

Krieger, D. (1975). Therapeutic Touch: the imprimatur of nursing. AJN. 75, 784–787.

Kreiger, D. (1976). Healing by the "laying-on" of hands as a facilitator of bioenergetic change: the response of in-vivo human hemoglobin. International Journal of Psychoenergetic Systems. 1, 121–129.

Leller, E. & Bzdek, V. M. (1986). Effects of therapeutic touch on tension headaches. Nursing Research. 35, 101–105.

Ligeikis-Clayton, C. & Oakes, D. M. (1997). If therapeutic touch works, prove it! RN. 60, 7, 9.

Mulloney, S. S. & Wells-Federman, C. (1996). Therapeutic touch: a healing modality. Journal of Cardiovascular Nursing. 10, 27–49.

Olson, M., Sneed, N., LaVia, M., et al. (1997).Stress induced immunosuppression and Therapeutic Touch. Alternative Therapies in Health & Medicine. 3, 68–74.

Peck, S. D. E. (1997). The effectiveness of therapeutic touch for decreasing pain in elders with degenerative arthritis. Journal of Holistic Nursing. 15, 176–198.

Quinn, J. (1982). An investigation of the effect of Therapeutic Touch done without physical contact on state anxiety of hospitalized cardiovascular patients. Dissertation Abstracts International. 43, 1797.

Rosa, L., et al. (1998). A close look at therapeutic touch. Journal of the American Medical Association. 279, 1005–1010.

Wirth, D. (1991). The effects of non-contact therapeutic touch on the healing rate of full thickness dermal wounds. Journal of Subtle Energies. 1, 1.

Further Reading

Knopf, A. (1995). Therapeutic Touch: a practical guide. New York: Knopf.

Krieger, D. (1993). Accepting your power to heal: personal practice of Therapeutic Touch. Santa Fe, NM: Bear and Co.

Krieger, K. (1992). The therapeutic touch: how to use your hands to help or to heal. 1st Fireside Ed. New York: Simon & Schuster.

Krieger, D. (1988). Living the Therapeutic Touch: healing as lifestyle. Wheaton, IL: Quest Books.

McCrae, J. (1992). Therapeutic Touch: a practical guide. New York: Knopf.

Quinn, J. (1996). Therapeutic Touch and a healing way. Alternative Therapies. 2, 68–75.

RESOURCES

American Holistic Nurses' Association
PO Box 2130
Flagstaff, AZ 86003-2130

Nurse Healers-Professional Associates, Inc.
175 Fifth Avenue, Suite 2755
New York, NY 10010
(212) 886-3776

Orcas Island Foundation
Box 86, Route 1
East Sound, WA 98245
(206) 376-4526

Pumpkin Hollow Farm
Box 135, RR 1
Craryville, NY 12521
(518) 325-3583

INTERNET

Office of Alternative Medicine
http://altmed.od.nig.gov/

Alternative Care
www.sky.net/~ngt/welcome.html

Complementary Modalities
www.ajn.org/ajn/5.4/a504026e.lt

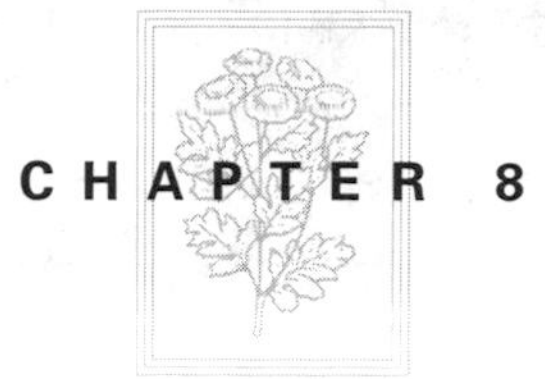

CHAPTER 8

BIOELECTROMAGNETIC APPLICATIONS

WHAT IS LIGHT THERAPY?

Light, sound, herbs, and massage are among the oldest healing tools. Even our ancestors understood that light affects sleep and wake patterns, energy level, and moods. We call our internal clock our circadian rhythm, and light profoundly influences how this rhythm works.

The body's circadian rhythm is regulated by the pineal gland's exposure to light and serves to coordinate biologic events in the body. Melatonin, the chief hormone produced by the pineal gland, is produced only during darkness. Its production is inhibited by light. Adequate melatonin ensures good sleep cycles with adequate REM sleep. Melatonin has sedative qualities and helps to reduce anxiety, panic disorders, and migraines. Melatonin is also a primary regulator of the immune system.

People who rotate shifts or sleep during daylight make less melatonin, and thus get poor quality sleep. Also, persons traveling between time zones upset their normal circadian rhythm. Research (Hyman, 1991) has demonstrated that shift workers have a higher incidence of heart disease, back pain, respiratory disorders, ulcers, depression, and sleep disorders. Shift workers also have a higher rate of error and accidents and often experience a significant loss of alertness and ability to make decisions.

Recent research has shown a connection between osteoporosis and melanoma and light. Osteoporosis and melanoma are connected to vitamin D; vitamin D is produced when the skin is exposed to sunlight. In turn, active vitamin D (activated by the kidneys) must be present in the gut to absorb calcium. It is suggested that 50% to 60% of the elderly population have a vitamin D deficiency that contributes to osteoporosis. Vitamin D also suppresses the growth of malignant melanoma cells. Therefore, a deprivation of sunlight could favor development of melanoma. These new findings lead us to question the belief that indoor living was better and safer for fair-skinned, freckled persons. A higher rate of melanoma occurs on the trunk of the body rather than the head and arms, which are commonly more exposed to sunlight.

Ninety percent of our time is spent indoors under inadequate lighting conditions. Even on a bright sunny day with windows uncovered, the average light exposure is only 500 lux (1 lumen/meter^2 [the international unit of illumination]). Night shift workers may only receive 50 lux during their shift. Outdoors, with average sunlight, the exposure is 50,000 lux.

Seasonal affective disorder (SAD), a cause of depression, occurs in northern climates during fall and winter when the days grow shorter. The symptoms of SAD are depression, excessive sleeping, "winter blues," a feeling of withdrawal, and decreased sex drive. Melatonin levels are also high in these people. Excess melatonin can cause fatigue and low energy levels.

Light therapy encompasses several different types:

- Full spectrum light (discussed here)
- Bright light therapy (2,000 to 5,000 lux) used to treat bulimia, menstrual disorders, and delayed sleep syndrome
- Ultraviolet light therapy experimentally used to treat high cholesterol and premenstrual syndrome
- Photodynamic therapy used to treat cancer
- Cold laser therapy used for pain control, to reduce inflammation, as an adjunct to percutaneous coronary angioplasty, and in dentistry to treat infections under the teeth.

What Is the History of Light Therapy?

In the 1950s, J. Downing, OD, PhD, after 20 years of research expanded the theory that light affected other areas of the brain besides the eye. Dr. Downing identified that light stimulated the cerebral cortex, which in turn, activated learning, thinking, creativity, memory, and body movements; the limbic system, which affects memory and emotions; and the brainstem to assist with coordination and balance.

In the 1970s, Dr. J. Nash Ott, a photobiologist, identified that healing or beneficial light must contain the full spectrum that occurs in natural sunlight. Most artificial lighting from incandescent and fluorescent lack the complete spectrum of balance. Ott and other researchers found that if certain wavelengths were absent in light, the body cannot fully absorb certain nutrients. It was determined that malillumination contributes to fatigue, tooth decay, depression, suppressed immune function, strokes, hair loss, alcoholism, drug abuse, Alzheimer's, and cancer (Ott, 1973). Recently, further studies have linked malillumination to loss of muscle tone and strength.

What Research, Reviews, and Comments Exist?

PRO

Yatham, et al (1997) support light therapy in the treatment of SAD, along with sumatriptan, a 5 HTID receptor agonist. The patients using this drug and light therapy showed the most improvement. Gysin, et al (1997) identified SAD in approximately 10% of the population, and in those who are depressed the percentage is higher. Bright light therapy appears to improve panic disorder, sleep disorders in the elderly, and bulimia. These authors suggest that true placebos for phototherapy need to be developed to increase the evaluation of research trials. Vasile, et al (1997) found a relative increase in regional cerebral blood flow (RCBF) in patients who improved using phototherapy. This finding suggests that an improvement in RCBF is associated with recovery from depression in SAD. Lee, et al (1997) found that short to medium (blue/green/yellow) wavelengths were essential for effectiveness in treating SAD. Red and ultraviolet wavelengths were relatively ineffective in treating SAD. Graw, et al (1997) found that there was reduction in the use of conventional antidepressants when light therapy was instituted for SAD. In addition, the light therapy reduced subsequent depressive episodes. Matias, et al (1996) states that although light therapy is an effective treatment for SAD, the exact mechanism of action is uncertain.

CON

Magnusson (1998) found that light therapy did not affect school attendance when used on students with SAD at three different colleges. Reichborn-Kjennerud and Lingjaerde (1996) found the light therapy had a poor outcome in treating SAD if there was one or more personality disorders, avoidance personality disorder, or many self-defeating personality disorders.

What Is Light Therapy Used to Treat or Improve?

- Depression associated with SAD
- Sleep disturbances
- Menstrual irregularities
- Mood swings, particularly if seasonal occurrence
- Delayed sleep phase syndrome

What Happens During a Visit?

Full spectrum lights are used (2,000 to 5,000 lux)*:

- Every morning for 30 minutes to 2 hours
- Sit 18 inches from light, keep head and eyes toward the light while reading or doing other tasks

Are There Any Risks Involved With Light Therapy?

There are no risks involved with light therapy. However, it is important to stress to patients that they should not self-diagnose and treat themselves without medical supervision.

What Training Is Required of the Practitioner?

No training is necessary. Light therapy can be self-administered. Lights and equipment can be purchased from The Sun Box Company (800-548-3968) or Apollo Light Systems, Inc. (800-545-9667).

The lights that are used should be 5,000 to 10,000 lux.

Bibliography

Anonymous. (1998). Light therapy. Health News. 4, 5.
Gimbel, T. (1994). Healing with color and light. NY: Fireside.
Graw, P., Gisin, B., & Wirz-Justice, A. (1997). Follow-up study of seasonal affective disorder in Switzerland. Psychopathology. 30, 208–214.
Gysin, F., Gysin, F., & Gross, F. (1997). Winter depression and phototherapy. The state of the art. Acta Medica Poutuguesa. 10, 887–893.
Hyman, J. W. (1991). The Light Book. NY: Ballantine Books.
Ibatoullina, E., Praschak-Reider, N., & Kasper, S. (1997). Severe atypical symptoms without depression in SAD: effects of bright light therapy. Journal of Clinical Psychiatry. 58, 495.

*Long-term exposure of full spectrum light containing ultraviolet (UV) can harm the eyes. Recent research suggest the UV may not be a necessary part of the light spectrum.

Lam, R. W., Terman, M., & Wirz-Justice, A. (1997). Light therapy for depressive disorders: indications and efficacy. Modern Problems of Pharmacopsychiatry. 25, 215–234.
Lee, T. M., Chan, C. C., Paterson, J. G., et al. (1997). Spectral properties of phototherapy for seasonal affective disorder: a meta-analysis. Acta Psychiatrica Scandinavica. 96, 117–121.
Matias, J., Manzano, J. M., Santalla, J. L., et al. (1996). Seasonal affective disorder and light therapy. Actas Luso-Espanolas de Neurologia. 24, 204–208.
Magnusson, A. (1998). Light therapy to treat winter depression in adolescents in Iceland. Journal of Psychiatry & Neuroscience. 23, 118–122.
Ott, J. (1973). Health & Light. Old Greenwick, CT: The Devin-Adair Co.
Reichborn-Kjennerud, T. & Lingjaerde, O. (1996). Response to light therapy in seasonal affective disorders: personality disorders and temperament as predictors of outcome. Journal of Affective Disorders. 41, 101–110.
Teicher, M. H., Glod, C. A., Magnus, E., et al. (1997). Circadian rest-activity disturbances in seasonal affective disorder. Archives of General Psychiatry. 54, 124–130.
Vasile, R. G., Sachs, G., & Anderson, J. L. (1997). Changes in regional cerebral blood flow following light treatment for seasonal affective disorder: responders vs. nonresponders. Biological Psychiatry. 42, 1000–1005.
Yatham, L. N., Lam, R. W., & Zis, A. P. (1997). Growth hormone response to sumatriptan challenge in seasonal affective disorder: effects of light therapy. Biological Psychiatry. 42, 24–29.

Further Reading

Amber, R. B. (1983). Color therapy. Santa Fe, NM: Aurora Press.
Liberman, J. (1993). Light: medicine of the future. Santa Fe, NM: Bear & Co. Publishing.

RESOURCES

College of Syntonic Optometry
1200 Robeson Street
Fall Rier, MA 02720-5508
(508) 673-1251

Environmental Health & Light Research Institute
16057 Tampa Palms Boulevard, Suite 227
Tampa, FL 33647
(800) 544-4878

Society for Light Treatment and Biological Rhythms
PO Box 478
Wilsonville, OR 97070
(503) 694-2404

INTERNET

Office of Alternative Medicine
http://altmed.od.nig.gov/

Natural Medicine Therapies
www.amrta.org/~amrta

MAGNETIC FIELD THERAPY

What Is Magnetic Field Therapy?

Magnetic Field Therapy (magnet field therapy, biomagnetic therapy, magnetotherapy, electromagnetic therapy) uses magnetic fields to treat and prevent disease. A magnetic field is generated whenever an electric current is passed through a wire, thus the term, electromagnetism (EM). The human body generates electromagnetic fields naturally, thus diagnostic tools such as magnetic resonance imaging (MRI) and Pet Scans were developed. EM fields vary in strength (Table 8-1). Researchers have identified that EM can affect the body in positive and negative ways, but it is still unclear how EM fields work in the body. The lower frequency forces may exert a physiologic effect by modifying the way hormones and growth factors interact with receptors on the surface of the body (Rubik, et al, 1995).

Magnets in all shapes and forms (shoe liners, belts, chair seats, mattress) are available. Sellers of these products claim that they can heal everything, allegedly by realigning the body's electromagnetic fields or improving circulation and cellular oxygenation. Unfortunately, few, if any, of these claims can be supported with clinical research.

Magnets have two poles: negative (North pole) and positive (South pole). Researchers claim that the negative pole has a calming effect and helps to normalize metabolic functioning. The positive pole has a stress effect and with prolonged exposure may interfere with metabolic functioning, producing O_2 free radicals and may encourage replication of latent microorganisms.

Magnet strength is measured in a gauss, which is a unit of measuring the intensity of magnetic flux or Tesla (1 tesla = 10,000 gauss). Every manufactured magnet has a gauss rating, but when the magnet is worn or applied to the skin, the gauss rating is much less.

What Is the History of Magnetic Field Therapy?

The use of magnets dates many thousands of years ago to China, Greece, Egypt, and India. In early Chinese medicine (see section for more information) there are references to how the person's energy (Chi) could be corrected by means of acupuncture, moxibustion (heat), and application of magnetic stones at specific sites on the body. Magnetic stones were most likely used because the Chinese saw their ability to move an object and thought that the magnetic stone could also move and restore human

TABLE 8-1 ELECTROMAGNETIC FIELD STRENGTH

Range	High	Medium	Low
Types	Gamma X-ray	Ultraviolet Infared	Microwaves Radio waves
Comments	Diagnose and treat disease Damage tissue	Can damage skin	?

energy. The Greeks used lodestones to treat disease because they associated the magnet with being able to move iron. Their philosophy is that the magnet has soul because it can move iron.

In Egypt, Cleopatra carried a magnet as an amulet on her forehead to preserve youth. Interestingly, the pineal gland (located behind the forehead), which produces melatonin and the gland's function, can be affected by electromagnetic fields. In India, Tibetan monks used bar magnets placed on the skull to improve concentration and learning capabilities.

In the 1770s, Dr. Franz Mesmer (this is where the term mesmerize comes from) used magnets placed on different parts of the body to cure disease. His friend, Mozart, used the magnet concept to cure disease in one of his musical operas.

In the United States, the father of magnetic therapy was Dr. C. J. Thacher. Dr. Thacher suggested that energy responsible for life comes from the magnetic force of the sun, which is conducted through the rich iron content of the blood. Diseases result when stressful lifestyles interfere with those magnetic forces. Dr. Thacher said all diseases and conditions including paralysis could be treated with magnets. Dr. Thacher was eventually considered a medical quack.

With the advent of many drugs to treat disease in the 20th Century, magnets were pushed back into the realm of quackery; but now that drugs such as antibiotics are not controlling and treating diseases, there is renewed interest in magnetic therapy.

What Research, Reviews, and Comments Exist?

PRO

Some of the best research regarding using EM to heal in pulsating bursts was done by Sharrard (1990). Sharrard found that EM sped healing of nonunion tibial fractures, those in which the bones did not fuse together.

Pennington, et al (1993) and Trock, et al (1994) found that EM fields could reduce the swelling of ankle sprains and the pain of osteoarthritis in the knee and spine. Salzberg, et al (1995) suggested that EM may accelerate the healing process of pressure sores with spinal cord injury. Szor and Topp (1998) reported a single case study of magnets placed over an abdominal wound that had been present for more than 1 year. Within 1 month after placing magnets over the wound, it healed. Hazlewood and Vallbona (1997) found that the pain associated with post-polio syndrome could be alleviated with magnets.

CON

Dexter (1997) demonstrated that magnetic therapy had no effect on severe obstructive sleep apnea and snoring at the Sleep Disorder Center in Wisconsin. Numerous companies market magnets to permanently treat these disorders. Harper and Wright (1977), in a brief review article, discussed their research to evaluate the pain thresholds of persons wearing a "real" magnet bracelet and a fake magnet bracelet. They found no difference in the experience of pain in their 16 subjects.

To date, if people are attempting to cure a serious disorder with a magnet, they need to realize that they may be wasting their time and money.

What Is Magnetic Therapy Used to Treat or Improve?

Magnetic field therapy has been used to treat:

- Arthritis
- Pain, acute and chronic
- Fibromyalgia
- Carpel tunnel syndrome
- Headaches
- Attention deficit disorders
- Enhance healing
- Infections and inflammations
- Speed the healing of sprains, strains, or fractures
- Diabetic neuropathy
- Gout
- Trigeminal neuralgia
- Toothache
- Seizures
- Multiple sclerosis
- Parkinson's disease

What Happens During Magnetic Therapy?

Magnetic therapy may be used by wearing magnetic belts, braces, or shoe inserts to decrease stress or enhance healing. Magnetic therapy may also use specifically designed ceramic, plastiform, or special earth chemical elements placed individually or in clusters above the organ or lymph nodes in distress. In Japan, small magnets are placed over acupuncture points. Patients may begin therapy in the practitioner's office and then with instruction, continue at home.

What Are Precautions for the Patient?

Several safety facts that persons using magnets need to understand include:

- Patients with pacemakers should not use magnets within 6 inches of pacers.
- Avoid dropping or banging magnets and do not heat a magnet above 500°F because strength is dissipated.
- Do not store different-sized magnets together because strength changes.
- Keep magnets away from bank cards because the magnetic strip on the card may be damaged, and computer hard drives and other magnetic media, such as diskettes, recording tapes, videos, and compact disks, to prevent damage or erasure of the contents.
- Magnets may affect battery-powered equipment.
- Keep magnets away from the MRI machine.
- Remove all magnets before surgery.
- Do not use in children younger than 5, or in frail elderly.
- Keep magnets away from persons who have metal plates, pins, or screws implanted in their body.

Are There Any Risks Involved With Magnetic Therapy?

The body's EM field may be affected by even the weakest magnet, so magnets should only be used by trained practitioners. Magnetic therapy can cause pain and have an affect on medication action in some people. EM therapy should not be used:

- During pregnancy
- For more than 8 to 10 hours continuously
- During or immediately after (wait at least 60 minutes) a meal

It is suggested that the positive magnetic pole never be applied to the body because it may cause seizures, insomnia, promote the growth of tumors, and promote addictive behavior. EM therapy may also produce acidosis, cellular edema, O_2 deficits, stress reactions, toxic metabolic end products of metabolism and O_2 free radicals.

Continued exposure to high frequency EM fields such as from alternating current (AC) can result in numerous medical problems. Research in 1979, later confirmed by a large study conducted by the New York State Department of Health, found that exposure to AC from electrical power lines affected neuro-hormones of the brain (Wolpay, 1987). Other studies have shown an increase in suicides, depression, chromosomal abnormalities, and learning difficulties (Becker, 1990; Smith & Best, 1989; Murphy, et al, 1993). More research is needed to determine the possible problems that may occur secondarily to repeated exposure to microwave ovens, hair dryers, curling irons, electric blankets, electric shavers, and electric heaters. The electrical technology of the 21st Century may be exerting subtle but important effects on biology.

What Training Is Required of the Practitioner?

Magnetic therapy may be performed by a skilled, educated practitioner or be self-administered.

Bibliography

Becker, R. O. (1990). Cross currents. The Promise of Electromedicine. The Perils of Electropollution. Los Angeles: Jeremy P. Tarcher. 208–210.

Dexter, D. (1997). Magnetic therapy is ineffective for the treatment of snoring and obstructive sleep apnea syndrome. Wisconsin Medical Journal 96, 35–37.

Harper, D. W. & Wright, E. F. (1977). Magnets as analgesics. Lancet 2, (8027), 47.

Hazlewood, C. & Vallbona, C. (1997). Magnets for analgesia in post polio syndrome. American Journal of Pain Management. Nov, 34, 54–55.

Murphy, J. C., et al. (1993). International Commission for Protection Against Environmental Mutagens and Carcinogens. Power frequency electric and magnetic fields: a review of genetic toxicology. Mutation Research. 296, 221-240.

Pennington, G. M., Danley, D. L., et al. (1993). Pulsed non-thermal, high-frequency electromagnetic energy (DIA-Pulse) in the treatment of grade 1 and grade 11 ankle sprains. Military Medicine. 158, (2), 101.

Rubik B., Becker, R. O., et al. (1995). Bioelectromagnetics applications in medicine. Alternative Medicine: Expanding Medical Horizons. Washington, DC: U.S. Government Printing Office. 45–65.

Salzberg, C. A., Cooper-Vastola, S. A., et al. (1995). The effects of non-thermal pulsed electromagnetic energy on wound healing of pressure ulcers in spinal cord injured patients. A double blind study. Ostomy Wound Manage. 41, (3), 42.

Sharrard, W. J. (1990). A double-blind trial of pulsed electromagnetic fields for delayed union of tibial fractures. Journal of Bone and Joint Surgery. British Volume. (London). 72, (3), 347.

Smith, C. & Best, S. (1989). Electromagnetic man: health and hazard in the electrical environment. London: J. M. Dent and Sons, Ltd.
Szor, J. K. & Topp, R. (1998). Use of magnet therapy to heal an abdominal wound: a case study. Ostomy Wound Manage. 44, (5), 24–29.
Trock, D. H., Bollet, A. J., & Markoll, R. (1994). The effect of pulsed electromagnetic fields in the treatment of osteoarthritis of the knee and cervical spine. Report of randomized, double-blind placebo controlled trials. Journal of Rheumatology. 21, (10), 1903.
Wolpay, J. (1987). Biological effects of power line fields. New York State Power-Lines Project

Further Reading

Becker, R. (1990). Cross Currents. Los Angeles: Jeremy P. Tarcher, Inc.
BEMI Currents. Journal of the Bio-Electro-Magnetics Institute. Reno, NE.
Davis, A. & Rawls, W. (1993). Magnetism and Its Effects of the Living System. Kansas City, MO: Acres U.S.A.
Lawrence R. & Rosch, P. (1998). Magnet therapy—The pain cure alternative. Rocklin, CA: Prima Health: Prima Publishing.
Philpott, W., Taplin, S. (1990). Biomagnetic handbook. Choctaw, OK: Enviro-Tech Products.

RESOURCES

Bio-Electro-Magnetics Institute
2490 West Moana Lane
Reo, NE 89509-3936
(702) 827-9099

Enviro-Tech Products
17171 Southeast 29th Street
Choctaw, OK 73020
(405) 390-3499

Dr. Wolfgang Ludwig
Silcherstrasse 21
Horb A.N.1
Germany
011-49-7451-8648 (Fax)

MagnetiCo, Inc.
4562 14th Street, NE
Calgary, Alberta,
Cananda T1Y 6C1
(403) 291-0085

Prometheus Italia SrL
Centro Commerciale, VR-EST
Viale del Lavoro 45
I-36037, S. Martino BA (VR), Italy

INTERNET

NIH Office of Alternative Medicine
http://altmed.od.nig.gov/

Alternative Medicine Connection
arxc.com/hotlinks.htlm

CHAPTER 9

BIOLOGIC TREATMENTS

CHELATION THERAPY

What Is Chelation Therapy?

Chelation comes from the Greek word *Cheli*, which means "to claw" or "to bind." Chelation therapy (oral and parenteral) is used to remove toxic metals from the body by binding them to another substance and then transporting them through the bloodstream to be eliminated by the kidneys. The process effectively removes calcium deposits from the arteries and other areas of the body where calcium may accumulate in abnormal levels, such as traumatized tendons, inflamed bursae, kidney stones, arthritic joints, and strained ligaments. Chelation does not remove calcium from areas where it is needed, such as bones and teeth. Chelation tends to strengthen the bones by reactivating dormant, healthy bone-forming cells. Oral chelating agents have been proven useful for minimizing the damage that can lead to bone disease. With regard to arteriosclerosis, chelation therapy can help remove calcium deposits that cause hardening of the arteries. Chelation therapy is only an approved method of treating heavy metal toxicities. Chelation is expensive, with each treatment costing approximately $100 to $150 and usually 20 to 30 treatments are required. Chelation therapy is not covered by most insurance companies; thus, if wanted, chelation therapy becomes an out-of-pocket expense.

What Is the History of Chelation Therapy?

The chelation process originated in 1893 with Alfred Werner, a French-Swiss chemist, who received the Nobel Prize in 1913 for developing the theories that later became the foundation for modern chelation chemistry. Werner's theories describing how metals bind to organic molecules resulted in the new field of chelation chemistry.

Modern chelation therapy has been around since World War II when Werner's theories were used by the U.S. government to develop antidotes for poison gas warfare. At the end of the war many physicians started using chelation therapy for other medical disorders.

Ethylene-dramine-tetra-acetate (EDTA) is a synthetic amino acid developed in Germany for the dye industry. It binds calcium, thus removing calcium from hard water. In 1950, Dr. N. Clark found that EDTA was effective in removing Ca^{++} deposits from the human body. From this use, a few physicians reasoned that EDTA could be used to treat symptoms of heavy metal toxicity. In the 1950s, the U. S. Navy began using EDTA to treat sailors exposed to lead-based paint who showed signs of toxicity. By the mid 1950s, chelation therapy was the preferred treatment in the United States for lead poisoning; it still is. Chelation therapy has been used safely on more than 500,000 patients. Dr. Clark hypothesized that because Ca^{++} plaque is a prominent component in atherosclerosis, EDTA could be an effective treatment for heart disease. Patients in his studies reported relief of chest pain and intermittent claudication. Many patients also reported improved memory, sight, hearing, sense of smell, and vigor. Unfortunately, the patent on EDTA expired in 1948, making it an inexpensive drug to manufacture. It seems unlikely that any pharmaceutical company will invest the dollars necessary to obtain U.S. Food and Drug Administration (FDA) approval.

What Research, Reviews, and Comments Exist?

PRO

Olszewer and Carter (1988), both working at Tulane University, documented that chelation therapy brought about significant improvement in 93.9% of patients suffering from coronary artery disease. In 1989, a study demonstrated that 99% of patients had improvement in their symptoms of intermittent claudication, and 30% had marked improvement, thus improving their quality of life and decreasing the likelihood of amputation. Cranton, in his textbook in 1989, said that chelation therapy has a profound effect on overall health. He suggests that chelation therapy:

- Slows the aging process
- Decreases allergies

- Decreases arthritis and muscle and joint aches
- Slows Alzheimer's disease progression, and in some persons, the disease does not progress for long periods
- Improves visual acuity
- Decreases progression in persons with macular degeneration

In 1993, Chappel suggested that billions of dollars could be saved in coronary artery bypass surgery if chelation therapy was performed first. In 1997, Lewin was still suggesting chelation therapy to reduce the symptoms of atherosclerosis. In a review article, Kidd (1998) reviews much research on chelation and suggests that with the positive research findings available on chelation and fish oils, they should be used together to revitalize the myocardium. Both complementary therapies used together may decrease the need for many bypass surgeries.

CON

Margolis at John's Hopkins School of Medicine (1995) found chelation therapy to be ineffective for the treatment of peripheral vascular disease. No improvement in symptoms was observed. Ernst (1997) systematically reviewed the randomized, placebo-controlled, double-blind trials on chelation therapy for peripheral artery occlusive disease (PAOD) (intermittent claudication) performed from 1992 to 1997 (four were found). The cumulative results in these studies clearly and conclusively demonstrate that chelation therapy does not ameliorate symptoms and does not change objective signs of the disease or the subjective well-being to a greater extent than placebo treatment. Ernst concluded that chelation therapy is associated with considerable risks and costs and should be considered obsolete and removed from the possible treatments of PAOD.

What Is Chelation Therapy Used to Treat or Improve?

Chelation therapy may improve:

- Atherosclerotic heart, blood vessel, and cerebral disease
- Pain and inflammation of arthritis
- Multiple arrhythmias (50% of arrhythmias improved in patients)
- Memory and concentration
- Vision (with vascular-related abnormalities or macular degeneration)
- Symptoms in patients with iron poisoning and iron storage disease (thalassemia)
- Detoxification from snake and spider bites

- Cancer survival
- Blood cholesterol levels (cholesterol in some patients decrease by 20%)
- The clearance of O_2 free radicals and possibly to slow the aging process
- Chronic disease that may be associated with amalgam fillings in teeth.

What Happens During a Visit?

Several agents can be used in chelation therapy. EDTA, a nontoxic agent, is only approved by the FDA for treatment of lead and heavy metal intoxication. EDTA binds with the toxic substances and then they are eliminated by the kidneys, so it is important to monitor renal function before and during therapy. EDTA:

- Lowers blood calcium levels and stimulates the parathyroid glands to produce parathormone. Parathormone removes calcium from abnormal locations (such as arteries) and deposits calcium in locations where it is needed (such as bones).
- Reduces the tendency for platelet aggregation and prevents thrombosis or clotting that blocks coronary arteries and leads to a heart attack.
- Stimulates enlargement of small blood vessels, causing blood to circulate around a blockage-capillary bypass.
- Is a powerful antioxidant that controls free radical damage caused by lipid peroxidation.
- Helps reestablish prostaglandin hormone balance. Prostaglandins, which are produced from fatty acids, are directly involved in the contraction and relaxation of arterial walls, and in blood clotting. Lipid peroxidation upsets the manufacture of these vital hormones. EDTA inhibits lipid peroxidation.
- Removes age-related cross-linkages in collagen and elastin that are responsible for skin-tone loss and wrinkling and improves tissue flexibility.
- Strengthens and improves the integrity of cellular and mitochondrial membranes.
- Removes abnormal metal ion deposits, such as copper and iron, that accumulate with age.
- Removes lead, cadmium, aluminum, mercury, and other toxic metals that interfere with enzyme function.

Deferoxamine is another agent that can be used, but the research is limited to animal models. Another agent is dexrazoxane (ICRF-187) approved for only parenteral use for reducing the incidence and severity of cardiomyopathy associated with doxorubicin administration in women with advanced breast cancer. Deferiprone is an oral iron-chelating agent that is being evaluated as a treatment for iron overload in thalassemia major. Deferiprone may worsen hepatic fibrosis, thus caution is advised.

Another product is the oral agent, penicillamine, used to treat heavy metal poisoning, rheumatoid arthritis, and Wilson's disease (a rare metabolic disease resulting in copper accumulation in the liver, red blood cells, and brain). Penicillamine, like EDTA, removes O_2 free radicals (see Nutritional Chapter), which probably helps relieve some of the symptoms of rheumatoid arthritis.

There are also available chelating nutrients:

- L-Gluthathione is a sulfur-containing amino acid composed of KL-cysteine, L-glutamic acid, and glycine. Gluthathione, a powerful antioxidant that inhibits the formation of free radicals, is a proven oral chelating agent. It protects the body against damage from cigarette smoke, radiation, chemotherapy, and x-rays. It is a detoxifier of harmful trace metals and drugs, and helps relieve blood and liver disorders. It also protects the heart by helping to keep the arterial walls free of debris.
- L-Carnitine prevents fatty build-up in the heart and arteries. It lowers blood fat levels and strengthens the heart. L-carnitine also enhances the effectiveness of antioxidant vitamins E and C, and normalizes abnormal heart rhythms.
- L-Methionine helps the body break down fats. It prevents fatty buildups in the liver and arteries. The amino acid also aids the digestive system by detoxifying harmful substances, preventing muscle weakness, revitalizing brittle hair, and deterring allergic chemical sensitivities and bone diseases.
- Allium Sativum lowers blood pressure by activating methyl allyl trisulfide. It also lowers cholesterol, reduces blood clot risk, and helps prevents heart attacks.
- Crataegus Oxyacantha is effective for reducing blood pressure, angina attacks, and serum cholesterol levels in addition to preventing cholesterol deposition on arterial walls.
- Other oral chelators, such as garlic, vitamin C, carrageenan, and zinc, can be used.

A complete history and physical examination are performed, noting all symptoms. Laboratory work and other diagnostic tests (electrocardiogram [EKG], stress test, doppler flow studies, kidney function tests) may be obtained to verify the diagnosis. Chelation therapy is ordered by allopathic or osteopathic physicians. A nurse may administer the products and monitor therapy.

- The product is administered intravenously (slowly over 2 to 3 hours) or orally (oral products have less effective results).
- Usually two to three treatments are performed a week, with a total of 20 to 30 treatments required.
- Dosage is individualized based on age, weight, kidney function, and disease presentation.
- There are yearly maintenance treatments performed after the initial therapy.

Are There Any Risks Involved With Chelation Therapy?

- Patient may experience side effects, such as weakness, dizziness, and gastrointestinal (GI) complaints, during treatments.
- Serious side effects can occur, such as arrhythmias, seizures, and renal tubular necrosis.
- Chelation therapy is contraindicated during pregnancy, lactation, and with severe kidney disease.

What Training Is Required of the Practitioner?

Chelation therapy is administered only by allopathic (medical) or osteopathic physicians. Board certification by the American Board of Chelation Therapists has been available since 1983.

Bibliography

Chappel, T. L. Preliminary findings from the meta-analysis study of EDTA chelation therapy. From a paper presented at the American College of Advancement in Medicine meeting. May 5–9, 1993. Houston, TX.

Elihu N., Anandasbapathy, S., & Frishman, W. H. (1998). Chelation therapy in cardiovascular disease: ethylenediaminetetraacetic acid, deferoxamine and dexrazoxane. Journal of Clinical Pharmacology. 38, 101–105.

Ernst, E. (1997). Chelation therapy for peripheral arterial occlusive disease. Circulation. 96, 1031–1033.

Grandjean, P., Guldager, B., et al. (1997). Placebo response in environmental disease. Chelation therapy of patients with symptoms attributed to amalgam fillings. Journal of Occupational and Environmental Medicine. 39, 707–714.

Kidd, P. M. (1998). Integrative cardiac revitalizatio: bypass surgery, angioplasty, and chelation. Benefits, risks, and limitations. Alternative Medicine Review. 3, 4–17.

Lewin, M. R. 91997). Chelation therapy for cardiovascular disease. Review and commentary. Texas Heart Institute Journal. 24, 81–89.

Margolis, S. (1995). Chelation therapy is ineffective for the treatment of peripheral vascular disease. Alternative Therapies in Health and Medicine. 1, 53–56.

Olivieri, N. F., Britteham, G. M., et al. (1998). Long-term safety and effectiveness of iron-chelation therapy with deferiprone for thalassemia major. New England Journal of Medicine. 339, 417–423.

Olszewer, E. & Carter, J. P. (1989). EDTA Chelation Therapy: A retrospective Study of 2870 patients. Textbook on EDTA Chelation Therapy, Cranton, E. M. (Ed.) Special Issue, Journal of Advancement in Medicine. 2 Nos. 1, 2. New York: Human Sciences Press, 183.

Olszewer, E., Carter, J. P. (1989). EDTA Chelation Therapy: a retrospective study of 2870 patients. Textbook on EDTA Chelation Therapy, Cranton, E. M. (Ed.), Special Issue, Journal of Advancement in Medicine 2 Nos. 1-2, New York: Human Sciences Press. 197–211.

Walker, M. & Gordon, G. (1982). The Chelation answer: how to prevent hardening of the arteries and rejuvenate your cardiovascular system. New York: M. Evans & Co., Inc.

Further Reading

Brecher, H. A. (1992). Something forever. New York: Healthsavers Press.

Cranton, E. (1990). Bypassing bypass. Troutdale, VA: Hampton Roads.

Cranton, E. (1989). A textbook on EDTA chelation therapy. Special Issue. Journal of Advancement in Medicine. Vol. 2, Nos. 1 & 2. New York: Human Sciences Press, Inc., Spring/Summer.

Halstead, B. (1979). The scientific basis of EDTA chelation therapy. Colton, CA: Golden Quill Publishers, Inc.

Julian, J. (1982). Chelation extends life. Hollywood, CA: Wellness Press.

Trowbridge, J. & Walker, M. (1992). The healing powers of chelation therapy. Stamford, CT: New Way of Life, Inc.

Walker, M. (1990). The chelation way. Garden City Park, NY: Avery Publishing Group, Inc.

RESOURCES

American Board of Chelation Therapy
70 West Huron Street
Chicago, IL 60610
(312) 266-7246

American College of Advancement in Medicine
PO Box 3427
Laguna Hills, CA 92654
(714) 583-7666

Great Lakes Association of Clinical Medicine, Inc.
70 West Huron Street
Chicago, IL 60610
(312) 266-7246

The Rheumatoid Disease Foundation
5106 Old Harding Road
Franklin, TN 37064
(615) 646-1030

INTERNET

Office of Alternative Medicine
http://altmed.od.nig.gov/

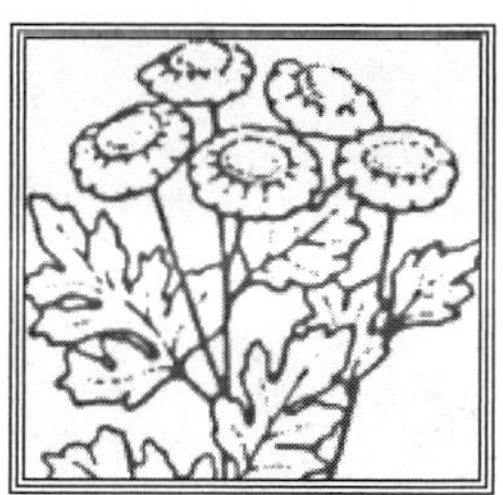

INDEX

*Page numbers in *italics* denote figures; those followed by *t* denote tables.

N

Q

R